PRINCIPLES *of* PHARMACOLOGY

Workbook

PRINCIPLES *of* PHARMACOLOGY

Workbook

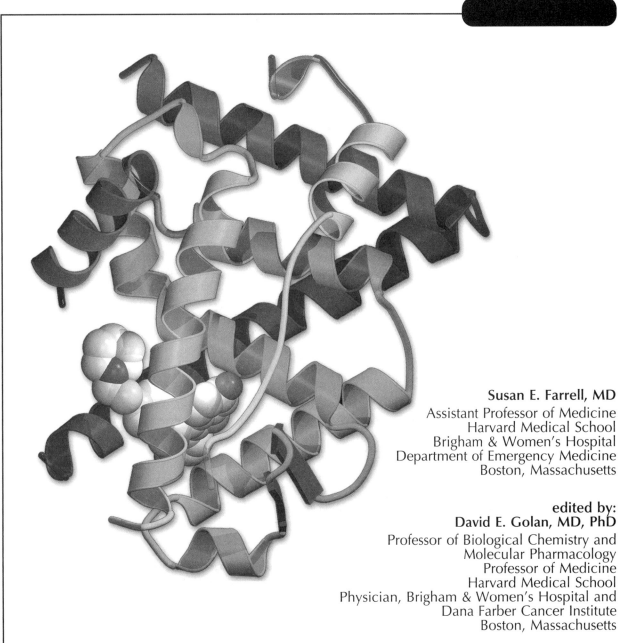

Susan E. Farrell, MD
Assistant Professor of Medicine
Harvard Medical School
Brigham & Women's Hospital
Department of Emergency Medicine
Boston, Massachusetts

edited by:
David E. Golan, MD, PhD
Professor of Biological Chemistry and
Molecular Pharmacology
Professor of Medicine
Harvard Medical School
Physician, Brigham & Women's Hospital and
Dana Farber Cancer Institute
Boston, Massachusetts

Wolters Kluwer | Lippincott Williams & Wilkins
Health

Philadelphia · Baltimore · New York · London
Buenos Aires · Hong Kong · Sydney · Tokyo

Acquisitions Editor: Donna M. Balado
Managing Editor: Stacey L. Sebring
Marketing Manager: Emilie Linkins
Production Editor: Sally Anne Glover
Designer: Doug Smock
Compositor: Maryland Composition, Inc.
Printer: Data Reproductions Corporation

9 8 7 6 5 4 3 2 1

DISCLAIMER

Care has been taken to confirm the accuracy of the information present and to describe generally accepted practices. However, the authors, editors, and publisher are not responsible for errors or omissions or for any consequences from application of the information in this book and make no warranty, expressed or implied, with respect to the currency, completeness, or accuracy of the contents of the publication. Application of this information in a particular situation remains the professional responsibility of the practitioner; the clinical treatments described and recommended may not be considered absolute and universal recommendations.

The authors, editors, and publisher have exerted every effort to ensure that drug selection and dosage set forth in this text are in accordance with the current recommendations and practice at the time of publication. However, in view of ongoing research, changes in government regulations, and the constant flow of information relating to drug therapy and drug reactions, the reader is urged to check the package insert for each drug for any change in indications and dosage and for added warnings and precautions. This is particularly important when the recommended agent is a new or infrequently employed drug.

Some drugs and medical devices presented in this publication have Food and Drug Administration (FDA) clearance for limited use in restricted research settings. It is the responsibility of the health care provider to ascertain the FDA status of each drug or device planned for use in their clinical practice.

To purchase additional copies of this book, call our customer service department at **(800) 638-3030** or fax orders to **(301) 223-2320**. International customers should call **(301) 223-2300**.

Visit Lippincott Williams & Wilkins on the Internet: http://www.lww.com. Lippincott Williams & Wilkins customer service representatives are available from 8:30 am to 6:00 pm, EST.

Dedication

To Ken: For your continuing love and patience.
To Effi-Anna and Sabine Katharine, my joys:
Another example of ''Never say 'I can't.' ''

PREFACE

This case-based workbook is written as a companion to the second edition of *Principles of Pharmacology: The Pathophysiologic Basis of Drug Therapy* edited by David E. Golan, Armen H. Tashjian, Jr., Ehrin J. Armstrong, and April W. Armstrong. In keeping with the philosophy of the text, the workbook contains clinical cases, questions, and explanations intended to promote the learning of pharmacology in the framework of human physiology, biochemistry, and pathophysiology. *The Principles of Pharmacology Workbook* consists of 54 chapters, corresponding to the chapters of the primary text. Each workbook chapter is anchored with bulleted learning objectives, followed by two case scenarios, the first identical to that presented in the primary text. Each clinical case is accompanied by five multiple-choice questions with extensive explanatory answers and figures from the textbook. More than 110 cases and 550 multiple-choice questions and answers are incorporated into the workbook content.

The workbook uses clinical examples to convey important therapeutic and adverse effects of drugs, understood in the context of a drug's mechanism of action. The format is intentionally designed to promote a mechanism-based understanding of pharmacology, with attention to clinical relevance. As such, one goal of the workbook is to facilitate a deeper understanding of the mechanistic basis of drug therapy in clinical medicine, rather than rote memorization of drug lists. A second goal is to facilitate students' review of pharmacology for Board examinations.

The workbook is also intended as a resource for reviewing and integrating knowledge of pharmacology with physiology, biochemistry, and pathophysiology. As such, it is an integrated tool for both course study and board exam preparation.

Susan E. Farrell, MD

ACKNOWLEDGMENTS

Many thanks to the text authors and editors of *Principles of Pharmacology: The Pathophysiologic Basis of Drug Therapy,* 2nd ed., who provided feedback for this work. Most thanks to David Golan for his continuing support, encouragement, and guidance.

CONTENTS

I

Fundamental Principles of Pharmacology

1

Drug-Receptor Interactions

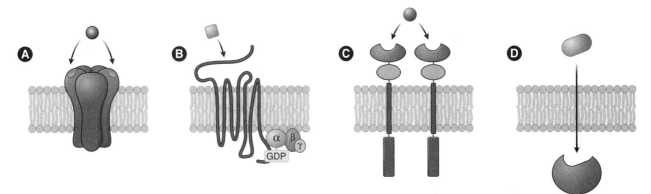

Figure 1-1. Four Major Types of Interactions Between Drugs and Receptors. Most drug-receptor interactions can be divided into four groups. **A.** Drugs can bind to ion channels spanning the plasma membrane, causing an alteration in the channel's conductance. **B.** Heptahelical receptors spanning the plasma membrane are functionally coupled to intracellular G proteins. Drugs can influence the actions of these receptors by binding to the extracellular surface or transmembrane region of the receptor. **C.** Drugs can bind to the extracellular domain of a transmembrane receptor and cause a change in signaling within the cell by activating or inhibiting an enzymatic intracellular domain (rectangular box) of the same receptor molecule. **D.** Drugs can diffuse through the plasma membrane and bind to cytoplasmic or nuclear receptors. This is often the pathway used by lipophilic drugs (e.g., drugs that bind to steroid hormone receptors). Alternatively, drugs can inhibit enzymes in the extracellular space without the need to cross the plasma membrane (not shown). GDP = guanosine diphosphate.

OBJECTIVES

- Understand the molecular basis for drug-receptor interactions and their subsequent cellular effects.

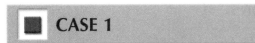

CASE 1

Intent on enjoying his newly found retirement, Mr. B. has made a point of playing tennis as often as possible during the past year. For the past 3 months, however, he has noted increasing fatigue. Moreover, he is now unable to finish a meal despite being an avid lifelong eater. Worried and wondering what these nonspecific symptoms mean, Mr. B. schedules an appointment with his doctor. On physical examination, the physician notes that Mr. B. has an enlarged spleen, extending approximately 10 cm below the left costal margin; the physical examination is otherwise within normal limits. Blood tests show an increased total white blood cell count (70,000 cells/mm^3), with an absolute increase in neutrophils, band forms, metamyelocytes, and myelocytes, but no blast cells (undifferentiated precursor cells). Cytogenetic analysis of metaphase cells demonstrates that 90% of Mr. B.'s myeloid cells possess the Philadelphia chromosome (indicating a translocation between chromosomes 9 and 22), confirming the diagnosis of chronic myeloid leukemia. The physician initiates therapy with imatinib.

QUESTIONS

1. How does the BCR-Abl receptor tyrosine kinase affect intracellular signaling pathways?

A. This kinase phosphorylates steroid hormones, causing them to upregulate growth transcriptional regulators of cell growth.

B. This kinase phosphorylates the tyrosine residue on the cytoplasmic tail of the receptor and opens plasma membrane channels to allow the entry of growth regulators.

C. This kinase removes phosphate groups from G protein receptors, allowing the adenylyl cyclase signaling pathway to become activated.

D. This kinase removes phosphate groups from DNA, allowing transcriptional regulators access to specific genes.

E. This kinase phosphorylates cytosolic proteins, leading to dysregulated cell growth.

2. How does imatinib interrupt the activity of the BCR-Abl protein?

A. Imatinib reverses the Philadelphia chromosomal mutation.

B. Imatinib prevents transcription of the Philadelphia chromosome.

C. Imatinib binds to the ATP-binding site of the BCR-Abl tyrosine kinase, denatures the protein, and destroys the kinase receptor.

D. Imatinib binds to the plasma membrane and prevents the BCR-Abl access to its target binding site.

E. Imatinib inhibits the ability of BCR-Abl to phosphorylate substrates.

Over the next month, the cells containing the Philadelphia chromosome disappear completely from Mr. B.'s blood, and he begins to feel well enough to compete in a seniors' tennis tournament. Mr. B. continues to take imatinib every day, and he has a completely normal blood count and no feelings of fatigue. He is not sure what the future will bring, but he is glad to have been given the chance to enjoy a healthy retirement.

3. Unlike imatinib, most of the older therapies for chronic myeloid leukemia (e.g., interferon-α) had significant "flu-like" adverse effects. Why did these older therapies cause significant adverse effects in most patients, whereas (as in this case) imatinib causes adverse effects in very few patients?

A. Older therapies target all myeloid cells.

B. Older therapies target the BCR-Abl protein kinase in normally functioning cells.

C. Older therapies target BCR-Abl production in all hematopoietic cells.

D. Older therapies target the Philadelphia chromosome throughout the body.

E. Older therapies target all future production of BCR-Abl protein kinase.

4. Why is imatinib a specific therapy for chronic myeloid leukemia?

A. Imatinib selectively binds the BCR-Abl protein of the tyrosine kinase receptor in abnormally growing hematopoietic cells.

B. Imatinib selectively degrades the Philadelphia chromosome in leukemic cells.

C. Imatinib selectively targets the tyrosine kinase–associated receptors.

D. Imatinib selectively binds to phosphatases, which phosphorylate tyrosine.

E. Imatinib selectively targets BCR-Abl synthesis in hematopoietic precursor cells.

5. When a drug interacts with its receptor, the magnitude of the cellular response may be greater than the magnitude of the immediate effect of the molecular drug-receptor interaction. This is referred to as:

A. tachyphylaxis

B. receptor recruitment

C. signal amplification

D. second messenger activation

E. heterologous desensitization

 CASE 2

A 62-year-old man is rushed to the hospital after ingesting a container of an organophosphate insecticide in a suicide attempt. On arrival in the emergency department, care providers note a strange odor emanating from the patient. The patient is unresponsive, and his physical examination is remarkable for profuse sweating, miotic pupils, and copious oral and bronchial secretions. He is noted to have diffuse muscle fasciculations, but is flaccid and paralyzed. When the patient is intubated, the physician notes copious amounts of strange-smelling watery secretions. The doctor subsequently develops tearing and bronchospasm. The patient's soaking clothes are removed and safely disposed of. The nurses also subsequently develop tearing and runny noses.

QUESTIONS

1. This patient's signs are consistent with excessive acetylcholine activity at both muscarinic and nicotinic receptors. Organophosphate insecticides cause toxicity by preventing the normal metabolism of acetylcholine. The most likely binding site of the organophosphate resides on:

A. a cell surface adhesion receptor

B. an extracellular enzyme

C. a tyrosine kinase receptor

D. a transcription regulator

E. an intracellular signal transduction enzyme

2. Based on their effect at cholinergic synapses, organophosphate insecticides would be considered:

A. noncompetitive, reversible antagonists

B. competitive, reversible antagonists

C. inverse agonists

D. direct agonists

E. indirect agonists

3. The oxygen–phosphorus bond formed between organophosphate insecticides and acetylcholinesterase is subject to a process of "aging," in which the bond results in permanent destruction of acetylcholinesterase function. The "aged" oxygen–phosphorus bond is:

A. an ionic bond

B. a hydrophobic interaction

C. a group of van der Waals interaction

D. covalent bond

E. hydrogen bond

4. Normally, acetylcholine acts at its nicotinic receptor at the neuromuscular junction to effect muscle cell depolarization and contraction. The nicotinic acetylcholine receptor is an example of:

A. a ligand-gated ion channel

B. a voltage-gated ion channel

C. a ligand-gated G protein–coupled receptor

D. a ligand-gated tyrosine kinase receptor

E. a voltage-gated extracellular enzyme

5. G protein–coupled receptors are composed of extracellular domains, transmembrane regions, and intracellular regions. Which of the following statements regarding G protein–coupled receptors is correct?

A. The extracellular domain consists of enzyme sites, which hydrolyze guanosine triphosphate to guanosine diphosphate after binding of the ligand.

B. The intracellular region is linked to a G protein, which affects signaling molecules after binding of the ligand.

C. The transmembrane region consists of five subunits, which release the G protein after binding of the ligand.

D. When the transmembrane region opens, it allows ions to pass through it.

E. The G protein–coupled receptors are specific to acetylcholine receptors.

2

Pharmacodynamics

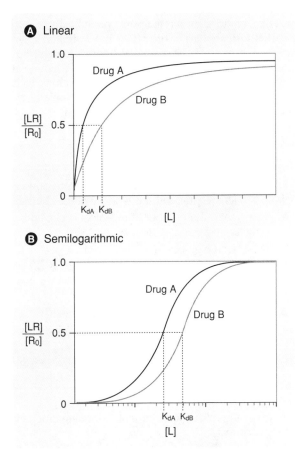

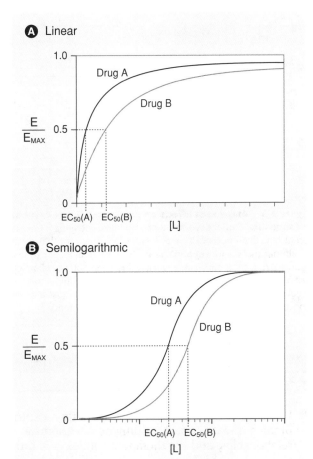

Figure 2-1. Ligand-Receptor Binding Curves. A. Linear graphs of drug-receptor binding for two drugs with different values of K_d. **B.** Semilogarithmic graphs of the same drug-receptor binding. K_d is the equilibrium dissociation constant for a given drug-receptor interaction—a lower K_d indicates a *tighter* drug-receptor interaction (higher affinity). Because of this relationship, Drug A, which has the lower K_d, will bind a higher proportion of total receptors than Drug B at any given drug concentration. Notice that K_d corresponds to the ligand concentration $[L]$ at which 50% of the receptors are bound (occupied) by ligand. $[L]$ is the concentration of free (unbound) ligand (drug), $[LR]$ is the concentration of ligand-receptor complexes, and R_o is the total concentration of occupied and unoccupied receptors. Thus,

$$\left[\frac{LR}{R_o}\right]$$

is the *fractional occupancy* of receptors, or the fraction of total receptors that are occupied (bound) by ligand.

Figure 2-2. Graded Dose–Response Curves. Graded dose–response curves demonstrate the effect of a drug as a function of its concentration. **A.** Linear graphs of graded dose–response curves for two drugs. **B.** Semilogarithmic graphs of the same dose-response curves. Note the close resemblance to Figure 2-1: the fraction of occupied receptors $[LR]/[R_o]$ has been replaced by the fractional effect E/E_{max}, where E is a quantifiable response to a drug (e.g., an increase in blood pressure). EC_{50} is the potency of the drug, or the concentration at which the drug elicits 50% of its maximal effect. In the figure, Drug A is more potent than Drug B because it elicits a half-maximal effect at a lower concentration than Drug B. Drugs A and B exhibit the same efficacy (the maximal response to the drug). Note that potency and efficacy are not intrinsically related—a drug can be extremely potent but have little efficacy, and vice versa. $[L]$ is drug concentration, E is effect, E_{max} is efficacy, and EC_{50} is potency.

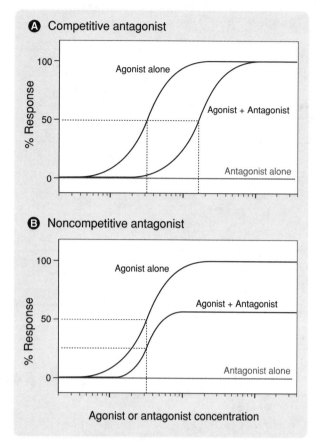

Figure 2-3. Antagonist Effects on the Agonist Dose–Response Relationship. Competitive and noncompetitive antagonists have different effects on potency (the concentration of agonist that causes a half-maximal response) and efficacy (the maximal response to an agonist). **A.** A competitive antagonist reduces the potency of an agonist without affecting agonist efficacy. **B.** A noncompetitive antagonist reduces the efficacy of an agonist. As shown here, most allosteric noncompetitive antagonists do not affect agonist potency.

OBJECTIVES

▮ Understand the molecular basis for drug-receptor binding and its impact on drug dose–response relationships, and the therapeutic index of a drug.

▮ Understand the actions of agonists and various antagonist classes, and their relationships to drug potency and efficacy.

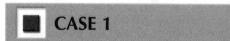 **CASE 1**

Admiral X. is a 66-year-old retired submarine captain with a 70 pack-year smoking history (two packs a day for 35 years) and a family history of coronary artery disease. Although he usually ignores the advice of his physicians, he does take the pravastatin prescribed to reduce his cholesterol level and aspirin to reduce his risk of coronary artery occlusion.

One day, while working in his woodshop, Admiral X. begins to feel tightness in his chest. The feeling becomes rapidly painful, and the pain begins to radiate down his left arm. He calls 911, and an ambulance transports him to the local emergency department. After evaluation, it is determined that Admiral X. is having an anterior myocardial infarction. Because the hospital has no cardiac catheterization laboratory and Adm. X has no specific contraindications to thrombolytic therapy (e.g., uncontrolled hypertension, history of stroke, or recent surgery), the physician initiates therapy with both a thrombolytic agent, tissue-type plasminogen activator (t-PA), and an anticoagulant, heparin. Improper dosing of both of these drugs can have dire consequences (hemorrhage and death) because of their low therapeutic indices, so Admiral X. is closely monitored, and the pharmacologic effect of the heparin is measured periodically by testing the partial thromboplastin time (PTT). Admiral X.'s symptoms resolve over the next several hours, although he remains in the hospital for monitoring. He is discharged after 4 days in the hospital; his discharge medications include pravastatin, aspirin, atenolol, lisinopril, and clopidogrel for secondary prevention of myocardial infarction.

QUESTIONS

1. Which of the following statements is correct regarding the relationship between the molecular interaction of a drug with its receptor and the potency of the drug?
   A. The greater the number of receptors occupied by a drug, the greater its potency.
   B. Drugs with high potency have a high EC_{50}.
   C. Drugs with high potency have a drug dose–response curve that lies to the right of less potent, but similar drugs.
   D. The presence of a competitive antagonist shifts the agonist dose–response curve to the right and decreases its potency.
   E. The greater a drug's potency, the higher its drug-receptor dissociation constant, K_d.

2. Which of the following statements regarding drug efficacy is correct?
   A. The efficacy of a drug is directly proportional to its drug-receptor binding dissociation constant.
   B. The maximal efficacy of an agonist is the condition at which receptor-mediated signaling by the drug is maximal.
   C. Highly efficacious drugs have high $ED_{50}s$ and low $LD_{50}s$.
   D. Highly efficacious drugs mediate their effect at a lower fraction of receptor binding.
   E. The presence of a competitive antagonist reduces the maximal possible response to drug-receptor binding, and hence reduces drug efficacy.

3. What properties of certain drugs, such as aspirin, allow them to be taken without monitoring of plasma drug levels, whereas other drugs, such as heparin, require such monitoring?

   A. Whereas aspirin is an oral agent, heparin is administered parenterally.

   B. Aspirin is available without prescription and can be taken safely without monitoring.

   C. Whereas aspirin exerts an irreversible pharmacologic effect, which does not need monitoring, the reversible effect of heparin must be monitored.

   D. Whereas aspirin causes a graded dose–response relationship, heparin causes a quantal dose–response relationship that must be monitored periodically.

   E. Whereas aspirin has a larger therapeutic index, heparin has a small therapeutic index.

4. Why does the fact that a drug has a low therapeutic index mean that the physician must use greater care in its administration?

   A. Drugs with a low therapeutic index can cause toxicity at a high ED_{50}.

   B. Drugs with a low therapeutic index can only cause toxicity over a small range of drug doses.

   C. Drugs with a low therapeutic index can cause irreversible effects after they are administered.

   D. Drugs with a low therapeutic index do not have therapeutic effects until the administered dose approaches the toxic dose.

   E. Drugs with a low therapeutic index have a greater degree of safety when administered at therapeutic doses.

5. The concept of "spare receptors" refers to:

   A. the up-regulation of receptors, enhancing the effect of a drug (agonist)

   B. the fact that the EC_{50} is greater than the K_d

   C. a maximal agonist response occurring with less than 100% receptor occupancy

   D. the fact that receptors are resistant to the presence of receptor antagonists

   E. the finding of enhanced potency despite the presence of receptor antagonists

■ CASE 2

Pittsburgh, PA; November 1988: A 34-year-old man is dropped off by a private car at the ambulance entry of an emergency department. He is disheveled and unresponsive and is rushed by security guards into the department. He is quickly placed on a cardiac monitor, and intravenous access is established. His vital signs reveal a heart rate of 26 bpm and he is apneic. He has no palpable blood pressure but has a palpable slow pulse at his femoral artery. Fresh needle track marks, consistent with recent injections, are present in his left antecubital fossa. Physicians suspect he is a victim of the current epidemic of "superpotent" heroin, "China White," which is sweeping Allegheny County. Despite oral intubation, mechanical ventilation, advanced cardiac life support measures, and large intravenous doses of an antidote, the patient dies.

QUESTIONS

1. In 1988, the Pittsburgh, PA area experienced an epidemic of heroin abusers dying from accidental overdoses of a short-acting synthetic opioid agonist, 3-methyl fentanyl, known on the street as China White. These synthetic analogues of fentanyl were estimated to have 6000 times the potency of morphine. Pharmaceutical fentanyl has 75 to 100 times the potency of morphine. If a semilogarithmic dose–response curve of these three opioid agonists were plotted, which agent would have the smallest EC_{50} and the left-most drug dose–response curve?

   A. morphine

   B. fentanyl

   C. 3-methyl fentanyl

   D. naloxone

   E. naltrexone

2. Heroin abusers sought out the "superpotent" China White in 1988 for the experience of the intense rush and the thrill of taking a potent drug with life-threatening effects. Many unsuspecting abusers injected 3-methyl fentanyl once and suffered cardiorespiratory arrest within minutes. Those who survived to receive medical care required large doses of naloxone. In many cases, patients experienced reversal of their opioid agonist effects within minutes of an initial administration of naloxone but then experienced resedation, requiring multiple repeated doses of naloxone. This effect of naloxone is a characteristic of:

   A. a reversible agonist drug effect

   B. a reversible competitive antagonist drug effect

   C. a noncompetitive antagonist drug effect

   D. a partial agonist drug effect

   E. an inverse agonist drug effect

3. Heroin is usually measured in doses of 25-mg bags. Unsuspecting users of China White, who might have achieved a desired "high" with three bags of heroin, died after injecting one bag of 3-methyl fentanyl. If 50% of China White users died after injecting one bag of 3-methyl fentanyl, which of the following statements is correct?

   A. Heroin is more potent than 3-methyl fentanyl.

   B. The therapeutic index for 3-methyl fentanyl is larger than that for heroin.

   C. The ED_{50} for 3-methyl fentanyl is 25 mg.

   D. The TD_{50} for 3-methyl fentanyl is 75 mg.

   E. The LD_{50} for 3-methyl fentanyl is 25 mg.

4. Based on the above case, which of the following statements is correct?

   A. The therapeutic index of 3-methyl fentanyl is high.

   B. The EC_{50} of 3-methyl fentanyl is high.

   C. The LD_{50} of 3-methyl fentanyl is high.

   D. The affinity of 3-methyl fentanyl for the μ opioid receptor is high.

   E. The K_d of 3-methyl fentanyl is high.

5. Which of the following is an example of the action of a chemical antagonist?

   A. Naloxone binds to the μ opioid receptor and prevents opioid agonist effects.

   B. Digoxin-specific antibodies bind to digoxin and prevent its action at the cardiac sodium-potassium pump.

   C. Fentanyl binds to the μ opioid receptor and prevents the action of morphine.

   D. β-Adrenergic receptor antagonists bind to the β1-adrenergic receptor and decrease tachycardia in the setting of hyperthyroidism.

   E. Mannitol osmotically draws water into the renal tubule and prevents its reabsorption.

3

Pharmacokinetics

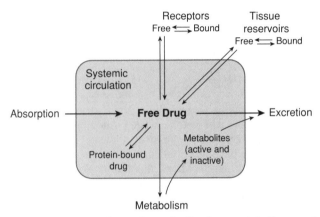

Figure 3-1. Drug Absorption, Distribution, Metabolism, and Excretion (ADME). The basic principles of pharmacokinetics affect the amount of free drug that ultimately reaches the target site. To elicit an effect on its target, a drug must be absorbed and then distributed to its target before being metabolized and excreted. At all times, free drug in the systemic circulation is in equilibrium with tissue reservoirs, plasma proteins, and the target site (which usually consists of receptors); only the fraction of drug that successfully binds to specific receptors has a pharmacologic effect. Note that metabolism of drug can result in both inactive and active metabolites; active metabolites may also be able to exert a pharmacologic effect, either on the target receptors or sometimes on other receptors. Adapted with permission from Hardman JG, Limbird LE, eds. Goodman & Gilman's The Pharmacological Basis of Therapeutics, 10th Ed, Figure 1-1, page 3. New York: The McGraw-Hill Companies, 2001.

OBJECTIVES

■ Understand the factors that affect drug absorption, distribution, metabolism, and excretion.

■ Understand how the pharmacokinetic characteristics of a drug can impact its therapeutic and potentially toxic effects.

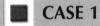

■ CASE 1

Mr. W. is a 66-year-old technology consultant who makes frequent trips abroad as part of his job in the telecommunications industry. His only medical problem is chronic atrial fibrillation, and his only chronic medication is warfarin. Mr.W. flies to Turkey for a consulting job. On the last night of the trip, he attends a large dinner featuring shish kebabs and other foods he does not often eat. The next day, he develops profuse, watery, foul-smelling diarrhea. A physician makes a diagnosis of traveler's diarrhea and prescribes a 7-day course of trimethoprim–sulfamethoxazole.

Mr. W. feels entirely well 2 days into the course of antibiotics, and 4 days later (while still taking his antibiotics), he entertains some clients at another lavish dinner. Mr. W. and his guests become intoxicated at the dinner, and Mr. W. stumbles and falls on the curb as he is leaving the restaurant. The next day, Mr. W. has a markedly swollen right knee that requires evaluation in a local emergency department. Physical examination and imaging studies are consistent with a moderate-sized hemarthrosis of the right knee, and laboratory studies show a markedly elevated International Normalized Ratio (INR) which is a standardized measure of prothrombin time and, in this clinical setting, a surrogate marker for plasma warfarin level. The emergency physician advises Mr. W. that his warfarin level is in the supratherapeutic (toxic) range and that this effect is likely attributable to adverse drug–drug interactions involving warfarin, antibiotics, and recent alcohol intoxication.

QUESTIONS

1. Which of the following could cause a patient with well-established therapeutic levels of a chronic medication to suddenly develop clinical manifestations of drug toxicity?
   A. The patient starts taking the medication with food.
   B. The patient starts taking another medication, which enhances hepatic first-pass metabolism of the chronic medication.
   C. The patient starts taking another medication, which increases the protein binding of the chronic medication.
   D. The patient starts taking another medication, which inhibits the hepatic metabolism of the chronic medication.
   E. The patient begins an aggressive exercise regimen, thereby increasing his muscle mass.

2. What was the cause of Mr. W.'s supratherapeutic warfarin level and subsequent bleeding?
   A. Trimethoprim–sulfamethoxazole inhibited the hepatic metabolism and clearance of warfarin.
   B. Trimethoprim–sulfamethoxazole enhanced the growth of gastrointestinal bacteria that normally degrade warfarin after its oral administration.
   C. Trimethoprim–sulfamethoxazole had an anticoagulant adverse effect.
   D. Trimethoprim–sulfamethoxazole competed with warfarin for binding at its receptor site of action.
   E. Trimethoprim–sulfamethoxazole prevented the renal secretion of warfarin.

3. How could Mr. W.'s situation have been avoided?
   A. The warfarin should have been discontinued while he was taking trimethoprim–sulfamethoxazole.
   B. The trimethoprim–sulfamethoxazole dose should have been decreased while he was taking warfarin.
   C. The warfarin dose should have been decreased while he was taking trimethoprim–sulfamethoxazole.
   D. The warfarin dose should have been decreased while he was drinking excessive ethanol at dinner.
   E. The trimethoprim–sulfamethoxazole dose should have been decreased while he was drinking excessive ethanol at dinner.

4. Drugs distribute within the body based on a four-compartment model and each drug's volume of distribution. Which of the following statements regarding the relationship between the administration of a drug and its distribution is correct?
   A. Drugs that exhibit high plasma protein binding tend to distribute rapidly into the protein-rich muscle compartment after intravenous administration.
   B. Drugs that have a large volume of distribution tend to distribute into all compartments after administration.
   C. Drugs tend to distribute into the fat compartment rapidly because it has the highest capacity for drug uptake and binding.
   D. Drugs that enter the vessel-rich compartment after administration tend to remain there and redistribute slowly to other compartments.
   E. Drugs that have a small volume of distribution tend to rapidly cross the blood–brain barrier.

5. Which of the following drug characteristics facilitates the transport of the drug across biologic membranes?
   A. nonpolar drug
   B. large molecular size drug
   C. ionized drug
   D. small diffusion gradient for drug
   E. hydrophilic drug

■ CASE 2

You are working in a local clinic. Your patient, Mr. S, is a 65-year-old man who you have been following closely over the past few weeks for progressively elevated blood pressure readings. You have just confirmed blood pressure readings of 145/105 mm Hg in Mr. S. this morning. You decide to begin a thiazide diuretic and a beta-receptor antagonist as antihypertensive therapy. As you try to choose between atenolol and propranolol for Mr. S., you recall that the thiazide you will prescribe is 98% plasma protein bound in the blood. You also consider the following facts about the two beta-receptor antagonists.

	Atenolol	Propranolol
Plasma protein binding	5%	95%
Urinary excretion of unchanged drug	85%	1%
Volume of distribution	39 L	270 L
β1/β2 selectivity	β1 selective	Nonselective

QUESTIONS

1. How does the differential plasma protein binding of atenolol versus propranolol affect your decision about therapy in this case?
   A. Atenolol is less highly protein bound, so it will have less ability to reach its receptor sites through the circulation.
   B. Atenolol is less highly protein bound, so it will be less likely to interfere with the plasma protein binding of thiazide.
   C. Propranolol is less highly protein bound, so it will be less likely to displace the thiazide from it plasma protein-binding sites.
   D. Propranolol is more highly protein bound, so it will be more likely to compete with the thiazide for binding at its end organ receptor sites.
   E. Propranolol is more highly protein bound, so it will require a lower administered dose to achieve an effect similar to that of atenolol.

2. Mr. S. is 65 years old, and you suspect that he has an age-related decrease in liver function. How does this fact impact your decision about the choice of therapy in this case?
   A. Atenolol is more highly metabolized by the liver, and the dose may need to be reduced to prevent drug accumulation and adverse effects.
   B. Atenolol is less highly metabolized by the liver, and the dose may need to be increased to be sure that therapeutic concentrations are achieved.
   C. Propranolol is less highly metabolized by the liver, and the dose may need to be increased to be sure that therapeutic concentrations are achieved.
   D. Propranolol is more highly metabolized by the liver, and the dose may need to be reduced to prevent liver failure.
   E. Propranolol is more highly metabolized by the liver, and the dose may need to be reduced to prevent drug accumulation and adverse effects.

3. You know that some drugs have undesirable CNS adverse effects. As you consider the pharmacokinetic parameters of atenolol versus propranolol, how does this information impact the likelihood of potential CNS adverse effects associated with each drug?
   A. Atenolol has a smaller volume of distribution and will not be able to achieve therapeutic concentrations in the CNS.
   B. Atenolol has a larger volume of distribution and will be more likely to cause CNS adverse effects.
   C. Propranolol has a larger volume of distribution and will be trapped in the fat compartment and less likely to cause CNS adverse effects.
   D. Propranolol has a larger volume of distribution and will be more likely to cause CNS adverse effects.
   E. Propranolol has a larger volume of distribution and will be more likely to reach therapeutic concentrations in the CNS.

4. You recall that Mr. S. has occasionally complained of asthma-like symptoms. How might this fact affect your choice of a beta-receptor antagonist?
   A. Atenolol is β_1 selective and will not be effective in controlling reactive airway disease.
   B. Atenolol is β_1 selective and may contribute to bronchospasm in patients with reactive airway disease.
   C. Propranolol is nonselective for β receptors and will not be effective in controlling reactive airway disease.
   D. Propranolol is nonselective for β receptors and will have reduced efficacy as an antihypertensive agent.
   E. Propranolol is nonselective for β receptors and may contribute to bronchospasm in patients with reactive airway disease.

5. The rate of metabolism and excretion of most drugs increases as the concentration of the drug increases in the systemic circulation. This is an example of:
   A. high extraction ratios
   B. saturation kinetics
   C. first-order kinetics
   D. zero-order kinetics
   E. high elimination half-life

4

Drug Metabolism

Table 4-1 **Pharmacologic Substrates, Inducers, and Inhibitors of Various Cytochrome P450 Enzymes**

P450 Enzyme	Substrates	Inhibitors	Inducers
P450 3A4	**Anti-HIV agents:** Indinavir Nelfinavir Ritonavir Saquinavir **Benzodiazepines:** Alprazolam Midazolam Triazolam **Calcium channel blockers:** Diltiazem Felodipine Nifedipine Verapamil **Immunosuppressants:** Cyclosporine Tacrolimus **Macrolide antibiotics:** Clarithromycin Erythromycin **Statins:** Atorvastatin Lovastatin **Others:** Loratadine Losartan Quinidine Sildenafil	**Antifungal agents (azoles):** Itraconazole Ketoconazole **Anti-HIV agents:** Delavirdine Indinavir Ritonavir Saquinavir **Calcium channel blockers:** Diltiazem Verapamil **Macrolide antibiotics:** Clarithromycin Erythromycin Troleandomycin (not azithromycin) **Others:** Cimetidine Grapefruit juice Mifepristone Nefazodone Norfloxacin	**Antiepileptics:** Carbemazepine Oxcarbazepine Phenobarbital Phenytoin **Anti-HIV agents:** Efavirenz Nevirapine **Rifamycins:** Rifabutins Rifampin Rifapentine **Others:** St. John's wort

(Continued)

OBJECTIVES

- Understand various pathways of drug metabolism.
- Understand how individual and pharmacologic factors can affect drug metabolism.

CASE 1

Ms. B. is a 32-year-old white woman who complains of sore throat and difficulty swallowing for the past 5 days. Physical examination reveals creamy white lesions on the tongue that are identified as oral thrush, a fungal infection. Her history includes sexual activity with multiple partners, inconsistent use of condoms, and continuous use of oral contraceptives

Table 4-1	**Pharmacologic Substrates, Inducers, and Inhibitors of Various Cytochrome P450 Enzymes** *(continued)*		
P450 Enzyme	**Substrates**	**Inhibitors**	**Inducers**
P450 2D6	**5-HT reuptake inhibitors:** Fluoxetine Paroxetine **Antiarrhythmic agents:** Flecainide Mexiletine Propafenone **Antidepressants:** Amitriptyline Clomipramine Desipramine Imipramine Nortiptyline **Antipsychotics:** Haloperidol Perphenazine Resperidone Venlafaxine **Beta-antagonists:** Alprenolol Bufuralol Carvedilol Metoprolol Penbutolol Propranolol Timolol **Opioids:** Codeine Dextromethorphan	**5-HT reuptake inhibitors:** Fluoxetine Paroxetine **Antiarrhythmic agents:** Amiodarone Quinidine **Antidepressants:** Clomipramine **Antipsychotics:** Haloperidol	None identified
P450 2C19	**Antidepressants:** Clomipramine Imipramine **Proton pump inhibitors:** Lansoprazole Omeprazole Pantoprazole **Others:** Propranolol R-warfarin	**Proton pump inhibitors:** Omeprazole **Others:** Fluoxetine Ritonavir Sertraline	Norethindrone Prednisone Rifampin
P450 2C9	**Angiotensin II receptor antagonists:** Irbesartan Losartan **Nonsteroidal anti-inflammatory drugs (NSAIDs)** Ibuprofen Suprofen **Others:** S-warfarin Tamoxifen	**Antifungal agents (azoles):** Fluconazole Miconazole **Others:** Amiodarone Phenylbutazone	Rifampin Secobarbital

(Continued)

| Table 4-1 | **Pharmacologic Substrates, Inducers, and Inhibitors of Various Cytochrome P450 Enzymes** *(Continued)* |

P450 Enzyme	Substrates	Inhibitors	Inducers
P450 2E1	**General anesthetics:** Enflurane Halothane Isoflurane Methoxyflurane Sevoflurane **Others:** Acetaminophen Ethanol	Disulfiram	Ethanol Isoniazid
P450 1A2	**Antidepressants:** Amitriptyline Clomipramine Clozapine Imipramine **Others:** R-warfarin Tacrine	**Quinolones:** Ciprofloxacin Enoxacin Norfloxacin Ofloxacin **Others:** Fluvoxamine	Char-grilled meat Cruciferous vegetables Insulin Omeprazole Phenobarbital Rifampin Tobacco

for the past 14 years. The presentation suggests a diagnosis of HIV-1 infection, which is confirmed by polymerase chain reaction (PCR) analysis. Ms. B. has a low CD4 T-cell count and is immediately started on a standard anti-HIV regimen that includes the protease inhibitor saquinavir. Her oral thrush resolves with a topical antifungal agent. Despite aggressive therapy, her CD4 cell count continues to decrease, and she presents to her physician several months later with fatigue and a persistent cough. Further investigation leads to a diagnosis of tuberculosis.

QUESTIONS

1. Many factors influence normal drug metabolism and transport. As her physician considers the most appropriate drug regimen to treat both Ms. B.'s acute tuberculosis and her underlying HIV disease, what factors might he consider?

    A. If oral thrush is present, it will prevent gastrointestinal absorption of oral contraceptives.

    B. The multidrug resistance protein 1 (MDR1) transporter will block the gastrointestinal absorption of antituberculous agents in patients with HIV infection.

    C. The metabolism of saquinavir will be enhanced by the administration of antituberculous agents.

    D. The metabolism of saquinavir will be enhanced by drinking grapefruit juice.

    E. The renal elimination of antituberculous drugs is prevented by saquinivir.

2. One of the first-line drugs in the treatment of tuberculosis is rifampin, which decreases the effectiveness of HIV protease inhibitors. What is the mechanism for this drug–drug interaction?

    A. Rifampin induces the activity of the P450 3A4 enzyme.

    B. Rifampin induces the production of glucuronic acid.

    C. Rifampin inhibits the activity of the MDR1 transporter.

    D. Rifampin competes with protease inhibitors for binding to P450 3A4.

    E. Rifampin diverts protease inhibitors to the kidney for rapid elimination.

3. Isoniazid is another drug commonly used in the treatment of patients with tuberculosis. Why does Ms. B.'s ethnic background give her physician reason for concern when considering the use of this drug?

    A. If Ms. B. is a "fast acetylator," she is at risk for supratherapeutic isoniazid concentrations.

    B. If Ms. B. is a "fast acetylator," she will have P450 3A4 enzyme induction.

    C. If Ms. B. is a "slow acetylator," she will develop supratherapeutic saquinivir concentrations.

    D. If Ms. B. is a "slow acetylator," she is at risk for isoniazid-associated drug toxicity.

    E. If Ms. B. is a "slow acetylator," she will be unable to absorb isoniazid from the gastrointestinal tract.

4. Some drugs are absorbed from the gastrointestinal tract and transported by the portal system to the liver, where they are metabolized. Their subsequent bioavailability may be lowered. This is called:
   A. conjugation/hydrolysis
   B. first-pass effect
   C. portal hypertension
   D. xenobiosis
   E. P450 enzyme induction

5. Oxidation/reduction reactions take place primarily within the:
   A. hepatocyte plasma membrane
   B. gastrointestinal epithelium
   C. endoplasmic reticulum
   D. cytosol
   E. hepatocyte nucleus

 CASE 2

Bessie B. is a 78-year-old woman who is brought to her family physician, Dr. Joy, by her daughter for an evaluation of excessive sleeping. Her family has noted her to be progressively confused and ''slow'' over the past week, falling asleep during dinner the past two evenings. This morning, she did not get up at her usual time to make the morning coffee, and her husband called their daughter to come over and help. Mrs. B.'s husband and daughter were able to wake her only with great difficulty to get dressed and come to the doctor. She slept in the car on the way. Mrs. B. has no complaints. She does state that she has been very tired, but she attributes it to planting this year's tomatoes in the garden, weeding the flowerbeds, and subsequently catching a cold and cough last week. There is no history of trauma or depression.

Mrs. B.'s medical history is remarkable for hypertension, stable coronary artery disease, a history of supraventricular tachycardia, and anxiety. She is allergic to penicillins and was recently started on an antibiotic for bronchitis. On physical examination her vital signs include a temperature of 98.6°F, a heart rate of 54 bpm, respiratory rate of 17 breaths/min., and blood pressure of 142/87 mm Hg. She is well nourished but appears somewhat tired. Her examination is normal except for her mental status. She appears slightly sedated, but she opens her eyes to voices and answers with slightly slurred speech. When Dr. Joy and her family are not directly interacting with her, she dozes. Dr. Joy reviews Mrs. B.'s medications, which include aspirin, alprazolam (a benzodiazepine), diltiazem (a calcium channel blocker), hydrochlorothiazide (a thiazide diuretic), lovastatin (an HMG-CoA reductase inhibitor), and clarithromycin (a macrolide antiobiotic).

QUESTIONS

1. Which of Mrs. B.'s medications might account for her drowsiness?
   A. aspirin
   B. alprazolam
   C. diltiazem
   D. lovastatin
   E. clarithromycin

2. Dr. Joy is concerned that Mrs. B. may be having a drug-drug interaction, which is causing altered metabolism and subsequent clinical toxicity (somnolence). As she reviews her medication list, she notes the recent addition of clarithromycin for the treatment of bronchitis. Clarithromycin is a macrolide antiobiotic. How do macrolides affect the normal metabolism of other drugs?
   A. Macrolide antibiotics competitively bind the active metabolites of prodrugs.
   B. Macrolide antibiotics irreversibly bind enzymes of conjugation.
   C. Macrolide antibiotics induce certain P450 enzymes.
   D. Macrolide antibiotics promote MDR1 transporter function.
   E. Macrolide antibiotics inhibit certain P450 enzymes.

3. Dr. Joy also considers Mrs. B.'s advancing age and suggests that some adjustments need to be made to her medication regimen. Which of the following statements regarding drug metabolism and age is correct?
   A. Neonates metabolize drugs using maternal enzymes passed through the placenta before birth.
   B. Neonates have enhanced enzyme function in the production of bilirubin.
   C. Elderly patients have a greater sensitivity to the metabolic effects of grapefruit juice.
   D. Elderly patients have enlarged livers but reduced blood flow to drug-metabolizing enzyme zones.
   E. Elderly patients have diminished hepatic drug-metabolizing enzyme activity.

4. One example of how drug metabolism is affected by racial or ethnic factors is:
   A. African Americans have a greater ability to metabolize β-receptor antagonists.
   B. Caucasian individuals have insufficient enzymatic ability to metabolize tricyclic antidepressants.
   C. More than 90% of Asians are ''fast acetylators'' in metabolizing rifampin.
   D. African Americans exhibit reduced enzyme activity to convert codeine to morphine.
   E. Asian Americans exhibit enhanced enzyme activity in the metabolism of warfarin.

5. Gray baby syndrome is a clinical syndrome of shock, pallor, and cyanosis that occurs in infants. The drug associated with the development of gray baby syndrome is:
   A. chloramphenicol
   B. warfarin
   C. oral contraceptives (used in the mother)
   D. psoralen
   E. isoniazid

5

Drug Toxicity

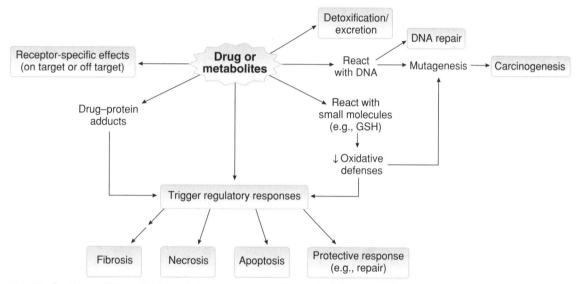

Figure 5-1. Mechanisms of Drug Toxicity. A drug or its metabolites or both interact with specific receptors to mediate on-target or off-target adverse effects. In addition, metabolites can be detoxified and excreted or can react with a variety of macromolecules, including DNA, small antioxidants such as glutathione (GSH), or cellular or plasma proteins. The formation of unrepaired or misrepaired DNA adducts is often mutagenic and may lead to cancer. The impairment of oxidative defenses can lead to inflammation and cell death (apoptosis or necrosis). The formation of drug–protein adducts can trigger immune responses that can damage cells and tissues. Regardless of the mechanism of damage, a gradation of acute responses from protective to apoptosis (programmed cell death) and necrosis can result, depending on the extent of damage and the temporal and dose relationships. Chronic inflammation and repair can also lead to tissue fibrosis.

OBJECTIVES

 Understand various mechanisms of drug toxicity.

■ CASE 1

Ms. G. is an 80-year-old piano teacher with progressively severe right leg pain over a period of 5 to 10 years. She has continued to teach in her studio but at the cost of increasing pain and fatigue. Imaging studies reveal severe osteoarthritis of the right hip. She is scheduled for elective replacement of the right hip with a prosthetic joint.

The total hip replacement is performed without immediate complications. During the first few days after the operation, Ms. G. is given low-molecular-weight heparin and warfarin as prophylaxis against deep vein thrombosis. Six days after the operation, she develops excruciating pain in the area of the operation. Right lateral hip and buttock swelling is noted on physical examination. A complete blood count reveals significant blood loss (decrease in hematocrit from 35% to 25%), and she is taken back to the operating room for evacuation of a large hematoma around the prosthetic joint. Although the hematoma does not appear to be grossly infected, cultures of the hematoma are positive for *Staphylococcus aureus*.

QUESTIONS

1. What was the rationale for co-administration of low-molecular weight heparin and warfarin in the immediate post-operative period?

   A. Low-molecular-weight heparin and warfarin are molecular enantiomers, which balance their anticoagulant effects when coadministered.

   B. Low-molecular-weight heparin competes with warfarin for sites of hepatic metabolism, and slows its metabolism to enhance its therapeutic effect.

   C. Low-molecular-weight heparin is administered to achieve anticoagulation until plasma warfarin concentrations reach a therapeutic anticoagulant level.

   D. Low-molecular-weight heparin is administered in the hospital, but warfarin can be administered at home.

   E. Coadministration of these drugs achieves an anticoagulant effect at lower drug dosages, while minimizing the drug-associated toxicity of each of the agents.

2. As anticoagulants, low-molecular weight heparin catalyzes the inactivation of factor Xa by antithrombin III, and warfarin inhibits the formation of clotting factors II, VII, IX, and X. Supratherapeutic anticoagulation and bleeding as a result of the coadministration of these drugs is an example of:

   A. a hypersensitivity reaction to a therapeutic drug

   B. an overdose of therapeutic drugs

   C. a pharmacokinetic drug–drug interaction

   D. a pharmacodynamic drug–drug interaction

   E. an "off-target" side effect of a therapeutic drug

3. Because prosthetic joint infections are difficult to treat successfully without removal of the prosthesis, Ms. G. is started on an aggressive 12-week course of combination antibiotics in which intravenous vancomycin and oral rifampin are administered for 2 weeks followed by oral ciprofloxacin and rifampin for 10 weeks. She tolerates the first 2 weeks of antibiotics without complications. What was the primary rationale for administration of vancomycin and rifampin followed by ciprofloxacin and rifampin for treatment of the *S. aureus* infection?

   A. A change in antibiotics will prevent the development of bacterial resistance to the agents.

   B. A more expensive drug (vancomycin) would be replaced by a less expensive drug (ciprofloxacin).

   C. One antibiotic combination would be replaced with another combination with greater synergistic antimicrobial effects.

   D. A more potentially allergenic antibiotic combination would be replaced with a less potentially allergenic combination.

   E. A less convenient intravenous formulation (vancomycin) would be replaced with a more convenient oral formulation (ciprofloxacin).

Thirty-six hours after switching her antibiotic from vancomycin to ciprofloxacin, she develops a high fever to 103°F and extreme weakness. Aspiration of the hip reveals only a scant amount of straw-colored (i.e., nonpurulent) fluid. Ms. G. is therefore admitted to the hospital for close observation.

Twelve hours after her admission, Ms. G. develops an extensive maculopapular rash over her chest, back, and extremities. Her ciprofloxacin and rifampin are discontinued and vancomycin is restarted. Gradually, over the next 72 hours, her temperature returns to normal and her rash begins to fade. There is no growth in the culture of the right hip aspirate. Ms. G. is continued on vancomycin as a single agent for the next 4 weeks without incident; rifampin is restarted, again without incident; and the 12-week antibiotic course is eventually completed using a combination of trimethoprim–sulfamethoxazole and rifampin.

4. Within hours of switching from vancomycin to ciprofloxacin, Ms. G. developed a high fever, weakness, and skin rash. These symptoms most likely represented:

   A. an infection with a ciprofloxacin-resistant bacteria

   B. an immediate hypersensitivity reaction to ciprofloxacin

   C. a delayed-type hypersensitivity reaction to ciprofloxacin

   D. a delayed-type hypersensitivity reaction to rifampin

   E. unopposed rifampin toxicity syndrome

Four months after her hip surgery, Ms. G. is back to teaching her piano students and making slow but steady progress in her rehabilitation program.

5. If Ms. G. was to develop a urinary tract infection next year, which of the following drugs would be contraindicated as therapy?

   A. vancomycin

   B. levofloxacin

   C. rifampin

   D. trimethoprim–sulfamethoxazole

   E. acetaminophen

 CASE 2

Friday, 9 PM: Jenna B. is a 17-year-old girl. She has a history of seizures since childhood, for which she takes phenytoin, an antiepileptic drug. This afternoon, she took a home pregnancy test, which was positive. She is terrified of telling her parents the news. She recently won a scholarship to a prestigious art school, and her parents are very excited about her future college plans. Desperate, Ms. B. ingests a bottle of acetaminophen in an overdose. She writes a suicide note to her parents and goes to bed.

QUESTIONS

1. How does acetaminophen cause toxicity in overdose?
   A. Acetaminophen binds to unintended alternate receptor sites in the liver.
   B. Acetaminophen is hepatically metabolized to a toxic metabolite.
   C. Acetaminophen acts as a hapten and induces an autoimmune hepatitis.
   D. Acetaminophen metabolites induce collagen deposition in the liver.
   E. Acetaminophen metabolism competitively blocks the normal metabolism of bile components and leads to cholestasis.

Saturday, 10 AM: Ms. B. awakes feeling terrible. She is very nauseated and vomits multiple times in her bathroom. Her mother finds her vomiting bilious liquid into the toilet, and Ms. B. breaks down in tears and tells her about the pregnancy and her drug ingestion of the night before. Her mother calls the pediatrician and rushes her to the emergency department at Children's Hospital.

2. Why was there a delay in time between Ms. B.'s ingestion of acetaminophen and the onset of her clinical symptoms of acetaminophen toxicity?
   A. Clinical symptoms do not occur until glutathione stores are depleted and the toxic metabolite begins to bind and induce damage to hepatocytes.
   B. Clinical symptoms are delayed when another drug (phenytoin) competes with acetaminophen for metabolic sites in the liver.
   C. Clinical symptoms are delayed because hepatic metabolism of drugs is slowed in pregnancy.
   D. Clinical symptoms do not occur until acetaminophen is able to form covalent bonds with hepatic metabolizing enzymes.
   E. Clinical symptoms are delayed when the stomach is full of drug tablets, which cannot be rapidly absorbed from the gastrointestinal tract.

3. Ms. B. takes phenytoin, an antiepileptic drug, which is hepatically metabolized and known to induce the activity of hepatic P450 enzymes. What might be the impact of chronic phenytoin use on her acetaminophen overdose?
   A. Ms. B.'s liver will be more efficient in metabolizing acetaminophen to its toxic metabolite, putting her at increased risk for liver toxicity.
   B. Ms. B.'s liver will be more efficient in conjugating the toxic metabolite to glucuronide, protecting her from liver toxicity.
   C. Ms. B.'s liver will be more efficient in conjugating the toxic metabolite to glutathione, protecting her from liver toxicity.
   D. Ms. B.'s liver will be unable to metabolize acetaminophen efficiently in the presence of phenytoin, protecting her from liver toxicity.
   E. Ms. B.'s liver will be unable to metabolize acetaminophen efficiently in the presence of phenytoin, putting her at increased risk for liver toxicity.

Saturday, 11AM: On arrival at Children's Hospital, Ms. B. is still retching and complaining of an ''aching'' upper abdominal discomfort. The pediatric emergency physician notes the following findings on examination: temperature, 99.3°F; pulse, 132 bpm; respiratory rate, 24 breaths/min. and blood pressure, 92/50 mm Hg. Ms. B. is pale and appears tired. Her mucous membranes are dry. She has moderate abdominal tenderness on palpation of the right upper quadrant. Intravenous access is initiated, and although laboratory studies (including complete blood count, electrolytes, blood urea nitrogen, creatinine, tests of liver damage and synthetic function, serum acetaminophen concentration, and pregnancy test) are still pending, an intravenous infusion of N-acetylcysteine is initiated as a loading dose and maintenance infusion.

4. The effect of chronic phenytoin use on acetaminophen metabolism in the liver is an example of:
   A. a hypersensitivity reaction to a therapeutic drug
   B. an overdose of therapeutic drugs
   C. a pharmacokinetic drug–drug interaction
   D. a pharmacodynamic drug–drug interaction
   E. an "off-target" side effect of a therapeutic drug

Sunday, 5PM: Ms. B. is completing her infusion of N-acetylcysteine. Her abdominal pain and nausea have resolved. Although the initial measurements of liver damage were elevated, these tests are normalizing. She and her parents meet with the child psychiatrist, and social worker.

5. Acetaminophen crosses the placenta. What is the potential impact of Ms. B.'s overdose on her pregnancy?
   A. If acetaminophen is conjugated by glucuronidation and sulfation, it will be trapped in the fetal kidneys.
   B. If acetaminophen reaches the fetal hepatic circulation, it will be conjugated to glutathione.
   C. If the fetal liver is developing during this period, teratogenic effects of acetaminophen will be realized.
   D. If the fetal liver is not developing during this period, no carcinogenic effect of acetaminophen will be realized.
   E. If the fetal hepatic P450 enzymes are functioning, the fetal liver will elaborate the toxic metabolite and cause fetal hepatotoxicity.

ANSWERS TO SECTION I

CHAPTER 1 ANSWERS

CASE 1

1. **The answer is E.** Normally, the receptor tyrosine kinases phosphorylate tyrosine residues on the cytoplasmic tail of the receptor, as well as on cytosolic signaling molecules. The mutant Philadelphia chromosome codes for a constitutively active receptor tyrosine kinase protein, BCR-Abl. **This kinase phosphorylates cytosolic proteins, leading to dysregulated cell growth** and chronic myeloid leukemia. This mutation is an example of a "gain-of-function" mutation, which allows ligand-independent activity and, in this case, uncontrolled cell growth.

2. **The answer is E. Imatinib inhibits the ability of BCR-Abl to phosphorylate substrates**. It binds to the ATP-binding site of the BCR-Abl tyrosine kinase and causes the protein to assume an enzymatically inactive conformation, which inhibits its kinase activity. This limits the intracellular signals for myeloid cell growth.

3. **The answer is A. Older therapies target all myeloid cells** and have effects on diverse cell processes. This leads to significant toxic adverse effects in many cells or tissues, which are affected by the chemotherapeutic drug's mechanism of action.

4. **The answer is A. Imatinib selectively binds the BCR-Abl protein in abnormally growing hematopoietic cells.** It is a chemotherapeutic agent, whose action is restricted to a specific cell-type distribution of a receptor. This accounts for its specificity and the low incidence of adverse effects in patients treated with imatinib. In contrast to receptor tyrosine kinases, tyrosine kinase–associated receptors do not have innate enzymatic activity, but rather, induce other cytosolic proteins to phosphorylate tyrosine residues.

5. **The answer is C. Signal amplification** refers to the ability of a cell to amplify the effects of receptor binding. For example, when a ligand binds to a G protein–cou-

pled receptor, the G protein molecule can bind to and activate many effector molecules, amplifying the cellular second messenger response to the ligand binding. Tachyphylaxis occurs when drugs have diminishing effects over time. The desensitization of the receptor and the cell can be homologous (only one type of receptor shows a diminished response to the agonist), or heterologous (two or more types of receptors show a coordinately diminished response).

CASE 2

1. **The answer is B.** The binding site of organophosphate insecticides is an **extracellular enzyme**, acetylcholinesterase. These chemicals bind to the active site of acetylcholinesterase and form an oxygen–phosphorus bond in the enzyme complex, which prevents the degradation of acetylcholine within the synaptic cleft. Because organophosphates nonselectively bind to acetylcholinesterase at both nicotinic and muscarinic sites, they can cause enhanced cholinergic neurotransmission at both of these cholinergic synapses. This results in a depolarizing neuromuscular blockade, as well as muscarinic symptoms of profuse sweating, miotic pupils, and copious oral and bronchial secretions. Cell surface adhesion receptors mediate cell to cell interactions and communication.

2. **The answer is E.** Organophosphate insecticides would be considered **indirect agonists** at cholinergic synapses. They do not bind directly to the acetylcholine receptor as direct agonists, but increase the concentration of acetylcholine within the synapse. In this way, they facilitate the agonist effect of acetylcholine at its receptor, where acetylcholine binds and induces a conformational change in the receptor-associated ion channel to increase membrane permeability for cations. Inverse agonists cause constitutively active receptor targets to adopt an inactive receptor conformation. Antagonists inhibit the ability of receptor targets to be activated by endogenous agonists.

3. **The answer is D.** The "aged" oxygen–phosphorus bond is a **covalent bond** that is essentially irreversible. The affected enzyme is destroyed, and subsequent acetylcholinesterase function is dependent on the regenera-

tion of new enzyme. The antidote to organophosphate poisoning, pralidoxime, reverses the oxygen–phosphorus bond but must be administered before aging occurs and the bond becomes covalent. An ionic bond occurs between atoms with opposite charges. Van der Waals forces result from the induced polarity on molecules as a result of shifting electron density, and create a weak attractive force between chemicals and their receptors. Hydrogen bonding is mediated by the interaction between positively and negatively polarized atoms.

4. **The answer is A.** The nicotinic acetylcholine receptor is an example of **a ligand-gated ion channel.** When two acetylcholine molecules bind to the postsynaptic receptor, a conformational change in the transmembrane channel occurs, allowing ion conductance through the channel. Voltage-gated ion channels change their state and conformation based on changes in the cell membrane potential.

5. **The answer is B. The intracellular region is linked to a G protein, which affects signaling molecules after binding of the ligand** to the extracellular domain of the receptor. The G protein diffuses away from the intracellular domain of the receptor to act on a number of effector molecules, including adenylyl cyclase, phospholipase C, and ion channels. Signals mediated by G proteins are usually terminated by the hydrolysis of GTP to GDP. The transmembrane region consists of a single polypeptide chain, which traverses the membrane seven times, connecting the extracellular ligand-binding site with the intracellular G protein linkage. It is not an ion channel. The G protein–coupled receptors are the most abundant class of receptors in the human body.

CHAPTER 2 ANSWERS

CASE 1

1. **The answer is D.** The potency (EC_{50}) of a drug is the concentration at which the drug elicits 50% of its maximal response. Highly potent drugs can elicit 50% of their maximal response at lower concentrations (or have small EC_{50}s). **The presence of a competitive antagonist shifts the agonist dose–response curve to the right and decreases its potency.** This is because the binding of a competitive antagonist alters the equilibrium for the binding of the agonist to its receptor and increases its apparent K_d. Agonists with low potency have a drug dose–response curve, which lies to the right of more potent but similar drugs. The greater a drug's potency, the lower its drug-receptor dissociation constant, K_d.

2. **The answer is B. The maximal efficacy of an agonist is the condition at which receptor-mediated signaling by the drug is maximal.** E_{max} is the maximal response produced by the agonist, at which additional drug will produce no additional response. This usually occurs when all receptors are occupied by the drug, with the exception of conditions when "spare receptors" are present. The presence of a noncompetitive antagonist reduces the maximal possible response to drug-receptor binding, and therefore reduces drug efficacy. This is because noncompetitive antagonists exert their effect by preventing the receptor from being activated, regardless of the presence or binding of the agonist drug. More potent drugs mediate their effect at a lower proportion of receptor binding. The ED_{50} is the median effective dose of a drug that produces a response in 50% of the population. The LD_{50} is the median lethal dose of a drug, causing a lethal effect in 50% of the population.

3. **The answer is E. Aspirin has a larger therapeutic index, while heparin has a small therapeutic index.** As such, aspirin elicits a therapeutic response over a wider range of doses without unacceptable adverse effects. In contrast, heparin has a therapeutic index of less than 2; it can cause toxicity and hemorrhage at doses that are less than twice the therapeutic dose. Therefore, its anticoagulant effect should be monitored closely. Graded dose–response relationships describe the effect of various drug doses in an individual. Quantal dose–response relationships describe the responses of a population to a given drug at a given dose.

4. **The answer is D. Drugs with a low therapeutic index do not have therapeutic effects until the administered dose approaches the toxic dose.** The therapeutic index is defined as TD_{50}/ED_{50}, where TD_{50} is the dose of a drug that causes a toxic response in 50% of the population, and ED_{50}, is the dose of a drug that causes a therapeutic effect in 50% of the population. The therapeutic index quantifies the relative safety margin of a drug. A drug with a low therapeutic index has a greater potential for toxicity as the administered dose is increased.

5. **The answer is C.** The concept of "spare receptors" refers to **a maximal agonist response occurring with less than 100% receptor occupancy.** In such a case, maximal efficacy of a drug is achieved at a lower dose of agonist drug despite the fact that receptors are not saturated. This is graphically represented as an EC_{50}, which is less than the K_d for the drug-receptor interaction. The presence of spare receptors allows the efficacy of a drug to be maintained even in the presence of low concentrations of antagonists. In contrast, the potency is reduced because a greater proportion of available receptors must be occupied by the agonist to achieve a 50% response.

CASE 2

1. **The answer is C. 3-methyl fentanyl** is the most potent of the three opioid agonists listed in this question. It would have the smallest EC_{50} and the left-most drug dose–response curve. Morphine would have the largest EC_{50} and right-most curve, and fentanyl would be in the middle. Naloxone and naltrexone are not opioid agonists, but antagonists.

2. **The answer is B.** Naloxone causes **a reversible competitive antagonist drug effect.** It competes with opioids for binding at the μ opioid receptor. By preventing opioid action at the active site, naloxone reverses the sedating and depressant effects of opioids. However, its half-life is approximately 1 hour, and resedation can occur through opioid action at μ opioid receptors that are no longer occupied by naloxone.

3. **The answer is E. The LD_{50} for 3-methyl fentanyl is 25 mg.** This is the dose of drug at which 50% of the users died.

4. **The answer is D. The affinity of 3-methyl fentanyl for the μ opioid receptor is high.** Fentanyl and its illicit analogues are highly potent opioid agonists. Abuse of these drugs is potentially lethal.

5. **The answer is B. Digoxin-specific antibodies bind to digoxin and prevent its action at the cardiac sodium-potassium pump.** This is an example of a chemical antagonist: the agonist effect of digoxin is prevented by "sequestration" of the drug by specific antibodies, which bind digoxin and remove it from its binding site on the cardiac myocyte. The binding of β-adrenergic receptor antagonists to the β1-adrenergic receptor, decreasing tachycardia in the setting of hyperthyroidism, is an example of physiologic antagonist action.

CHAPTER 3 ANSWERS

CASE 1

1. **The answer is D. The patient starts taking another medication, which inhibits the hepatic metabolism of the chronic medication.** This change in drug metabolism will alter the steady-state plasma concentrations of the chronic medication, and may lead to symptoms of clinical toxicity. In contrast, some changes can lead to a decrease in a chronic drug's availability and therapeutic effect. For example, taking the chronic medication with food may reduce its gastrointestinal absorption. Taking another medication that enhances hepatic first-pass metabolism may reduce the amount of the active drug available to the systemic circulation after absorption. Increasing muscle mass may alter the volume of distribution of the chronic medication and reduce the amount of free drug available to act at its receptor sites.

2. **The answer is A. Trimethoprim–sulfamethoxazole inhibited the hepatic metabolism and clearance of warfarin.** This increased the steady-state concentration of warfarin and caused supratherapeutic warfarin concentrations. In addition, ethanol also inhibited the metabolism of warfarin. These factors led to an excessive warfarin level and bleeding.

3. **The answer is C. The warfarin dose should have been decreased while the patient was taking trimethoprim–sulfamethoxazole.** In addition, excessive ethanol should be avoided when its metabolism competes with the normal metabolic pathways of chronic medications. Chronic warfarin therapy should not be abruptly discontinued.

4. **The answer is B. Drugs that have a large volume of distribution tend to distribute into all compartments after administration.** The volume of distribution represents the fluid volume that would be required to contain the total amount of absorbed drug if it were at a uniform concentration throughout that volume. The distribution of a drug is achieved through the circulatory system. Drugs that exhibit high plasma protein binding tend to stay within the vascular compartment and have a small volume of distribution. The vessel-rich compartment is the first extravascular compartment in which drug concentration increases. However, because of the high vascularity of this compartment, drug redistribution from this compartment also occurs rapidly. Although the fat compartment has the highest capacity for drug uptake, it is the least vascular. Therefore, drug uptake into and redistribution from the fat compartment occur at a slower rate.

5. **The answer is A. Nonpolar drugs,** lipophilic drugs, and drugs of small molecular size tend to cross biologic membranes easily. Polar, ionized drugs, and drugs with small diffusion gradients do not cross membranes as easily and may require transmembrane protein transporters to facilitate their transport across biologic membranes.

CASE 2

1. **The answer is B. Atenolol is less highly protein bound, so it is less likely to interfere with the plasma protein binding of the thiazide.** In contrast, propranolol, which exhibits high protein binding, displaces the thiazide from its plasma protein binding sites, increasing the concentration of free thiazide and its diuretic effect. Drugs that are more highly bound to plasma proteins have a smaller volume of distribution, but may require larger administered doses to reach the free drug concentrations necessary to achieve their therapeutic effect.

2. **The answer is E. Propranolol is more highly metabolized by the liver, and the dose may need to be reduced to prevent drug accumulation and adverse effects.** Alternatively, the frequency of proprano-

lol dosing could be reduced to limit drug accumulation and adverse effects. In contrast, atenolol is 85% excreted by the kidneys in an unchanged form, and impaired liver function would not be expected to alter its dose. However, renal insufficiency could lead to an accumulation of atenolol.

3. **The answer is D. Propranolol has a larger volume of distribution and will be more likely to cause CNS adverse effects**, including drowsiness, lethargy, coma, and seizures at toxic levels. Because of its lipophilic nature and large volume of distribution, propranolol also distributes to the fat compartment, which can act as a depot reservoir for continued slow redistribution of the drug to other compartments. In contrast, atenolol is more hydrophilic and has a smaller volume of distribution. It is unlikely to cause CNS adverse effects.

4. **The answer is E. Propranolol is nonselective for β receptors and may contribute to bronchospasm in patients with reactive airway disease.** Because bronchial smooth muscle relaxation is mediated by β_2 receptors, a nonselective beta-receptor antagonist might contribute to bronchospasm in Mr. S.

5. **The answer is C. First-order kinetics** refers to a rate of metabolism and excretion of a drug that is directly proportional to the concentration of the drug in the systemic circulation. As the concentration of a drug increases, its rate of metabolism also increases proportionally. In other words, its clearance mechanisms do not become saturated under normal therapeutic circumstances. In contrast, some drugs demonstrate saturation kinetics such that their clearance mechanisms become saturated at or near the therapeutic concentration of the drug. As the drug concentration increases, the clearance rate does not increase but remains constant. This is a characteristic of zero-order kinetics. In such a case, increasing drug concentrations can lead to toxic effects. Organs with high extraction ratios contribute significantly to drug clearance from the plasma. The elimination half-life is the amount of time over which a drug concentration in plasma decreases to half of its original concentration.

CHAPTER 4 ANSWERS

CASE 1

1. **The answer is C. The metabolism of saquinavir will be enhanced by the administration of antituberculous agents**, which induce the activity of P450 enzymes responsible for saquinavir's metabolism. The multidrug resistance protein 1 (MDR1) transporter actively transports drugs back into the intestinal lumen and can limit the bioavailability of a number of drugs, including HIV-1 protease inhibitors and digoxin. The metabolism of saquinavir could be reduced by drinking grapefruit juice. Grapefruit juice contains psoralen derivatives that inhibit the P450 3A4 enzymes (as well as the MDR1 transporter in the small intestine).

2. **The answer is A. Rifampin induces the activity of P450 3A4** (as well as P450 2C19, P450 2C9, and P450 1A2), probably by increasing the expression of the enzyme protein that is responsible for the metabolism of many drugs, including protease inhibitors. Concurrent administration of rifampin with saquinivir would enhance the metabolism of saquinivir. This would limit the bioavailability and subsequent therapeutic efficacy of the protease inhibitor. Macrolide antibiotics such as erythromycin inhibit the activity of the MDR1 transporter.

3. **The answer is D. If Ms. B. is a "slow acetylator" she is at risk for isoniazid-associated drug toxicity.** Isoniazid metabolism is by conjugation, mediated by N-acetyl transferase, an enzyme whose expression is genetically variable. Forty-five percent of whites and blacks in the United States (and some northern Europeans) synthesize this enzyme at a decreased rate. This results in "slow" acetylation of certain drugs, particularly isoniazid. The consequence is a reduced rate of isoniazid metabolism, higher serum concentrations of the free drug, which inhibits P450 enzymes and puts the patient at risk for drug–drug interactions and toxicity. Saquinivir is metabolized by oxidation, not conjugation.

4. **The answer is B. First-pass effect** is the phenomenon by which orally administered drugs are absorbed and carried directly to the liver, where they undergo metabolism before they reach the systemic circulation and their target organs. If hepatic metabolism is extensive, the amount of active drug reaching the systemic circulation may be insufficient, necessitating alternative methods of administration, including parenteral or transdermal administration.

5. **The answer is C.** Oxidation/reduction reactions take place primarily within the **endoplasmic reticulum** of hepatocytes and some other tissue cells. Conjugation and hydrolysis reactions take place in the cytosol and the endoplasmic reticulum.

CASE 2

1. **The answer is B. Alprazolam**, a benzodiazepine, can cause sedation.

2. **The answer is E. Macrolide antibiotics inhibit certain P450 enzymes.** They are metabolized by the enzyme, and the product subsequently forms a complex with the active site of the enzyme. This effect slows the metabolism of many other drugs, including alprazolam (causing excessive sedation), diltiazem (causing bradycardia), and lovastatin (putting the patient at risk for statin-associated muscle breakdown). Macrolide antibiotics also inhibit the MDR1 transporter function, contributing to enhanced gastrointestinal absorption of some drugs, including digoxin.

3. **The answer is E. Elderly patients have diminished drug-metabolizing hepatic enzyme activity,** smaller liver mass, and reduced hepatic blood flow. All of these factors contribute to a reduced capacity to metabolize drugs in elderly patients. Because elderly patients tend to be given multiple medications, it is necessary to check for drug–drug interactions and to adjust medication doses appropriately. Neonates have the capacity to carry out most oxidative reactions. Their drug-metabolizing enzyme systems mature over the first 2 weeks of life. Neonatal jaundice is caused by a deficiency of the bilirubin-conjugating enzyme, UDP-GT. Grapefruit juice contains psoralen derivatives, which inhibit both P450 3A4 and MDR1 activity.

4. **The answer is D.** Some genetic aspects of race or ethnicity can affect drug metabolism. This may be based on differences in the activity of certain enzymes or in polymorphisms in the genes encoding certain enzymes. For example, **African Americans exhibit reduced ability to convert codeine to morphine.** This is because of a higher percentage (compared to white and Asian persons) of functionally inactive P450 2D6 enzymes, which are responsible for this conversion, as well as the metabolism of β-receptor antagonists and cyclic antidepressants. Asian Americans tend to exhibit reduced metabolism of warfarin. This is due to a genetic variation in the expression of hepatic drug-metabolizing enzymes. More than 90% of Asians are "fast acetylators" in metabolizing isoniazid.

5. **The answer is A. Chloramphenicol** is an antibiotic that was once prescribed for the treatment of *Hemophilus influenza* infection in infants. Its oxidation metabolite is toxic, and if it is not conjugated appropriately for elimination, it can build up in the plasma. Toxic levels of this metabolite cause gray baby syndrome.

CHAPTER 5 ANSWERS

CASE 1

1. **The answer is C. Low-molecular weight heparin is administered to achieve anticoagulation until plasma warfarin concentrations reach a therapeutic anticoagulant level.** The therapeutic effect of warfarin depends on its inhibition of hepatic synthesis of clotting factors. This effect is not fully achieved for several days after the initiation of warfarin therapy. Low-molecular weight heparin causes more rapid anticoagulation and is often administered as a "bridge" to full anticoagulation with warfarin. Low-molecular weight heparin should be discontinued after therapeutic levels of warfarin have been achieved.

2. **The answer is D.** Supratherapeutic anticoagulation and bleeding as a result of the coadministration of these drugs is an example of **a pharmacodynamic**

drug–drug interaction. Toxic pharmacodynamic drug interactions occur when two drugs activate complementary pathways, leading to an exaggerated biological effect. In this case, both low-molecular weight heparin and warfarin caused excessive anticoagulation through different mechanisms, leading to hemorrhage. Pharmacokinetic drug interactions occur when one drug alters the absorption, distribution, metabolism, or excretion of another drug, changing the concentration of that drug available to cause its biologic effect. "Off-target" side effects of a therapeutic drug occur when the drug binds to an unintended target or receptor.

3. **The answer is E. A less convenient intravenous formulation (vancomycin) would be replaced with a more convenient oral formulation (ciprofloxacin).** Ciprofloxacin, a fluoro quinolone, is generally well tolerated and less likely than vancomycin to cause hypersensitivity reactions or toxicity. Unfortunately, Mrs. G. developed a hypersensitivity reaction to it. Both antibiotic combinations should be synergistic in their effect. Vancomycin is more expensive than oral ciprofloxacin, but this would not be the primary reason behind the choice of drug regimens.

4. **The answer is C.** Mrs. G.'s symptoms represent **a delayed-type hypersensitivity reaction to ciprofloxacin.** This T-cell–mediated immune response occurs on reexposure to a foreign antigen, which triggers a cytokine release, leading to fever, rash, and hypotension. Type I immediate hypersensitivity reactions result from IgE-mediated mast cell degranulation on reexposure to a sensitizing antigen. The release of histamine and inflammatory mediators results in urticaria, bronchospasm, vasodilation, and hypotension.

5. **The answer is B. Levofloxacin**, a fluoroquinolone, would be contraindicated, given the patient's hypersensitivity reaction to ciprofloxacin.

CASE 2

1. **The answer is B. Acetaminophen is hepatically metabolized to a toxic metabolite.** Under normal dosage conditions, acetaminophen is primarily metabolized through conjugation (> 90%). The metabolic pathway through the P450 enzymes is a minor component of acetaminophen metabolism (5% to 7%). The reactive intermediate it produces is immediately conjugated to glutathione and is renally excreted. In overdose, the normal conjugation pathways are saturated, and more acetaminophen is available to be metabolized by the P450 enzymes to this reactive metabolite. When glutathione stores are depleted, the toxic metabolite is free to react with hepatocytes, causing a toxic hepatitis and hepatocellular death. An "off-target" effect occurs when a drug causes toxicity by binding to alternate, unintended receptor sites.

2. **The answer is A. Clinical symptoms do not occur until glutathione stores are depleted and the**

toxic metabolite begins to bind and induce damage to hepatocytes. After a single overdose, the onset to clinical toxicity may be delayed by 12 to 18 hours.

3. **The answer is A. Ms. B.'s liver enzymes will be more efficient in metabolizing acetaminophen to its toxic metabolite, putting her at increased risk for liver toxicity.** Phenytoin induces the activity of the P450 enzymes, but conjugation is unaffected. As a result, any acetaminophen that is available for oxidative metabolism by the P450 enzymes will be more efficiently metabolized to the reactive toxic intermediate. The risk of liver toxicity will be increased.

4. **The answer is C.** The effect of chronic phenytoin use on acetaminophen metabolism in the liver is an example of **a pharmacokinetic drug–drug interaction**.

Phenytoin use induces the oxidative metabolism of acetaminophen by the P450 enzyme system.

5. **The answer is E. If the fetal hepatic P450 enzymes are functioning, the fetal liver will elaborate the toxic metabolite resulting in fetal hepatotoxicity.** Fetal liver enzyme function begins between the 16th and 20th week of gestation. After this time, any excess acetaminophen that crosses the placenta and enters the fetal liver can be metabolized to the toxic metabolite. Delayed treatment of pregnant patients with acetaminophen overdose is associated with fetal demise. Teratogens are substances that induce defects in the fetus. Carcinogens are substances that cause DNA mutations, which over time can lead to a neoplastic transformation of cells. Acetaminophen is neither a teratogen, nor a carcinogen. Normally, the majority of acetaminophen is conjugated by glucuronidation and sulfation, and is renally excreted.

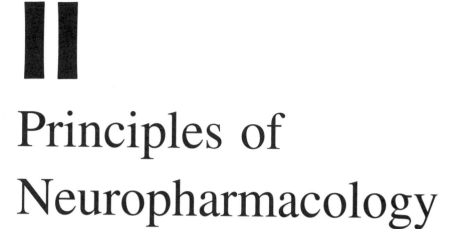

II

Principles of Neuropharmacology

6

Principles of Cellular Excitability and Electrochemical Transmission

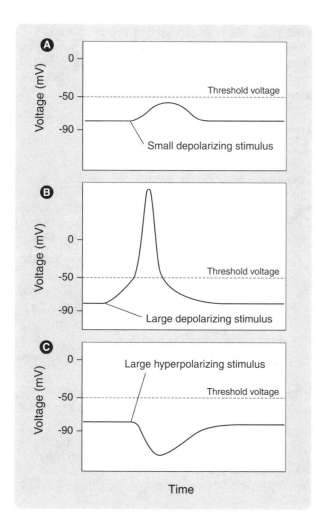

Figure 6-1. The Action Potential. A. In the example shown, a resting cell has a membrane potential of approximately −80 mV. If a small depolarizing stimulus is applied to the cell (e.g., a stimulus that opens a few voltage-gated Ca^{2+} channels), the membrane slowly depolarizes in response to the influx of Ca^{2+} ions. After the stimulus ends and the Ca^{2+} channels close, the membrane returns to its resting potential. The time course of the voltage change is determined by the membrane capacitance. **B.** If a larger depolarizing stimulus is applied to the cell, such that the membrane potential exceeds its "threshold" voltage, the membrane rapidly depolarizes to about +50 mV and then returns to its resting potential. This event is known as an action potential; its magnitude, time course, and shape are determined by voltage-gated Na^+ and K^+ channels that open in response to membrane depolarization. **C.** In comparison, application of a hyperpolarizing stimulus to a cell does not generate an action potential, regardless of the magnitude of hyperpolarization.

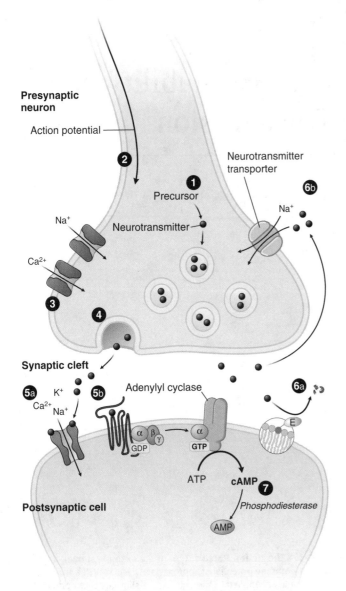

Figure 6-2.   Steps in Synaptic Transmission. Synaptic transmission can be divided into a series of steps that couple electrical depolarization of the presynaptic neuron to chemical signaling between the presynaptic and postsynaptic cells. **1.** Neuron synthesizes neurotransmitter from precursor and stores the transmitter in vesicles. **2.** An action potential traveling down the neuron depolarizes the presynaptic nerve terminal. **3.** Membrane depolarization activates voltage-dependent Ca^{2+} channels, allowing Ca^{2+} entry into the presynaptic nerve terminal. **4.** The increased cytosolic Ca^{2+} enables vesicle fusion with the plasma membrane of the presynaptic neuron, with subsequent release of neurotransmitter into the synaptic cleft. **5.** Neurotransmitter diffuses across the synaptic cleft and binds to one of two types of postsynaptic receptors. **5a.** Neurotransmitter binding to ionotropic receptors causes channel opening and changes the permeability of the postsynaptic membrane to ions. This may also result in a change in the postsynaptic membrane potential. **5b.** Neurotransmitter binding to metabotropic receptors on the postsynaptic cell activates intracellular signaling cascades; the example shows G protein activation leading to the formation of 3',5'-adenosine monophosphate (cAMP) by adenylyl cyclase. In turn, these signaling cas-

OBJECTIVES

■ Understand the physiology of cellular excitability and electrochemical transmission.

■ CASE 1

Karl B. is a 47-year-old man who works for the Virginia state government. He is traveling to Japan to meet with several CEOs to discuss the prospective openings of their companies' satellite offices in Roanoke. While visiting Yamaguchi, his hosts take him to dinner at an expensive restaurant where the specialty is fugu fish. Mr. B. is impressed because he has heard that this special dish is not available in the United States and is an expensive delicacy in Japan.

Before the meal is over, Mr. B. notes an unusual and delightful sensation of tingling and numbness in his mouth and around his lips. His hosts are pleased that he is experiencing the desired effect of fugu fish ingestion.

QUESTIONS

1. The Japanese tiger pufferfish, *Fugu rubripes*, contains a neurotoxin, tetrodotoxin, which is concentrated in the fish's liver, gonadal organs, and skin. Tetrodotoxin binds to and blocks the sodium channel. Which of the following statements regarding sodium flux across the cell membrane is correct?

   A. The permeability of the neuronal cell membrane at rest is greatest for sodium ions

   B. The resting membrane potential most closely approximates the Nernst potential for sodium ions ($+61$ mV).

   C. The exchange of three sodium for two potassium ions across the cell membrane is an energy-dependent process.

   D. When sodium channels open to allow sodium flux across the cell membrane, the membrane potential peaks at 0 mV.

   E. The intracellular sodium ion concentration is greater than the extracellular sodium ion concentration.

cades can activate other ion-selective channels. **6.** Signal termination is accomplished by removal of transmitter from the synaptic cleft. **6a.** The transmitter can be degraded by enzymes (E) in the synaptic cleft. **6b.** Alternatively, transmitter can be recycled into the presynaptic cell by reuptake transporters. **7.** Signal termination can also be accomplished by enzymes (e.g., phosphodiesterase) that degrade postsynaptic intracellular signaling molecules (e.g., cAMP).

2. How does the action of tetrodotoxin alter the resting membrane potential?

A. The membrane potential becomes more positive.

B. The membrane potential becomes more negative.

C. The membrane potential approaches the Nernst potential for sodium.

D. The membrane potential is unaffected by sodium channel blockade.

E. The membrane potential approaches the Nernst potential for calcium.

3. What will be the effect of sodium channel blockade on the cellular action potential?

A. The action potential will be shortened.

B. The action potential will be blunted.

C. The action potential will be inhibited.

D. The action potential will be prolonged in duration.

E. The action potential will be of greater magnitude.

Mr. B. is fascinated and somewhat fearful of the potential toxic effects of tetrodotoxin as they are described to him by his knowledgeable hosts. However, his hosts assure him that the sushi chef at this fine restaurant is fully licensed to prepare fugu fish and is certified by the Japanese government. Still, back at his hotel, thoughts of the meal make Mr. B. nauseated.

4. What would be the clinical effect of tetrodotoxin poisoning at the neuromuscular junction?

A. flaccid muscle paralysis

B. tetanic muscle contraction

C. muscle cell inflammation and breakdown

D. muscle contraction followed by prolonged relaxation

E. uncontrolled muscle fasciculations

Mr. B. is relieved when he awakens the next morning, feeling well and energized. He tests his muscles and his strength is as good as ever! However, he decides that he will politely forgo seafood for the rest of the business trip and ask for Kobe beef instead.

5. Why is cellular repolarization a slower process than depolarization?

A. Depolarization is fast because of the rapid opening and closing of potassium channels.

B. Depolarization is fast because of the rapid opening and closing of the ATP-dependent sodium/potassium pump.

C. Repolarization is prolonged because of the inactivation of delayed rectifier potassium channels.

D. Repolarization is prolonged because of the slow rate of closing of calcium channels.

E. Repolarization is prolonged because of the slower opening and closing of delayed rectifier potassium channels.

 CASE 2

James M., a previously healthy 33-year-old man, lives in a basement apartment in West Philadelphia. One night while sleeping on his couch, he feels a sudden sharp, pinprick-like pain on the right side of the back of his neck. The pain awakens him, and he brushes at the back of his neck. He notices that he has crushed some type of black insect, perhaps a spider. He falls back to sleep. Two hours later, Mr. M. is again awakened, now by a gradually increasing pain and tightness in his neck. Within 30 minutes, he feels progressive tightness spreading from his chest into his abdomen and a terrible diffuse abdominal pain, which radiates around to his flanks. He also feels sweaty and hot and has a generalized headache and stiff neck.

On arrival at the local emergency department, Mr. M. is restless, in obvious discomfort, and complaining of waves of pain. His vital signs reveal a temperature of 100.3°F, a pulse of 139 bpm, a respiratory rate of 22 breaths/min., and a blood pressure of 189/103 mm Hg. The examining physician notes that Mr. M. is diaphoretic and seems to have diffuse muscle tightness. His conjunctivae are injected. There is a small red area on the back of his neck. His abdomen is diffusely tender and rigid to palpation. When Mr. M. relates the story of the neck pain and the ''black bug,'' the physician entertains the possibility that Mr. M. has been bitten by a black widow spider.

QUESTIONS

1. The female black widow spider, *Latrodectus mactans*, elaborates a neurotoxic venom, which is composed of several active components. Alpha-latrotoxin binds to presynaptic receptors. It causes the persistent opening of presynaptic cation channels and calcium flux across the neuronal plasma membrane. Which of the following statements regarding calcium channels is correct?

A. The neuronal plasma membrane is most permeable to calcium ions.

B. In cardiac cells, voltage-gated calcium channels are involved in the depolarization phase of the action potential.

C. Leak channels allow calcium ions to passively enter the cell.

D. The sodium/calcium exchanger transports intracellular calcium and sodium to the outside of the cell.

E. When calcium channels are in the inactivated state, the neuron cannot be stimulated to depolarize and produce an action potential.

2. What is the role of calcium in cell membrane function?

 A. Calcium influx prevents the plasma membrane from becoming permanently depolarized.

 B. Calcium is required to maintain the sequestration of neurotransmitters within presynaptic vesicles.

 C. Calcium influx triggers the rapid neuronal action potential and its propagation.

 D. Calcium influx triggers the exocytosis of neurotransmitter-containing synaptic vesicles.

 E. Calcium extrusion from presynaptic cells facilitates neurotransmitter uptake.

3. How could the effect of *Lactrodectus* venom on presynaptic neuronal calcium channels have contributed to Mr. M.'s clinical presentation?

 A. Calcium channel binding inhibited normal cellular activation.

 B. Calcium influx caused massive release of neurotransmitters.

 C. Calcium influx hyperpolarized the cell membrane.

 D. Calcium channel binding destroyed the channel and caused neuronal cell apoptosis.

 E. Calcium channel binding limited exocytosis of vesicles.

Mr. M. is treated with intravenous benzodiazepines and opioid analgesics with some relief. However, he has persistent muscle tightness, tachycardia, and hypertension. Twenty-four hours after admission, he is treated with one vial of *Latrodectus* antivenin, with relief of his symptoms within several hours. After 3 days, he is discharged home, but he states that he will be sleeping in his car for the time being!

4. Which of the following factors contributes to maintenance of the resting potential of the cell membrane?

 A. A lipid bilayer membrane, which is highly permeable to anions.

 B. Cations are extracellular and anions are intracellular in biologic cells

 C. Transmembrane ion channels, which open very transiently to allow ion passage

 D. Transmembrane ion pumps, which maintain ion gradients

 E. Intracellular vesicles, which sequester excess ions

5. Which of the following pairs (ion channel : function) is correct?

 A. voltage-gated sodium channels: cause vesicle exocytosis

 B. voltage-gated sodium channels: responsible for repolarization

 C. voltage-gated potassium channels: responsible for repolarization

 D. voltage-independent potassium channels: responsible for repolarization

 E. voltage-gated calcium channels: open during the rapid phase of depolarization

7

Principles of Nervous System Physiology and Pharmacology

OBJECTIVES

- Understand how abnormal neurotransmitter function contributes to disease.
- Understand how pharmacologic interventions can treat some nervous system diseases.

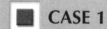

CASE 1

Martha P. is a 66-year-old woman with a 4-year history of worsening Parkinson's disease, a neurologic disorder resulting from the progressive degeneration of nigrostriatal neurons that use dopamine as a neurotransmitter.

QUESTIONS

1. Which of the following functions is controlled by the dopaminergic neurons of the nigrostriatal tract?
   A. arousal and alertness
   B. initiation of movement
   C. hunger and thirst
   D. temperature regulation
   E. emotions

2. What could be a clinical effect of dopaminergic neuron degradation in Parkinson's disease?
   A. inability to move one side of the body
   B. inability to tolerate cold temperatures
   C. inability to get out of a deep armchair
   D. emotional lability and inappropriate laughing and crying
   E. drug-craving behavior

While visiting her physician, Ms. P. registers an unusual complaint: "It seems that my Sinemet doesn't work as well when I take it with meals." Ms. P. explains that she has recently started a new "low-carb" diet that has increased her protein intake at the expense of high-carbohydrate foods. Concerned, she asks, "Could my diet have anything to do with this?"

3. Why does protein consumption interfere with the action of levodopa?
   A. Protein components bind the large neutral amino acid transporter and reverse its normal transport of levodopa into the central nervous system.
   B. Proteins bind to levodopa in the circulation and prevent its diffusion into the central nervous system.
   C. Proteins enhance the function of dopamine decarboxylase and the peripheral conversion of levodopa to dopamine.
   D. Protein components compete with levodopa for transport across the blood–brain barrier.
   E. Protein prevents the normal gastrointestinal absorption of levodopa.

Ms. P.'s physician explains that levodopa, a component of Sinemet, helps replace a chemical in her brain that is produced in insufficient quantities because of the loss of certain neurons in her brain.

4. Levodopa is used in the treatment of Parkinson's disease. What is the relationship of this compound to dopamine?
   A. Levodopa is a dopamine analogue that upregulates dopamine receptors.
   B. Levodopa is metabolized by dopamine β-hydroxylase to dopamine in the central nervous system.
   C. Levodopa is a dopamine analogue that is preferentially bound by the dopamine receptor antibody.
   D. Levodopa is a monoamine oxidase inhibitor that reduces dopamine degradation in the central nervous system.
   E. Levodopa is L-dopa, which is metabolized by dopamine decarboxylase to dopamine in the central nervous system.

Peripheral capillary

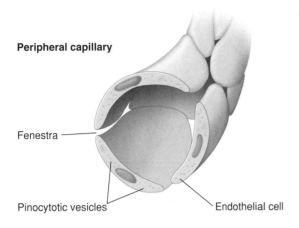

Fenestra

Pinocytotic vesicles

Endothelial cell

Brain capillary

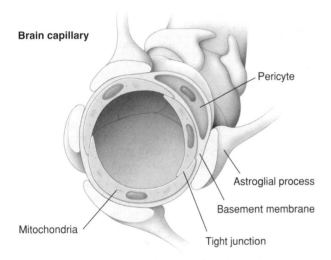

Pericyte

Astroglial process

Basement membrane

Mitochondria

Tight junction

Figure 7-1. **Features of capillaries in the central nervous system compared to the peripheral vasculature.** In the periphery, capillary endothelial cells have gaps (termed *fenestrae*) between them and use intracellular pinocytotic vesicles to facilitate the transcapillary transport of fluid and soluble molecules. In contrast, CNS vessels are sealed by tight junctions between the endothelial cells. The cells have fewer pinocytotic vesicles and are surrounded by pericytes and astroglial processes. In addition, capillary endothelial cells in the CNS have more mitochondria than those in systemic vessels; these mitochondria may reflect the energy requirements necessary for CNS endothelial cells to transport certain molecules into the CNS and transport other molecules out of the CNS.

Although many factors could lead to the decreased effectiveness of her medication, Ms. P.'s doctor confirms her suspicion that her high-protein diet could be interfering with the medication's ability to reach her brain. He recommends that she moderate her protein intake and, if necessary, take a higher dose of Sinemet after a high-protein meal. On her follow-up visit Ms. P. is happy to report that her medication is more effective now that she is eating less protein.

5. Which of the following might be a clinical effect of taking too much levodopa?
   A. drowsiness and lethargy
   B. gastrointestinal ileus
   C. inhibition of the vomiting center
   D. loss of balance and a sensation of spinning
   E. psychosis

 CASE 2

In 2001, the *New England Journal of Medicine* reported a case of a 16-year-old Cambodian male who was admitted to Massachusetts General Hospital with confusion and facial grimacing after drinking a traditional herbal tea for relief of upper respiratory symptoms and diarrhea. During his hospital evaluation, the patient had episodes of agitation and muscle fasciculations. An electroencephalogram showed no evidence of seizure activity. On the second hospital day, the patient's jaw clenched, and he became rigid and unresponsive for 10 minutes. His pulse rate was 180 bpm, respiratory rate was 60 breaths/min., and blood pressure was 160/90 mm Hg. An antidote was administered intravenously with resolution of his symptoms within several minutes. Toxicologic analysis of the patient's urine via high-performance liquid chromatography and gas chromatography–mass spectrometry revealed the presence of strychnine.

Strychnine is a white, odorless, bitter crystalline powder that was historically used as a rodenticide as early as the 16th century. Strychnine has also been used as a poisonous adulterant in illicit drugs such as heroin and cocaine. Strychnine poisoning has been reported after ingesting the strychnos nut or "Slang Nut," a traditional Cambodian herbal remedy, derived from the fruit of the tree *Strychnos nux vomica*.

QUESTIONS

1. Strychnine poisoning typically presents with intermittent muscle spasms and rigidity, which can look like seizure activity. However, in contrast to generalized cerebral seizures, the strychnine-poisoned patient usually has an awake mental status between episodes of muscle activity. Given this presentation, which of the following neurotransmitter effects is a result of strychnine poisoning?
   A. inhibition of glycine activity in the spinal cord
   B. enhancement of GABA activity in the cerebral hemispheres
   C. enhancement of glutamate activity in the peripheral muscles
   D. inhibition of acetylcholine activity at the parasympathetic postganglionic neurons
   E. inhibition of histamine activity in the cerebral hemispheres

2. This patient was administered an intravenous antidote, which reversed his muscle rigidity. Given the mechanism of action of strychnine, which of the following therapies might be most therapeutic in this case?
- **A.** levodopa
- **B.** a monoamine oxidase inhibitor
- **C.** a benzodiazepine
- **D.** phenytoin
- **E.** an antihistamine

3. Glutamate is an excitatory amino acid neurotransmitter. It exerts it effect primarily by:
- **A.** preventing the synthesis of dopamine
- **B.** promoting the release of enkephalins
- **C.** inhibiting adenosine receptors
- **D.** opening ligand-gated ion channels
- **E.** preventing the reuptake of catecholamines

4. Donepezil is a therapeutic agent used to enhance alertness in patients with dementia. It acts by enhancing the central nervous system activity of:
- **A.** dopamine
- **B.** acetylcholine
- **C.** caffeine
- **D.** scopolamine
- **E.** serotonin

5. Many drugs exert their central nervous system effects by crossing the blood–brain barrier. Agents that cross the blood–brain barrier more easily tend to be:
- **A.** of high molecular weight
- **B.** highly polarized
- **C.** hydrophilic
- **D.** lipophilic
- **E.** acidic

8

Cholinergic Pharmacology

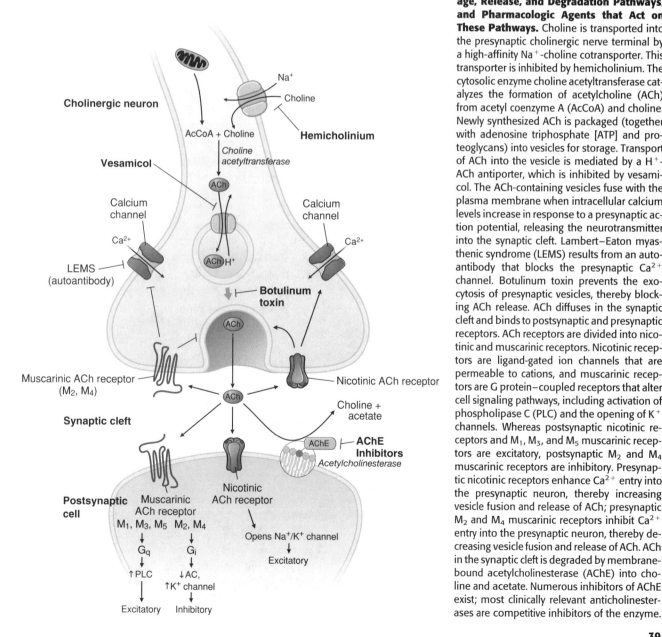

Figure 8-1. Acetylcholine Synthesis, Storage, Release, and Degradation Pathways, and Pharmacologic Agents that Act on These Pathways. Choline is transported into the presynaptic cholinergic nerve terminal by a high-affinity Na^+-choline cotransporter. This transporter is inhibited by hemicholinium. The cytosolic enzyme choline acetyltransferase catalyzes the formation of acetylcholine (ACh) from acetyl coenzyme A (AcCoA) and choline. Newly synthesized ACh is packaged (together with adenosine triphosphate [ATP] and proteoglycans) into vesicles for storage. Transport of ACh into the vesicle is mediated by a H^+-ACh antiporter, which is inhibited by vesamicol. The ACh-containing vesicles fuse with the plasma membrane when intracellular calcium levels increase in response to a presynaptic action potential, releasing the neurotransmitter into the synaptic cleft. Lambert–Eaton myasthenic syndrome (LEMS) results from an autoantibody that blocks the presynaptic Ca^{2+} channel. Botulinum toxin prevents the exocytosis of presynaptic vesicles, thereby blocking ACh release. ACh diffuses in the synaptic cleft and binds to postsynaptic and presynaptic receptors. ACh receptors are divided into nicotinic and muscarinic receptors. Nicotinic receptors are ligand-gated ion channels that are permeable to cations, and muscarinic receptors are G protein–coupled receptors that alter cell signaling pathways, including activation of phospholipase C (PLC) and the opening of K^+ channels. Whereas postsynaptic nicotinic receptors and M_1, M_3, and M_5 muscarinic receptors are excitatory, postsynaptic M_2 and M_4 muscarinic receptors are inhibitory. Presynaptic nicotinic receptors enhance Ca^{2+} entry into the presynaptic neuron, thereby increasing vesicle fusion and release of ACh; presynaptic M_2 and M_4 muscarinic receptors inhibit Ca^{2+} entry into the presynaptic neuron, thereby decreasing vesicle fusion and release of ACh. ACh in the synaptic cleft is degraded by membrane-bound acetylcholinesterase (AChE) into choline and acetate. Numerous inhibitors of AChE exist; most clinically relevant anticholinesterases are competitive inhibitors of the enzyme.

OBJECTIVES

■ Understand acetylcholine physiology, including its synthesis, release, metabolism, and effects at muscarinic and nicotinic receptors.

■ Understand how pharmacologic agents can modify acetylcholine function, resulting in both therapeutic and potentially toxic effects.

 CASE 1

The year is 1744. Virginian settlers capture Chief Opechan-canough, warrior chief of the Powhatans and uncle to Poca-hontas. Opechancanough is considered a master tactician and has a reputation as a brutal warrior. One colonial correspondence portrays a different picture of the captured chief, however:

"The excessive fatigues he encountered wrecked his constitution; his flesh became macerated; his sinews lost their tone and elasticity and his eyelids were so heavy that he could not see unless they were lifted by his attendants . . . he was unable to walk; but his spirit, rising above the ruins of his body, directed [his followers] from the litter on which he was carried by his Indians."

While Opechancanough is confined to a prison in Jamestown, it is discovered that, after a period of inactivity, he is able to raise himself from the ground to a standing position.

It is thought that the story of Opechancanough provides the earliest recorded description of myasthenia gravis, a neuromuscular disease resulting from the autoimmune production of antibodies directed against cholinergic receptors at the neuromuscular junction. In 1934, almost two centuries later, the English physician Mary Broadfoot Walker encounters several patients with similar symptoms of muscle weakness, which remind her of the symptoms of patients with tubocurare poisoning.

QUESTIONS

1. Why do tubocurare poisoning and myasthenia gravis produce similar symptoms?
   A. Both conditions are characterized by weakness due to choline deficiency.
   B. Both conditions are characterized by weakness due to a lack of presynaptic acetylcholine (ACh) release.
   C. Both conditions are characterized by paralysis associated with antibody-mediated destruction of ACh.
   D. Both conditions are characterized by weakness due to a diminished number of available postsynaptic N_M receptors.
   E. Both conditions are associated with weakness due to increased ACh degradation.

Given her findings, Dr. Walker administers an antidote, physostigmine, to her immobile patients. The results are startling: Within minutes, her patients are able to rise and walk across the room. Dr. Walker has discovered the first truly effective medication for myasthenia gravis. Despite the significance of her accomplishment, it is largely ridiculed by the scientific community because the treatment improves the symptoms of myasthenia gravis too rapidly and effectively to be believable. It is not until many years later that the scientific community comes to accept her findings.

2. How does physostigmine improve the symptoms of myasthenia gravis?
   A. Physostigmine enhances the release of presynaptic Ach.
   B. Physostigmine prevents the degradation of ACh.
   C. Physostigmine prolongs the duration of ACh binding at the N_M receptor.
   D. Physostigmine prevents the reuptake of ACh.
   E. Physostigmine promotes rapid recovery and availability of N_M receptors.

3. Under what conditions is it potentially dangerous to administer physostigmine to patients presenting with muscle weakness?
   A. botulinum poisoning
   B. tubocurare poisoning
   C. organophosphate poisoning
   D. bethanechol ingestion
   E. succinylcholine allergy

4. Which of the following is another potential therapeutic use of physostigmine?
   A. scopolamine poisoning
   B. muscarine poisoning
   C. pralidoxime poisoning
   D. pilocarpine poisoning
   E. nicotine poisoning

5. Which of the following is a sign of ACh agonism at its postsynaptic muscarinic receptor?
   A. urinary retention
   B. muscle fasciculations
   C. bradycardia
   D. tachycardia
   E. dry mucous membranes

 CASE 2

In 2004, an unlicensed Florida doctor, Bach McComb, injected himself and three patients with an unapproved preparation of botulinum toxin as an anti-wrinkle treatment. Within hours, he presented to a hospital with diffuse muscle weakness and difficulty breathing. He subsequently became paralyzed and required prolonged mechanical ventilation to support his respirations. The other patients suffered similar adverse effects. In 2005, McComb plead guilty to federal charges of administering unapproved drugs.

QUESTIONS

1. How does botulinum toxin cause muscle weakness and prolonged paralysis?
   A. Botulinum toxin prevents the entry of ACh into presynaptic storage vesicles.
   B. Botulinum toxin degrades ACh within presynaptic storage vesicles.
   C. Botulinum toxin blocks calcium channels and calcium-mediated exocytosis of presynaptic storage vesicles.
   D. Botulinum toxin binds irreversibly to the SNARE proteins and blocks the fusion of presynaptic storage vesicles with the cell membrane.
   E. Botulinum toxin degrades synaptobrevin and prevents the fusion of presynaptic storage vesicles with the cell membrane.

2. Given the mechanism of action of botulinum toxin, if botulinum-poisoned patients are administered physostigmine, as in the case of Chief Opechancanough, which of the following could be a resulting clinical effect?
   A. improved muscle strength
   B. coma
   C. sweating and diarrhea
   D. muscle fasciculations followed by paralysis
   E. pupillary dilatation

3. If a botulinum-poisoned patient were given physostigmine, with the above effects, what would be an appropriate therapy?
   A. atropine
   B. more physostigmine
   C. succinylcholine
   D. methacholine
   E. pralidoxime

4. The effects of physostigmine in a botulinum-poisoned patient are mediated at which of the following receptors?
   A. M_1
   B. M_2
   C. M_3
   D. M_4
   E. N_M

5. Neurotransmission through the autonomic ganglia is complex. The primary postsynaptic ganglionic response is mediated by the rapid depolarization of nicotinic ACh receptors, but is modulated by muscarinic ACh M_1, dopaminergic, α-adrenergic, and peptidergic transmission. As a result, the effect of ganglionic blockade largely depends on the relative predominance of sympathetic and parasympathetic tone at the end organ. Which of the following statements regarding the effect of ganglionic blockade on end organ function is correct?
   A. Autonomic ganglionic blockade causes vasoconstriction and hypertension.
   B. Autonomic ganglionic blockade causes vasodilation and hypotension.
   C. Autonomic ganglionic blockade causes urinary incontinence.
   D. Autonomic ganglionic blockade causes bradycardia.
   E. Autonomic ganglionic blockade causes vomiting and diarrhea.

9

Adrenergic Pharmacology

 CASE 1

The year is 1960. Ms. S. has felt depressed for a number of years. She has tried several different medications to alleviate her feelings of hopelessness and lack of motivation, but nothing seems to help. Recently, however, her doctor has prescribed iproniazid, a new medication reported to be of benefit in many cases of depression. He tells her that researchers think the drug acts by inhibiting an enzyme in the brain called MAO (MAO one of the enzymes responsible for catecholamine degradation.) Because it is a new drug, its potential adverse effects are not well defined, so her doctor advises Ms. S. to report any unusual effects of the medication.

Hopeful, but not expecting significant changes, Ms. S. begins taking the medication. Within a few weeks, she begins to feel motivated and energetic for the first time in 20 years. Exuberant at her newly found sense of energy, Ms. S. reclaims her past life as a debutante and socialite by hosting a gala wine and cheese reception. The best and brightest of the city are invited, and the party is looking to be a success. As she stands up to give thanks to her attendees, Ms. S. celebrates with a large swig of her favorite 1954 Chianti. By the end of the party, Ms. S. has a severe headache and nausea. Recalling her doctor's warning, she has a friend rush her to the nearest hospital. In the emergency department, the attending physician records a blood pressure of 230/160 mm Hg.

QUESTIONS

1. What is the mechanistic explanation for the interaction of MAO inhibitors with red wine and aged cheese?
   A. Aged cheese contains small amounts of amphetamine, which cannot be metabolized in the presence of MAOIs, and displaces vesicular norepinephrine (NE).
   B. Red wine and aged cheese directly block the inhibitory action of MAO inhibitors (MAOIs).
   C. Red wine and aged cheese contain tyramine, which cannot be metabolized in the presence of MAOIs, and displaces vesicular NE.
   D. Ethanol in red wine prevents the reuptake of catecholamines, which cannot be metabolized in the presence of MAOIs.
   E. Red wine and aged cheese contain tyramine, which acts directly on postsynaptic adrenergic receptors, and cannot be metabolized in the presence of MAOIs.

Recognizing that Ms. S. is experiencing a hypertensive emergency, the doctor quickly administers phentolamine. Ms. S.'s blood pressure quickly normalizes, and the doctor's subsequent clinical investigation identifies a new, and now famous, drug–food interaction involving MAOIs.

2. What is the mechanism of action of phentolamine, and what was its clinical effect in this circumstance?
   A. Nonselective α-adrenergic antagonist; blocks catecholamine-induced vasoconstriction, and decreases blood pressure
   B. Nonselective α-adrenergic antagonist; prevents tyramine-induced displacement of NE, and decreases anxiety
   C. Nonselective α-adrenergic antagonist; facilitates catechol-O-methyltransferase (COMT)-mediated metabolism of catecholamines, and decreases blood pressure
   D. Nonselective α-adrenergic agonist; causes vasodilation and sedation
   E. Nonselective α-adrenergic agonist; competes with catecholamines to reduce vasoconstriction, and decreases blood pressure

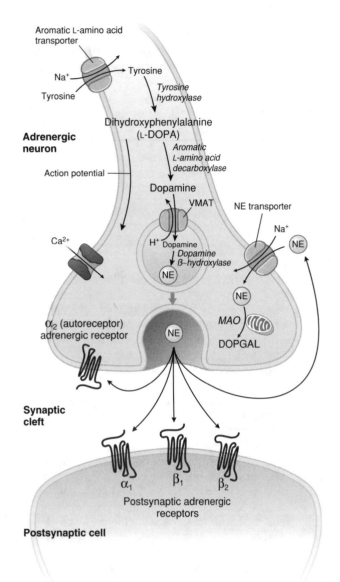

Figure 9-1. Catecholamine Synthesis, Storage, Release, and Reuptake Pathways. The endogenous catecholamines dopamine, norepinephrine (NE), and epinephrine are all synthesized from tyrosine. The rate-limiting step in catecholamine synthesis, the oxidation of cytoplasmic tyrosine to dihydroxyphenylalanine (L-DOPA), is catalyzed by the enzyme tyrosine hydroxylase. Aromatic L-amino acid decarboxylase then converts L-DOPA to dopamine. Vesicular monoamine transporter (VMAT) translocates dopamine (and other monoamines) into synaptic vesicles. In adrenergic neurons, intravesicular dopamine-β–hydroxylase converts dopamine to NE. NE is then stored in the vesicle until release. In adrenal medullary cells, NE returns to the cytosol, where phenylethanolamine N-methyltransferase (PNMT) converts NE to epinephrine. The epinephrine is then transported back into the vesicle for storage (not shown). α-Methyltyrosine inhibits tyrosine hydroxylase, the rate-limiting enzyme in catecholamine synthesis (not shown). Released NE can stimulate postsynaptic α_1-, β_1-, or β_2-adrenergic receptors or presynaptic α_2-adrenergic autoreceptors. Released NE can also be taken up into presynaptic terminals by the selective NE transporter. NE in the cytoplasm of the presynaptic neuron can be further taken up into synaptic vesicles by VMAT (not shown) or degraded to 3,4-dihydroxyphenylglycoaldehyde (DOPGAL) by mitochondrion-associated monoamine oxidase (MAO).

3. Why didn't the physician use a β-adrenergic receptor antagonist to treat Ms. S.'s hypertension?
   A. β-Adrenergic receptor antagonists could block the CNS effects of catecholamines and worsen Ms. S.' depression.
   B. β-Adrenergic receptor antagonists could block the reuptake of catecholamines by the NE transporter and cause psychosis.
   C. β-Adrenergic receptor antagonists could block catecholamine stimulation at the heart, but allow persistent catecholamine-induced vasoconstriction at the α-adrenergic receptors.
   D. β-Adrenergic receptor antagonists could delay the normal metabolism of tyramine.
   E. β-Adrenergic receptor antagonists could block catecholamine stimulation at the heart and cause asystole.

4. Ms. S.'s hypertensive crisis was caused by the tyramine–MAOI interaction. Which of the following physiologic actions could prevent this interaction?
   A. Inhibition of the vesicular monoamine transporter
   B. Inhibition of the vesicular acetylcholine transporter
   C. Induction of the aromatic L-amino acid transporter
   D. Inhibition of tyrosine hydroxylase
   E. Induction of the NE transporter

5. Hexamethonium is a sympathetic ganglionic blocker. It blocks the:
   A. postsynaptic β-adrenergic receptor
   B. presynaptic acetylcholine release
   C. postsynaptic ganglionic acetylcholine receptor
   D. skeletal muscle acetylcholine receptor
   E. presynaptic α-adrenergic receptor

■ **CASE 2**

A 25-year-old man is brought to the emergency department by police when bystanders call 911 to report a confused and combative man knocking over shelves in a local convenience store. The patient is wildly agitated and tries to assault police officers and care providers on arrival at the hospital. His examination is remarkable for a temperature of 105°F, a heart rate of 162 bpm, and a blood pressure of 207/134 mm Hg. His pupils are dilated, and his skin is diaphoretic. When the patient is undressed, several crack cocaine vials fall out of his pants pockets.

QUESTIONS

1. What mechanism of action of cocaine produced this patient's symptoms?
   A. Cocaine is a direct agonist at both α- and β-adrenergic receptors.

B. Cocaine inhibits the NE transporter and prevents reuptake of synaptic catecholamines, which are thus available to act at both α- and β-adrenergic receptors.

C. Cocaine is taken up into the synaptic vesicles of sympathetic neurons by vesicular monoamine transporter (VMAT) and displaces NE, which can then act at both α- and β-adrenergic receptors.

D. Cocaine inhibits MAO and prevents the metabolism of catecholamines, which are able to act at both α- and β-adrenergic receptors.

E. Cocaine causes upregulation and increased sensitivity of both α- and β-adrenergic receptors.

The patient is placed on a cardiac monitor, and intravenous access is established. The cardiac monitor shows a sinus tachycardia at a rate of 162 bpm. Aggressive cooling methods are begun, and the emergency physician searches for evidence of coexisting trauma. The nurse asks if the patient should be administered metoprolol, a β-adrenergic receptor antagonist, to control the patient's tachycardia.

2. If a β-adrenergic receptor antagonist is administered to this patient, which of the following clinical effects could result?

A. Hyperglycemia

B. Bronchodilation if the patient has a history of asthma

C. Increase in blood pressure

D. Tachycardia

E. Hypothermia

3. Which of the following agents will act directly to decrease this patient's elevated blood pressure?

A. methylphenidate, an amphetamine analogue

B. phenylephrine, an α₁-adrenergic receptor agonist

C. phentolamine, a non-selective α-adrenergic receptor antagonist

D. yohimbine, an α₂-adrenergic receptor antagonist

E. terbutaline, a β₂-adrenergic receptor agonist

4. Clonidine has been used as an antihypertensive agent. What is its mechanism of action in reducing blood pressure?

A. Clonidine is a direct β₂-adrenergic receptor agonist that enhances vasodilation.

B. Clonidine is a direct α₂-adrenergic receptor antagonist that decreases NE release and sympathetic tone.

C. Clonidine is a direct α₂-adrenergic receptor agonist that decreases NE release and sympathetic tone.

D. Clonidine is a direct α₁-adrenergic receptor antagonist that decreases vasoconstriction.

E. Clonidine is a direct β₁-adrenergic receptor antagonist that decreases cardiac output.

5. Serotonin syndrome is a clinical syndrome characterized by restlessness, tremor, and seizures. It is caused by excess serotonin concentration at its receptors. Serotonin syndrome can be precipitated by the concomitant use of drugs that enhance synaptic serotonin concentrations. Which of the following drug combinations could cause serotonin syndrome?

A. clonidine and cocaine

B. phenelzine and phenylephrine

C. amitriptyline and phenylephrine

D. duloxetine and iproniazid

E. imipramine and metaproterenol

10

Local Anesthetic Pharmacology

OBJECTIVES

▪ Understand the mechanism of action by which local anesthetics diminish sensory, motor, and autonomic impulse transmission.

▪ Understand the physiology of pain transmission and how various local anesthetics are administered to reduce pain perception.

▪ Recognize categories of local anesthetics, their pharmacology, therapeutic uses, and potential toxicities.

■ CASE 1

E.M. is a 24-year-old graduate student in organic chemistry. While working in the lab one evening, he spills a beaker of hydrofluoric acid (HF) in the fume hood. Although he reflexively jerks his hand away, some of the liquid falls on the fingertips of his left hand. Some minutes later, E.M. feels a stinging pain, which increases in intensity and is followed by a burning, throbbing ache. Realizing the corrosiveness of the acid, E.M. begins rinsing his hand with water and a magnesium sulfate solution (the magnesium chelates the toxic fluoride ions). He also telephones 911 and is transported to the emergency department.

The resident notes that the acid has penetrated the nail beds of the affected fingers and that E.M. is in severe pain. She commends him on his timely and appropriate actions and decides on treatment with calcium gluconate (another fluoride chelator) to neutralize the remaining HF, in conjunc-

tion with a digital nerve block to reduce the pain. Lidocaine without epinephrine is injected into the fingers, followed by calcium gluconate. E.M. first notices a relief of the stinging, although the ache takes somewhat longer to fade. By the time his wounds are dressed, he cannot feel any sensation in his fingers. Over the next 2 weeks, E.M.'s wounds heal spontaneously, and the pain, now well controlled with ibuprofen, abates. He is able to plunge back into lab work, but his brush with serious injury affects him in an unforeseen way: He begins to contemplate applying to medical school.

QUESTIONS

1. Which of the following mechanisms of action is responsible for the pain-relieving effect of lidocaine?

   A. Lidocaine binds to an intracellular site on the voltage-gated sodium channel, inhibits its activation, and blocks the propagation of action potentials in motor fibers.

   B. Lidocaine binds to an intracellular site on the voltage-gated calcium channel, inhibits its opening, and blocks the propagation of action potentials in nociceptive C-fibers.

   C. Lidocaine binds to an intracellular site on the voltage-gated sodium channel, inhibits its activation, and blocks the propagation of action potentials in nociceptive A- and C-fibers.

   D. Lidocaine binds to the extracellular pore of the sodium channel, blocks sodium entry, and inhibits the activation of nociceptive A- and C-fibers.

   E. Lidocaine binds to an extracellular site on the sodium channel, blocks sodium entry, and inhibits the activation of nociceptive, sensory, motor, and autonomic fibers.

A Poorly hydrophobic local anesthetic

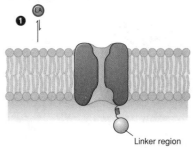

Linker region

B Moderately hydrophobic local anesthetic

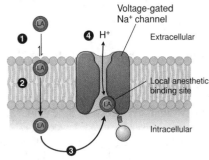

Voltage-gated Na⁺ channel

Extracellular

Local anesthetic binding site

Intracellular

C Extremely hydrophobic local anesthetic

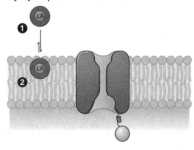

Figure 10-1. Local Anesthetic Hydrophobicity, Diffusion, and Binding. Local anesthetics (LAs) act by binding to the cytoplasmic (intracellular) side of the voltage-gated Na⁺ channel. The hydrophobicity of a local anesthetic determines how efficiently it diffuses across lipid membranes and how tightly it binds to the Na⁺ channel, and therefore governs its potency. **A.** Poorly hydrophobic LAs are unable to cross the lipid bilayer efficiently: **1.** neutral LA cannot adsorb to or enter the neuronal cell membrane because the LA is very stable in the extracellular solution and has a very high activation energy for entering the hydrophobic membrane. **B.** Moderately hydrophobic LAs are the most effective agents: **1.** neutral LA adsorbs to the extracellular side of the neuronal cell membrane; **2.** LA diffuses through the cell membrane to the cytoplasmic side; **3.** LA diffuses and binds to its binding site on the voltage-gated sodium channel; **4.** after it is bound, LA can switch between its neutral and protonated forms by binding and releasing protons. **C.** Extremely hydrophobic LAs become trapped in the lipid bilayer: **1.** neutral LA adsorbs to the neuronal cell membrane **2.** where it is so stabilized that it cannot dissociate from or translocate across the membrane.

2. Why did E.M. initially experience a "stinging pain" before the sensation of a "dull aching pain," and why did the "stinging pain" resolve more quickly than the "dull pain" after lidocaine administration?

   A. "Stinging pain" correlates with the highly localized, first pain sensation that is rapidly transmitted by my-

elinated Aδ-fibers, and is least sensitive to the inhibitory effects of local anesthetics.

   B. "Stinging pain" correlates with the diffusely localizable, second pain sensation that is slowly transmitted by nonmyelinated C-fibers, and is less sensitive to the inhibitory effects of local anesthetics.

   C. "Stinging pain" correlates with the initial highly localized impulses of myelinated Aδ-fibers, which subsequently become desensitized and then transmit a delayed "dull aching pain," which is highly sensitive to the effects of local anesthetics.

   D. "Stinging pain" correlates with the highly localized, first pain sensation that is rapidly transmitted by myelinated Aδ-fibers, and is highly sensitive to the inhibitory effects of local anesthetics.

   E. "Stinging pain" correlates with the diffusely localizable, first pain sensation that is rapidly transmitted by nonmyelinated C-fibers, and is less sensitive to the inhibitory effects of local anesthetics.

3. Lidocaine is a commonly used local anesthetic of the amide-linked class. It has a rapid onset of action and a medium duration of action. Which of the following characteristics explains its pharmacokinetic effects?

   A. Low hydrophobicity prevents lidocaine from being "trapped" within the neuronal cell membrane; an amide linkage prevents its degradation by esterases.

   B. Low pKa allows a larger fraction of drug to be in a neutral form and able to penetrate the neuronal membrane; an amide linkage maintains a low pKa near the area of administration.

   C. Very high hydrophobicity allows lidocaine to easily penetrate the neuronal cell membrane; an amide linkage allows tighter binding at the binding site on the sodium channel.

   D. High pKa allows a larger fraction of the drug to be in a neutral form and able to penetrate the neuronal membrane; an amide linkage prevents its degradation by esterases.

   E. Moderate hydrophobicity allows lidocaine to penetrate the neuronal cell membrane and remain near the area of administration; an amide linkage prevents its degradation by esterases.

4. Epinephrine is sometimes administered with lidocaine. How does the coadministration of epinephrine affect lidocaine's local anesthetic effect?

   A. Epinephrine-induced vasoconstriction maintains a low pH in the area of lidocaine administration, facilitating its penetration into the neuronal cell.

   B. Epinephrine-induced vasoconstriction helps to maintain the concentration of lidocaine in the area of administration by slowing its rate of removal.

   C. Epinephrine prevents the unbinding of lidocaine from its intracellular site on the sodium channel.

D. Epinephrine inactivates tissue esterases to prevent the degradation of lidocaine.

E. Epinephrine makes local sodium channels more sensitive to the effects of lidocaine.

5. Amide-linked local anesthetics are primarily metabolized by:
A. pseudocholinesterases
B. hepatic microsomal cytochrome P450 enzymes
C. renal dipeptidases
D. tissue esterases
E. hepatic conjugation with glutathione

 CASE 2

Sally S. brings her 3-year-old daughter, Jessica, to their family physician for an evaluation after Jessica trips in the playground and cuts her forehead. The physician notes a 3.5-cm linear laceration on Jessica's forehead and recommends suturing the wound in order to achieve the best cosmetic effect. Jessica is terrified of needles, and the physician asks his nurse to apply a topical gel of LET (lidocaine/epinephrine/tetracaine) to the wound to provide anesthesia.

QUESTIONS

1. Lidocaine and tetracaine are both local anesthetics. Epinephrine is a smooth muscle constrictor. Which of the following statements regarding these agents could account for their effectiveness as a combination topical anesthetic formulation?
A. Tetracaine is an ester-linked anesthetic, so the use of the amide-linked lidocaine prevents its degradation by local tissue esterases and prolongs the duration of action of this formulation.
B. Lidocaine counteracts the vasoconstricting effect of epinephrine, limiting local tissue ischemia caused by this formulation.
C. Lidocaine is moderately hydrophobic, so it competes with tetracaine for penetration of the neuronal cell membrane and decreases the time to onset of action of this formulation.
D. Tetracaine is more hydrophobic than lidocaine, so it prolongs the duration of action and increases the potency of this formulation.
E. Tetracaine is more hydrophobic than lidocaine and is unable to diffuse away from the neuronal cell membrane, and its inhibition of calcium channels potentiates the inhibition of sodium channel provided by lidocaine.

Ms. S. is concerned that these drugs may cause some toxicity such as a loss of motor function (this happened to her after receiving a central nerve blockade during her labor with Jessica). She has also heard that topical anesthetics can cause abnormal heart rhythms and seizures.

2. Ms. S. was given a combined spinal/epidural local anesthetic to lessen her labor pain. She did experience some relief of painful contractions but 20 minutes later developed numbness and paralysis in her legs. Which of the following statements could explain her paralysis?
A. Local anesthetic injected into the cerebrospinal fluid penetrated the spinal cord, inhibiting the normal transmission of motor impulses, causing lower extremity paralysis.
B. Local anesthetic injected into the cerebrospinal fluid inhibited normal glutamate transmission in the spinal cord, causing lower extremity paralysis.
C. Local anesthetic injected into the cerebrospinal fluid diffused proximally and caused respiratory arrest.
D. Local anesthetic injected into the epidural space preferentially inhibited the normal transmission of motor impulses, causing lower extremity paralysis.
E. Local anesthetic injected into the cerebrospinal fluid inhibited the normal production of substance P, causing lower extremity paralysis.

3. Local anesthetic toxicity can involve the cardiovascular, pulmonary, dermal, immunologic, and central nervous systems. Which of the following combinations (adverse effect : related mechanism) is correct?
A. hypersensitivity : amide-linked metabolites with allergenic properties
B. cardiac conduction blockade : sodium channel blockade in the cardiac conduction system
C. seizures : excessive blockade of glutamate receptors
D. reduced cardiac contractility : enhanced release of sodium from the sarcoplasmic reticulum
E. hypersensitivity : inhibition of calcium channels in the plasma membrane

4. Ms. S. wants to know why Jessica must wait for 30 minutes after the application of the LET gel before the skin on her forehead will be numb enough for the family physician to suture the wound.

What is the major barrier to the penetration of topical local anesthetic into its site of action?
A. stratum corneum
B. stratum basale
C. epineurium
D. perineurium
E. endoneurium

5. Painful tissue injury causes nociceptors to fire at a high rate in the area of damage. This rapid firing of impulses allows the administration of local anesthetic in the area of damage to preferentially block nociceptor activation to a greater extent than other sensory or motor impulses. This phenomenon is called:
A. epineurial activation
B. hypersensitivity
C. hydrophobicity
D. phasic inhibition
E. tonic inhibition

11

Pharmacology of GABAergic and Glutamatergic Neurotransmission

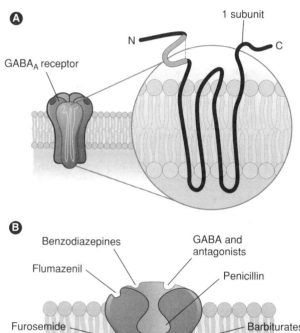

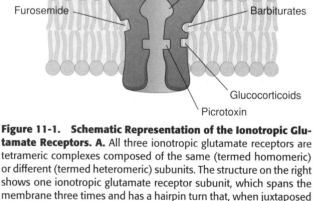

Figure 11-1. Schematic Representation of the Ionotropic Glutamate Receptors. A. All three ionotropic glutamate receptors are tetrameric complexes composed of the same (termed homomeric) or different (termed heteromeric) subunits. The structure on the right shows one ionotropic glutamate receptor subunit, which spans the membrane three times and has a hairpin turn that, when juxtaposed with homologous turns from the other three subunits, forms the lining of the ion channel's pore. **B.** Major binding sites on the α-amino-3-hydroxy-5-methyl-4-isoxazole propionic acid (AMPA)/ kainate and N-methyl-D-aspartic acid (NMDA) classes of ionotropic glutamate receptors are shown. Although there is indirect evidence for the location of many of the drug-binding sites that are schematically indicated in this diagram, the definitive localization of these sites remains to be determined.

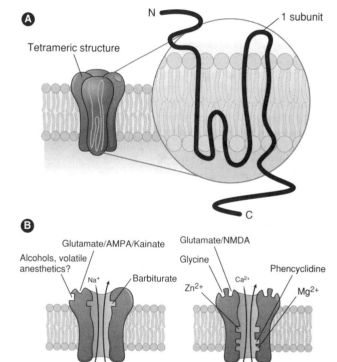

Figure 11-2. Schematic Representation of the GABA$_A$ Receptor. A. The pentameric structure of the GABA$_A$ receptor. Each receptor is made up of five subunits, and each subunit is of one of three predominant subtypes: α, β, or γ. Activation requires the binding of two GABA molecules to the receptor, one to each of the two α subunits. Each subunit of the GABA$_A$ receptor has four membrane-spanning regions and a cysteine loop in the extracellular N-terminal domain (depicted as a dashed line). **B.** Major binding sites on the GABA$_A$ receptor. Although there is indirect evidence for the location of many of the drug-binding sites that are schematically indicated in this diagram, the definitive localization of these sites remains to be determined.

OBJECTIVES

■ Understand the physiology of GABAergic and glutamatergic neurotransmission.

■ Understand how pharmacologic agents can modify gamma-aminobutyric acid (GABA) activity, resulting in therapeutic and potentially toxic effects.

■ Understand how pharmacologic agents affecting glutamate activity may become effective therapies for some neurologic diseases.

CASE 1

S.B., a 70-year-old man is having trouble sleeping. He recalls that his sister has been prescribed phenobarbital, a barbiturate, to control her epileptic seizures, and that barbiturates are sometimes also prescribed as sleeping pills. He decides to take ''just a few'' with some alcohol to help him sleep. Shortly afterward, Mr. B. is rushed to the emergency department after his sister finds him minimally responsive. On examination, he is difficult to arouse and dysarthric, with an unsteady gait and impaired attention and memory. His respiratory rate is approximately 6 shallow breaths per minute. The patient is subsequently intubated to protect him from aspirating gastric contents.

QUESTIONS

1. Barbiturates act to control epileptic seizures and to induce sleep. What is their mechanism of action in causing these effects?
   A. Barbiturates increase the frequency of chloride channel opening at the GABA$_A$ receptor.
   B. Barbiturates increase the duration of chloride channel opening at the GABA$_B$ receptor.
   C. Barbiturates decrease the activation of the kainate receptor by glutamate.
   D. Barbiturates increase the duration of chloride channel opening at the GABA$_A$ receptor.
   E. Barbiturates increase the activation of the N-methyl-D-aspartic acid (NMDA) receptor by glutamate.

2. This patient ingested a barbiturate with ethanol and developed profound central nervous system (CNS) and respiratory depression. What is the interaction of barbiturates with ethanol to cause this effect?
   A. Both agents enhance GABA$_A$-mediated chloride influx and inhibit glutamate excitatory effects at its receptors.
   B. Both agents inhibit norepinephrine (NE) synthesis throughout the CNS.

C. Barbiturates enhance GABA$_A$-mediated chloride influx, while ethanol inhibits the glutamate excitatory effects at the α-amino-3-hydroxy-5-methylisoxazole-4- propionic acid (AMPA) receptor.
   D. Both agents increase the synthesis and release of GABA.
   E. Both agents enhance GABA's affinity for the GABA$_A$ receptor and inhibit glycine excitatory effects at its receptors.

Activated charcoal is administered through a nasogastric tube to limit further absorption of phenobarbital. The patient also receives intravenous sodium bicarbonate to alkalinize his urine to a pH of 7.5 to facilitate renal drug excretion. Three days later, he has recovered sufficiently to return home.

3. This patient's older age may have contributed to the degree of phenobarbital-induced CNS depression he experienced. How does the patient's age affect the extent of CNS depression caused by barbiturates?
   A. Elderly patients have a greater ratio of body fat to muscle and are unable to accumulate lipophilic drugs.
   B. Elderly patients exhibit reduced hepatic clearance of barbiturates.
   C. Elderly patients exhibit reduced renal clearance of phenobarbital.
   D. Elderly patients who ingest an overdose of sedative drugs exhibit single compartment kinetics of drug distribution.
   E. Elderly patients have enhanced gastrointestinal absorption of barbiturates.

4. Which of the following is a sign of barbiturate poisoning?
   A. pulmonary shunting
   B. tachypnea
   C. amnesia to recent events
   D. absence seizures
   E. suppression of adrenal glucocorticoid release

5. How do the pharmacokinetics and metabolism of barbiturates modulate their clinical effect?
   A. Highly lipophilic barbiturates cross the blood–brain barrier rapidly, resulting in a rapid and sustained effect in the CNS.
   B. Orally administered barbiturates undergo first-pass hepatic metabolism to more potent, long-acting active metabolites.
   C. Barbiturates induce the hepatic P450 CYP enzymes responsible for their metabolism, enhancing their efficacy at lower doses.

D. The clinical effect of barbiturates in the CNS is terminated by redistribution of the drug to other highly perfused organs.

E. Barbiturates with an acidic pKa, such as phenobarbital, cannot be orally administered because of the risk of gastric mucosal irritation.

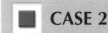 **CASE 2**

Fly agaric, (*Amanita muscaria*), belongs to the mushroom class containing ibotenic acid and muscimol. These species of mushrooms have been used for centuries by various cultures as a component of religious and ritualistic ceremonies. Ingestion of large quantities of this mushroom can cause mixed symptoms of neurotoxicity, including jerking movements, seizures, and mild hallucinations, as well as ethanol-like intoxication and mild sedation.

QUESTIONS

1. Ibotenic acid is the chemical in *A. muscaria* responsible for jerking movements and seizures. Which of the following sites of action could explain the effects of ibotenic acid?
   A. Blockade of presynaptic neuronal calcium channels
   B. Blockade of presynaptic neuronal sodium channels
   C. Activation of the GABA$_B$ receptor
   D. Activation of the benzodiazepine binding site on the GABA$_A$ receptor complex
   E. Activation of the NMDA receptor

2. Ibotenic acid is decarboxylated to muscimol, which is the chemical in *A. muscaria* responsible for intoxication and sedation. Which of the following sites of action could explain the effects of muscimol?
   A. Antagonism of the benzodiazepine binding site on the GABA$_A$ receptor complex
   B. Activation of presynaptic neuronal sodium channels
   C. Activation of the AMPA receptor

   D. Activation of the GABA$_A$ receptor
   E. Blockade of the GABA$_B$ receptor

3. Why are some GABA agonists effective as sedatives while others are used as antiepileptic agents, and others are considered general anesthetics?
   A. GABA agonists with different clinical effects target only GABA$_A$ receptors in the CNS, not GABA$_B$ receptors.
   B. GABA agonists have different clinical effects based on the magnitude of their administered dose.
   C. GABA agonist sedatives and antiepileptics are administered orally while general anesthetics are administered intravenously.
   D. GABA agonists with more specific clinical effects show variable efficacy in their opening of chloride channels.
   E. GABA agonists with more specific clinical effects show greater selectivity in their binding to GABA receptors with specific subunit compositions.

4. Which of the following is an effect of ionotropic glutamate receptor activation?
   A. Potassium channels open, and potassium influx is enhanced.
   B. Sodium and calcium channels open, and sodium and calcium influx is enhanced.
   C. Magnesium channels open, and magnesium influx is enhanced.
   D. Phospholipase C is activated, and the influx of neurosteroids is enhanced.
   E. Chloride channels open, and chloride efflux is enhanced.

5. Glutamate antagonists may be effective in the treatment and/or prevention of:
   A. spinal cord transection
   B. sequelae of ischemic stroke
   C. dementia
   D. schizophrenia
   E. muscle atrophy

12

Pharmacology of Dopaminergic Neurotransmission

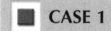

OBJECTIVES

- Understand dopamine physiology, including its synthesis, release, metabolism, and effects.

- Understand how pharmacologic agents can modify dopamine function, resulting in both therapeutic and potentially toxic effects.

■ CASE 1

Mark S. is a 55-year-old man who goes to see his physician because he notices a tremor in his right hand that has developed gradually over a number of months. He finds he can keep the hand quiet if he concentrates on it, but the shaking quickly reappears if he is distracted. His handwriting has become small and difficult to read, and he has trouble using a computer mouse. His wife complains that he never smiles anymore and that his face is becoming expressionless. She also says that he walks more slowly and he has trouble keeping up with her. As Mr. S. enters the examination room, his doctor notices that he is walking hunched over and has a short, shuffling gait. The doctor finds on physical examination that Mr. S. has increased tone and cogwheel rigidity in his upper extremities, particularly on the right side, and that he is significantly slower than normal at performing rapid alternating movements. The physician determines that Mr. S.'s symptoms and signs most likely represent the early stages of Parkinson's disease, and she prescribes a trial of levodopa.

QUESTIONS

1. How does the selective loss of dopaminergic neurons result in symptoms such as those that Mr. S. is experiencing?
    A. Loss of dopaminergic neurons in the circumventricular organs contributes to the inhibition of cortical control of movement.
    B. Loss of dopaminergic neurons in the tuberoinfundibular pathway causes the release of gamma-aminobutyric acid (GABA) and movement inhibition.
    C. Loss of dopaminergic neurons in the striatum causes the release of GABA and movement inhibition.
    D. Loss of dopaminergic neurons in the substantia nigra contributes to reduced activity of the direct pathway and movement inhibition.
    E. Loss of dopaminergic neurons in the substantia nigra contributes to reduced activity of the indirect pathway and movement inhibition.

2. What will be the effect of levodopa on the course of Mr. S.'s disease?
    A. Levodopa will prevent the progression of—but not reverse—Mr. S.'s current symptoms.
    B. Levodopa/carbidopa will restore damaged dopaminergic neurons and will reverse Mr. S.'s disease.
    C. Levodopa/carbidopa will dramatically improve Mr. S.'s symptoms.
    D. Levodopa will promote the synthesis of dopamine within the central nervous system (CNS) and slow the progression of Mr. S.'s disease.
    E. Levodopa/carbidopa will promote the development of alternative pathways for the control of movement and will stabilize Mr. S.'s symptoms.

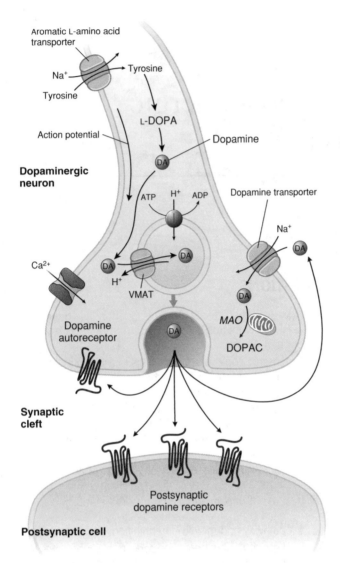

Figure 12-1. Dopaminergic Neurotransmission. Dopamine (DA) is synthesized in the cytoplasm and transported into secretory vesicles by the action of a nonselective monoamine-proton antiporter (vesicular monoamine transporter [VMAT]) that is powered by the electrochemical gradient created by a proton ATPase. Upon nerve cell stimulation, DA is released into the synaptic cleft, where the neurotransmitter can stimulate postsynaptic dopamine receptors and presynaptic dopamine autoreceptors. DA is transported out of the synaptic cleft by the selective, Na^+-coupled dopamine transporter (DAT). Cytoplasmic DA is retransported into secretory vesicles by VMAT or degraded by the enzyme monoamine oxidase (MAO). ADP = adenosine diphosphate; ATP = adenosine triphosphate; DOPAC = dihydroxyphenylacetic acid; L-DOPA = levodopa.

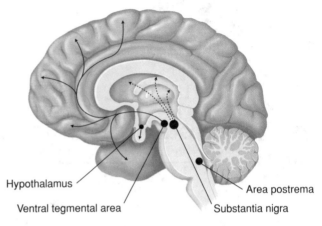

Figure 12-2. Central Dopamine Pathways. Dopaminergic neurons originate in a number of specific nuclei in the brain. Neurons that originate in the hypothalamus and project to the pituitary gland (arrow) are tonically active and inhibit prolactin secretion. Neurons that project from the substantia nigra to the striatum regulate movement (dashed arrows). Dopaminergic neurons that project from the ventral tegmental area to the limbic system and prefrontal cortex are thought to have roles in the regulation of mood and behavior (arrows). The area postrema contains a high density of dopamine receptors, and stimulation of these receptors activates the vomiting centers of the brain.

3. How will Mr. S.'s response to levodopa change over time?
   A. He will develop sensitization to levodopa and require less frequent dosages.
   B. He will develop tolerance to levodopa and require increasing dosages.
   C. He will develop intermittent "on" and "off" periods, requiring "drug holidays" from levodopa.
   D. As dopaminergic neurons regenerate, he will require less frequent levodopa administration.
   E. He will develop tolerance to levodopa and require continuous infusions of the drug.

4. The efficacy and long-term adverse effects associated with the pharmacologic treatments for Parkinson's disease influence the choice of therapy at different stages of the disease. Which of the following statements regarding the choice of therapy for Parkinson's is correct?
   A. Because of its efficacy, levodopa therapy should be initiated as soon as the diagnosis of Parkinson's disease is confirmed.
   B. Because of its adverse effects, levodopa therapy should be delayed until all other potential therapeutic options have been exhausted.
   C. Dopamine agonist therapy should be delayed until the patient has developed tolerance to the effects of levodopa.
   D. Inhibitors of dopamine metabolism should be administered as soon as the diagnosis of Parkinson's disease is confirmed.
   E. Dopamine agonist therapy is an effective initial treatment for Parkinson's disease in young patients.

5. Benztropine and trihexyphenidyl do not directly affect dopamine concentrations or dopaminergic receptor activation. How do they exert a beneficial effect in patients with Parkinson's disease?

A. These agents block cholinergic activation of dyskinetic muscle cells.

B. These agents block excitatory N-methyl-D-aspartic acid (NMDA) receptors in the striatum.

C. These agents modify striatal cholinergic interneurons, which regulate the direct and indirect pathways.

D. These agents enhance the excitatory NMDA receptors, which stimulate the direct pathway.

E. These agents block the cholinergic inhibition of the indirect pathway.

 CASE 2

A 23-year-old woman is brought to the emergency department by ambulance after her friends noted her to be acting bizarrely paranoid at a party. The patient is confused and cannot give any history. She is repetitively grinding her teeth and biting her lower lip, movements known as bruxisms. Her examination is remarkable for a heart rate of 123 bpm and a blood pressure of 150/95 mm Hg. Her skin is moist, and her pupils are dilated. She is awake but delirious and moderately agitated. Her friends report that she told them she had ingested one "hit" of ecstasy, a designer amphetamine.

QUESTIONS

1. How does the mechanism of action of the amphetamines relate to this patient's clinical symptoms?

A. Amphetamines displace dopamine from presynaptic vesicles and cause CNS stimulation.

B. Amphetamines block the action of dopamine in the mesocortical system and cause a flattened affect.

C. Amphetamines have a direct agonist effect on dopaminergic neurons in the area postrema and cause hallucinations.

D. Amphetamines prevent the release of dopamine from presynaptic neurons in the mesolimbic system and cause paranoid schizophrenia-like symptoms.

E. Amphetamines have monoamine oxidase (MAO) inhibitory activity, causing an increased concentration of tyrosine, which leads to paranoid delusions.

2. Amphetamine users often exhibit repetitive motor movements, similar to the bruxisms of this patient. What might be the etiology for these movement abnormalities?

A. Excessive dopamine in the mesolimbic system

B. Excessive dopamine in the ventral tegmental area

C. Excessive dopamine in the striatum

D. Depletion of dopamine in the mesolimbic system

E. Depletion of dopamine in the striatum

3. The patient's friends report that she has a history of depression and is taking a prescription antidepressant medication, tranylcypromine, a MAO inhibitor. Considering this patient's therapeutic use of tranylcypromine, what potential adverse effects is she at risk for by concurrently taking ecstasy?

A. Bradycardia

B. Muscle rigidity and subsequent parkinsonian symptoms

C. Loss of peripheral vascular tone

D. Liver failure

E. Seizures

4. Antipsychotic agents are used to treat the symptoms of schizophrenia. Their potency of D2 dopaminergic receptor blockade is also associated with their adverse effects, notably extrapyramidal effects. Which of the following is an example of an extrapyramidal effect?

A. shuffling gait

B. orthostatic hypotension

C. sedation

D. galactorrhea

E. neuroleptic malignant syndrome

5. Neuroleptic malignant syndrome is the most severe adverse effect associated with the D2 receptor antagonism of antipsychotic agents. Which of the following agents is most likely to cause this rare, but life-threatening syndrome?

A. clozapine

B. haloperidol

C. amantadine

D. quetiapine

E. chlorpromazine

 CASE 3

Robin L., a 34-year-old woman who is 11 weeks' pregnant, has severe nausea and vomiting related to pregnancy. She visits her obstetrician and is started on prochlorperazine, an antiemetic, to control her symptoms.

QUESTIONS

1. Prochlorperazine is a phenothiazine. How do its actions control the symptoms of nausea?

A. Blockade of D3 receptors in the mesocortical system

B. Blockade of D2 receptors in the mesolimbic system

C. Blockade of D2 receptors in the area postrema

D. Blockade of muscarinic receptors in the GI tract

E. Stimulation of D2 receptors in the nigrostriatal system

2. Twelve hours after Ms. L. takes her second dose of the medication, she develops frightening symptoms of facial and neck tightness. She finds it difficult to open her mouth and feels her neck is "pulling" her head to the right. Her husband drives her to the emergency department, where the attending physician diagnoses her as suffering from an acute dystonic reaction, an adverse effect of phenothiazine use.

How do Ms. L.'s symptoms relate to the mechanism of action of the phenothiazines?

A. Blockade of D2 receptors in the pituitary causes prolactin secretion and a false-positive pregnancy test

B. Blockade of D2 receptors in the mesocortical system causes positive schizophrenia-like symptoms of hysteria

C. Blockade of D2 receptors in the mesolimbic system causes a flattened affect and alogia

D. Blockade of D2 receptors in the nigrostriatal system causes altered muscle tone

E. Blockade of peripheral α-adrenergic receptors causes hypotension and stroke

The physician administers diphenhydramine and benztropine, drugs with antihistamine and antimuscarinic activity. Within 30 minutes, Ms. L. feels that her muscle tightness is less, and she is able to open her mouth and turn her head more easily. She is discharged home with a prescription for a nonantipsychotic antiemetic drug for control of her nausea, as well as prescriptions for diphenhydramine and benztropine for the next several days to prevent recurrence of this adverse effect.

13

Pharmacology of Serotonergic and Central Adrenergic Pharmacology

OBJECTIVES

- Understand the biochemistry and physiology of central adrenergic and serotonergic neurotransmission as they relate to affective disorders.

- Understand the pharmacology, indications for, and adverse effects of agents used to treat patients with various affective disorders.

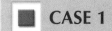

CASE 1

Mary R. is a 27-year-old office worker who presents to her primary care physician, Dr. Lee, with an 18-lb weight loss over the previous 2 months. Ms. R. tearfully explains that she is plagued by near-constant feelings of sadness and by a sense of helplessness and inadequacy at work. She feels so terrible that she has not had a good night of sleep in more than 1 month. She no longer enjoys living and has recently become scared when new thoughts of suicide enter her mind. Ms. R. tells Dr. Lee that she had felt like this once before but that it passed. Dr. Lee asks her about her sleep patterns, appetite levels, ability to concentrate, energy level, mood, interest level, and feelings of guilt. He asks her specific questions about thoughts of suicide, particularly whether she has formed a specific plan and whether she has ever attempted suicide. Dr. Lee explains to Ms. R. that she has major depressive disorder, likely caused by a chemical imbalance in her brain, and he prescribes the antidepressant fluoxetine.

QUESTIONS

1. Ms. R.'s diagnosis of major depressive disorder is based on the presence of which of the following symptoms?
   A. prior suicide attempt
   B. feeling tired and sleeping all day
   C. paranoid thoughts that her boss is critical of her work
   D. fear that she is going to die
   E. symptoms lasting 2 months

2. What is the mechanism of action of fluoxetine in alleviating the symptoms of depression?
   A. Fluoxetine prevents the metabolism of serotonin.
   B. Fluoxetine prevents the reuptake of serotonin.
   C. Fluoxetine is an agonist at postsynaptic serotonin receptors.
   D. Fluoxetine enhances the release of serotonin from presynaptic vesicles.
   E. Fluoxetine enhances the synthesis of serotonin from tryptophan.

Two weeks later, Ms. R. calls to indicate that the medicine is not working. Dr. Lee encourages her to continue taking the medicine, and after 2 more weeks, Ms. R. begins to feel better.

3. Why is there a delay in the onset of fluoxetine's therapeutic effect?
   A. It takes several weeks for fluoxetine to upregulate the sensitivity of postsynaptic serotonin receptors.
   B. It takes several weeks for fluoxetine to increase serotonin synthesis.
   C. It takes several weeks for fluoxetine concentrations in the central nervous system to become therapeutic.
   D. It takes several weeks for autoreceptors to become desensitized to the increased synaptic serotonin concentrations caused by fluoxetine.
   E. It takes several weeks for presynaptic vesicles to store and release the increased concentrations of serotonin promoted by fluoxetine therapy.

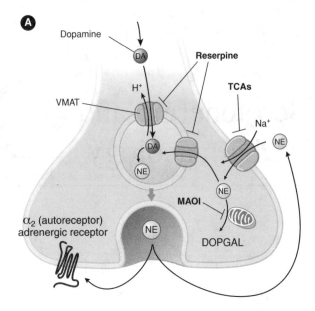

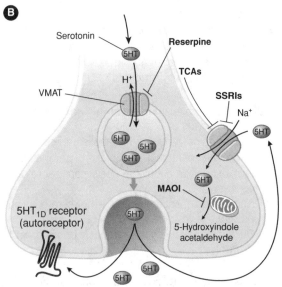

Figure 13-1. Sites and Mechanisms of Action of Antidepressant Drugs. The sites of action of antidepressant drugs and of reserpine (which can induce depression) are indicated in noradrenergic neurons (**A**) and serotonergic neurons (**B**). Monoamine oxidase inhibitors (MAOIs) inhibit the mitochondrial enzyme monoamine oxidase (MAO); the resulting increase in cytosolic monoamines leads to increased vesicular uptake of neurotransmitter and to increased release of neurotransmitter during exocytosis. Tricyclic antidepressants (TCAs) and heterocyclic antidepressants inhibit both the norepinephrine transporter (NET) and the serotonin (5HT) transporter (SERT), causing increased levels of both norepinephrine (NE) and 5HT in the synaptic cleft. Selective serotonin reuptake inhibitors (SSRIs) specifically inhibit the SERT-mediated reuptake of 5HT. TCAs, heterocyclics, and SSRIs increase the duration of neurotransmitter action in the synaptic cleft, leading to increased downstream signaling. Reserpine, which can induce depression in humans and in animal models, blocks the VMAT (vesicular monoamine transporter)-mediated uptake of monoamines into synaptic vesicles, which ultimately destroys the vesicles. DOPGAL = 3,4-dihydroxyphenylglycoaldehyde.

Ms. R. no longer feels sad and demoralized; the feelings of helplessness and inadequacy that previously plagued her have diminished. In fact, when she returns to see Dr. Lee 6 weeks later, she reports feeling much better. She no longer needs much sleep and is always full of energy. She is now convinced that she is the most intelligent person in her company. She proudly tells Dr. Lee that she has recently purchased a new sports car and gone on a large shopping spree. Dr. Lee tells her that she may be having a manic episode and, in consultation with a psychiatrist, prescribes lithium and tapers the fluoxetine. Ms. R. is hesitant to take the new medication, arguing that she feels fine and that she is concerned about the adverse effects of lithium.

4. What caused Mr. R.'s hypomania?
  A. hypersensitivity to fluoxetine
  B. cure of her depression
  C. tolerance to fluoxetine
  D. overdose of fluoxetine
  E. use of fluoxetine

5. After her hypomanic episode Ms. R. is continued on lithium as a mood stabilizer. Which of the following is a potential adverse effect of lithium therapy?
  A. psychosis
  B. thyroid goiter
  C. sexual dysfunction
  D. orthostatic hypotension
  E. migraine headaches

■ CASE 2

Jeanne K. is a 43-year-old unemployed woman with a history of depression. This evening, she has been drinking rather heavily with her boyfriend, Jack N. After nearly a case of beer, they have a quarrel, and Mr. N. storms out of the house. Ms. K. is feeling truly despondent about her situation and finishes off her bottle of antidepressant pills with the rest of her beer. When Mr. N. returns home 20 minutes later, Ms. K. appears intoxicated and drowsy on the sofa, and he goes to bed. One hour later, when Mr. N. awakens to urinate, he tries to make up with Ms. K. but finds her unresponsive on the sofa and calls 911 for help.

On arrival in the emergency department, Ms. K. is only slightly more responsive, moaning when the nurse inserts a peripheral intravenous catheter and places her on a cardiac monitor. She admits that she took an overdose of her pills because she was "mad at Jack." Her vital signs reveal a temperature of 99°F, heart rate of 122 bpm, respiratory rate of 14 breaths/min., and blood pressure of 96/58 mm Hg. When the resident physician examines Ms. K., she notes that her pupils are dilated at 6 mm, her lips and mucous membranes are very dry, and her skin is dry and flushed. Ms. K.'s 12-lead ECG shows a sinus tachycardia with a prolonged QT and widened QRS intervals.

QUESTIONS

1. What antidepressant drug can cause anticholinergic symptoms and cardiac conduction abnormalities as aspects of its toxicity?
   A. selegiline
   B. paroxetine
   C. amitriptyline
   D. bupropion
   E. sumatriptan

The resident correctly interprets the 12-lead ECG as showing quinidine-like conduction abnormalities and urgently institutes therapy to stabilize Ms. K. In addition, she orally intubates Ms. K. to protect her airway and minimize the risk of aspiration.

2. The antidepressant drug that Ms. K. ingested can cause cardiac conduction delays, which can deteriorate into life-threatening ventricular tachycardia and fibrillation. At which site is it acting to cause these effects?
   A. cardiac sodium channels
   B. alpha$_1$- adrenergic receptors
   C. presynaptic autoreceptors
   D. amphetamine receptors
   E. cardiac potassium channels

Ms. K. survives an unstable 24 hours in the intensive care unit, and is extubated two days after her admission. During her recovery, a psychiatrist is consulted to advise how best to treat her depression and alcohol use. After much discussion of her current work status and home situation with Mr. N., she decides to enter Alcoholics Anonymous and agrees to try another antidepressant medication. The psychiatrist suggests a new atypical antidepressant.

3. Which of the following agents is considered an atypical antidepressant?
   A. dexfenfluramine
   B. imipramine
   C. tyramine
   D. ondansetron
   E. mirtazapine

4. Lithium is a mood stabilizer used for the treatment of bipolar affective disorder. It is a monovalent cation with similar electrochemical properties to sodium and potassium. Lithium toxicity can occur in patients who have:
   A. hepatic failure
   B. renal insufficiency
   C. cerebrovascular disease
   D. hypothyroidism
   E. chronic obstructive pulmonary disease

5. The rate-limiting enzymatic step in serotonin synthesis is:
   A. tyramine hydroxylase
   B. tryptophan hydroxylase
   C. aromatic L-amino acid decarboxylase
   D. serotonin transportase
   E. catechol-O-methyltransferase

14

Pharmacology of Abnormal Electrical Neurotransmission in the Central Nervous System

OBJECTIVES

- Understand the molecular mechanisms of abnormal electrical neurotransmission responsible for clinical seizure activity.

- Understand the pharmacology of, indications for, and adverse effects of agents used to treat patients with various seizure disorders.

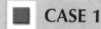

CASE 1

Jon arrives in the emergency department with his brother Rob at 9:12 PM. Because his brother is still too lethargic to speak, Jon relays most of the story to the attending physician. The two had been watching television when Jon noticed that his 40-year-old brother seemed to be daydreaming. Never missing an opportunity to tease, Jon began chiding his brother for ''spacing out.'' But instead of the boisterous laugh that he was so used to, Jon observed only a confused, almost fearful stare.

Jon recalls that, almost suddenly, his brother's right hand began to bend into an awkward position. The stiffening then spread to involve his right arm, followed by both the right arm and right leg, and finally the entire body, almost as if he were attempting to contract every muscle in his body. This sustained contraction lasted for about 15 seconds and was followed by shaking movements of all four limbs that lasted another 30 seconds or so. The frequency of the shaking slowed after several minutes, and Rob then became limp, began breathing very heavily, and remained unresponsive. Rob regained consciousness on the way to the emergency department.

QUESTIONS

1. What is the significance of the order of the spread of the seizure from the hand, to the arm, and then to the leg?
   A. This order of spread is consistent with an aura.
   B. This order of spread is consistent with the spread of synchronous activity across the motor homunculus.
   C. This order of spread is consistent with the presence of a space-occupying lesion in the brain.
   D. This order of spread is consistent with the spread of synchronous activity to the reticular activating system.
   E. This order of spread is consistent with thalamocortical involvement of synchronous activity.

2. The generalized seizure included a tonic phase (stiffening) followed by a clonic phase (shaking). What is the basis of these two phases of seizure activity at the molecular level?
   A. Asynchronous sodium channel opening causes disequilibrium between gamma-aminobutyric acid (GABA) and glutamate activity, resulting in tonic-clonic activity.
   B. Lack of glutamate excitation results in tonic activity, and sporadic bursts of GABA inhibition result in intervening clonic activity.
   C. Loss of GABA input results in tonic activity, and an oscillation between GABA inhibitory and glutamate excitatory impulses results in clonic activity.
   D. Excessive GABA inhibitory impulses are overridden by oscillating glutamate excitatory impulses, resulting in tonic–clonic activity.
   E. Excessive intracellular calcium influx holds glutamate channels in the active state, resulting in tonic activity, and periodic extrusion of intracellular calcium restores normal glutamate activity in oscillating bursts.

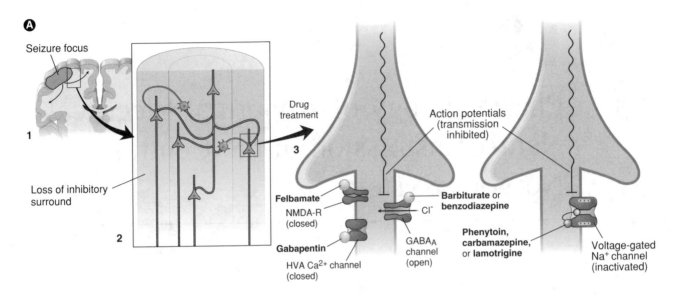

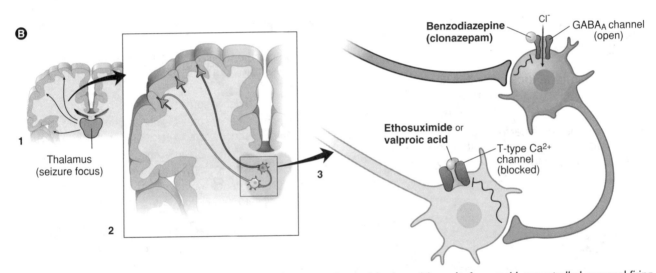

Figure 14-1. Mechanisms of Pharmacotherapy for Seizures. A. The partial seizure (**1**) results from rapid, uncontrolled neuronal firing and a loss of surround inhibition (**2**). Antiepileptic drugs act at four molecular targets to enhance inhibition and prevent spread of synchronous activity (**3**): Barbiturates and benzodiazepines prevent seizure spread by acting on the GABA$_A$ receptor to potentiate GABA-mediated inhibition. Na$^+$ channel inhibitors such as phenytoin, carbamazepine, and lamotrigine prevent rapid neuronal firing by selectively prolonging Na$^+$ channel inactivation in rapidly firing neurons. Felbamate suppresses seizure activity by inhibiting the N-methyl-D-aspartic acid (NMDA) receptor and thereby decreasing glutamate-mediated excitation. Gabapentin decreases release of excitatory neurotransmitter by inhibiting the high-voltage-activated (HVA) calcium channel. **B.** The absence seizure (**1**) is caused by a self-sustaining cycle of activity generated between thalamic and cortical cells (**2**). Antiepileptic drugs prevent this synchronous thalamocortical cycle (**3**) by acting at two molecular targets: Clonazepam, a benzodiazepine, potentiates GABA$_A$ channels in the reticular thalamic nucleus, thus decreasing the activation of the inhibitory reticular neurons and decreasing the hyperpolarization of the thalamic relay neurons. T-type calcium channel inhibitors such as ethosuximide and valproic acid prevent the burst activity of thalamic relay neurons that is required for synchronous activation of cortical cells.

At the hospital, a magnetic resonance imaging scan shows a small neoplasm in Rob's left temporal lobe. Because the neoplasm appears to be benign, Rob, following the advice of his physician, decides not to undergo surgery.

3. Given the current understanding of the molecular mechanisms underlying seizures, by what mechanisms could a focal neoplasm result in a seizure?

    A. A focal neoplasm could alter the local neuronal environment and compromise the normally protective mechanisms that prevent abnormal synchronous discharge.

    B. A focal neoplasm always secretes potassium, which compromises the normal ion channel function and promotes abnormal synchronous discharge.

    C. A focal neoplasm secretes tumor glutamate factors, which inhibit normal GABA inhibitory function and allow abnormal synchronous discharge.

    D. A focal neoplasm compresses normal sodium channels and facilitates the transmission of abnormal synchronous discharge across the corpus callosum.

E. A focal neoplasm is able to generate abnormal synchronous discharges within its tissues.

The potential benefits and risks of various anticonvulsant drugs, including phenytoin, carbamazepine, valproic acid, and lamotrigine, are discussed, and it is decided to start Rob on a regimen of carbamazepine to prevent further seizures.

4. What is the mechanism of action common to phenytoin, carbamazepine, valproic acid, and lamotrigine in preventing seizures?
   A. All of these agents inhibit calcium channels.
   B. All of these agents enhance potassium efflux from neurons.
   C. All of these agents limit glutamate binding to its receptors.
   D. All of these agents enhance GABA inhibitory tone.
   E. All of these agents have sodium channel blocking effects.

5. Based on his clinical circumstances, why was carbamazepine the antiepileptic drug chosen for Rob?
   A. Carbamazepine has less adverse effects and potential drug interactions than phenytoin.
   B. Carbamazepine is more effective in treating absence seizures.
   C. Carbamazepine enhances its own metabolism so that patients can gradually reduce their initial dosage.
   D. Carbamazepine has an inactive metabolite, which lessens the risk of toxicity associated with this drug.
   E. Carbamazepine is a once-a-day injectable drug.

■ CASE 2

Jessie is a 10-year-old girl who was diagnosed with dyskinetic cerebral palsy at the age of 3 years. Her cerebral palsy manifests as writhing, choreoathetoid movements of her hands and feet, which make it difficult for her to sit or stand. She wears specially fitted orthotic braces on her feet and legs, and uses a wheelchair to maneuver through the halls at her school. When Jessie was 5 years old, she experienced her first seizure, which was of the generalized tonic–clonic subtype. She has been maintained on phenytoin and has had fairly good control of her seizures for the past several years. They tend to occur only in relation to infectious illnesses or excessive fatigue.

Last week while on a family trip visiting relatives in Florida, Jessie developed a cough and low-grade fever. She was diagnosed with pneumonia at an urgent care clinic and was started on erythromycin for her pulmonary symptoms. Over the past 4 days, her fever resolved, and her cough improved. However, yesterday, her mother and father noted her to be unusually drowsy. They attributed it to the recent travel home.

Today at school, her physical therapist thought Jessie seemed less coordinated than her baseline. Jessie had trouble holding her upper body still in her wheelchair and seemed to be unsteady while she was seated. She also complained of dizziness during her routine physical therapy. Jessie's mother made an urgent appointment for her to be seen by her neurologist, Dr. Black. Dr. Black noted Jessie to have nystagmus and truncal ataxia in addition to much decreased limb coordination. A serum phenytoin level was ordered and returned elevated at 34 μg/mL (normal, 10–20 μg/mL).

QUESTIONS

1. Phenytoin is a first-line antiepileptic drug for the treatment of partial and generalized seizures. However, it has an extensive adverse effect profile. In addition to Jessie's symptoms of dizziness, drowsiness, nystagmus, and ataxia, which of the following is also a potential adverse effect of phenytoin therapy?
   A. pancreatitis
   B. aplastic anemia
   C. gingival hyperplasia
   D. absence seizures
   E. abnormal bleeding

2. Jessie's phenytoin dose remained unchanged, yet she developed toxic serum concentrations and clinical symptoms of toxicity. What is the most likely cause of this?
   A. Erythromycin inhibited the hepatic P450 metabolism of phenytoin.
   B. Erythromycin altered the normal gastrointestinal flora and enhanced absorption of phenytoin.
   C. Erythromycin displaced phenytoin from plasma albumin, allowing a greater concentration of free drug to enter the central nervous system.
   D. Erythromycin altered the blood–brain barrier, facilitating the entry of phenytoin into the central nervous system.
   E. Erythromycin prevented renal elimination of phenytoin.

3. Phenytoin is a sodium channel blocker that prolongs the period of inactivation of neuronal sodium channels. It acts in a use-dependent manner. What does this mean in relation to its therapeutic effects?
   A. Phenytoin blocks T-type calcium channels only during waking periods and prevents absence seizures.
   B. Phenytoin blocks sodium channels only in the activated state and prevents partial seizures.
   C. Phenytoin blocks sodium channels in slow-wave cycles and prevents generalized seizures.
   D. Phenytoin blocks sodium channels in rapidly firing neurons and prevents partial and secondary generalized seizures.
   E. Phenytoin blocks sodium channels in slowly firing neurons and prevents absence seizures.

4. Which of the following statements regarding the treatment of absence seizures is correct?

   A. Carbamazepine inhibits T-type calcium channel opening in thalamocortical cells.

   B. Gabapentin inhibits GABA metabolism and enhances GABA-mediated inhibition of absence seizure activity.

   C. Ethosuximide prolongs sodium channel inactivation in thalamocortical cells.

   D. Valproic acid limits T-type calcium channel activation and enhances GABA-mediated inhibition of absence seizures.

   E. Ethosuximide inhibits the high voltage–activated calcium channel opening in thalamocortical cells.

5. What are the similarities and differences of benzodiazepines and barbiturates as antiepileptic therapies?

   A. Benzodiazepines and barbiturates both prevent the metabolism of GABA, but only barbiturates are associated with aplastic anemia.

   B. Benzodiazepines and barbiturates both bind to the GABA receptor complex, but only barbiturates are able to bind both the sodium channel and T-type calcium channels.

   C. Benzodiazepines and barbiturates both enhance GABA-mediated inhibition, but only barbiturates are able to enhance the activity at the GABA receptor in the absence of GABA.

   D. Benzodiazepines and barbiturates both cause sedation as a adverse effect, but only barbiturates cause acute withdrawal symptoms on withdrawal of the drug.

   E. Benzodiazepines and barbiturates both enhance GABA-mediated inhibition, but only benzodiazepines can exacerbate absence seizures.

15

General Anesthetic Pharmacology

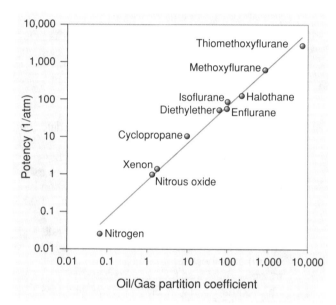

Figure 15-1. The Meyer-Overton rule. Molecules with a larger oil/gas partition coefficient (λ(oil/gas)) are more potent general anesthetics. This log–log plot shows the very tight correlation between lipid solubility (λ(oil/gas)) and anesthetic potency over five orders of magnitude. Note that even such gases as xenon and nitrogen can act as general anesthetics when breathed at high enough partial pressures. The equation describing the line is: Potency = λ(oil/gas) / 1.3. Recall that Potency = 1/MAC.

OBJECTIVES

■ Understand the pharmacodynamic and pharmacokinetic principles of inhaled anesthetics.

■ Understand the pharmacology, therapeutic uses, and adverse effects of general anesthetics.

■ **CASE 1**

Matthew is a 7-year-old, 20-kg boy who has been undergoing multidrug chemotherapy for aggressive osteosarcoma of his right femur. The time has now come for a surgical resection.

• 8:00 PM (night before the operation): Dr. Snow, the anesthesiologist, provides reassurance and revisits the importance of fasting after midnight to prevent aspiration of gastric contents while under general anesthesia.
• 6:30 AM: Matthew clings to his mother and appears anxious, cachectic, and in some pain. His vital signs are stable with an elevated pulse of 120 bpm and a blood pressure of 110/75 mm Hg. An oral dose of midazolam (a benzodiazepine; see Chapter 11 Pharmacology of GABAergic and glutamatergic neurotransmission) is given to relieve anxiety and to allow Matthew to separate from his parents.
• 7:00 AM: Dr. Snow injects a small amount of lidocaine subcutaneously (a local anesthetic; see Chapter 10 Local Anesthetic Pharmacology) before inserting an intravenous catheter (which he carefully conceals from Matthew until the last possible moment). Through the catheter, Dr. Snow delivers an infusion of morphine sulfate (an opioid; see Chapter 16 Pharmacology of Analgesia) for analgesia.
• 7:30 AM: Dr. Snow rapidly induces anesthesia with an intravenous bolus of 60 mg (3 mg/kg) of thiopental (a barbiturate; see Chapter 11). Within 45 seconds, Matthew is in a deep anesthetic state. The doctor adds a dose of intravenous succinylcholine (a depolarizing muscle relaxant; see Chapter 8 Cholinergic Pharmacology) to facilitate endotracheal intubation, and Matthew is placed on artificial respiration.
• 7:32 AM: A mixture of inhaled general anesthetics consisting of 2% isoflurane, 50% nitrous oxide, and 48% oxygen is provided through the ventilator to maintain the anesthetic state.

QUESTIONS

1. Dr. Snow used a mixture of inhaled isoflurane and nitrous oxide. What is the advantage of using a mixture of two anesthetics?
   A. Isoflurane minimizes potential nitrous oxide-induced hypotension.
   B. Isoflurane facilitates more rapid induction, while nitrous oxide facilitates more rapid recovery.
   C. Isoflurane allows for more potent anesthesia, while nitrous oxide minimizes potential isoflurane-induced hepatotoxicity.
   D. Isoflurane facilitates more rapid induction and recovery, while nitrous oxide allows for more potent anesthesia.
   E. Isoflurane allows for more potent anesthesia, while nitrous oxide facilitates more rapid induction and recovery.

- 7:50 AM: Matthew shows no response, either through movement or increased sympathetic tone (e.g., increased heart rate, increased blood pressure), to the first surgical incision.
- 8:20 AM: Dr. Snow notices with a start that Matthew's pulse has fallen to 55 bpm and his blood pressure to 85/45 mm Hg. Berating himself for forgetting to turn down the inspired partial pressure of the anesthetic as its mixed venous partial pressure increased, Dr. Snow reduces the inspired isoflurane level to 0.8% while keeping the nitrous oxide level at 50%. Within 15 minutes, Matthew's pulse and blood pressure rebound.

2. Dr. Snow forgot to decrease the inspired partial pressure of the anesthetic as its mixed venous partial pressure increased. Why is it necessary to reduce the inspired partial pressure of isoflurane shortly after successful induction?
   A. As the alveolar partial pressure equilibrates with the inspired partial pressure of the anesthetic, anesthetic will diffuse from the bloodstream into the exhaled air.
   B. As the CNS' partial pressure equilibrates with the alveolar partial pressure, no further uptake of inspired anesthetic into blood can occur.
   C. As the cardiac muscle partial pressure equilibrates with the higher inspired partial pressure of the anesthetic, arrhythmias can occur.
   D. As the CNS' partial pressure equilibrates with the higher inspired partial pressure of the anesthetic, cardiopulmonary depression can occur.
   E. As the CNS' partial pressure equilibrates with the higher inspired partial pressure of the anesthetic, hepatotoxicity can occur.

- 12:35 PM: After a long surgery, Dr. Snow stops the isoflurane and nitrous oxide and turns on pure oxygen for a few minutes.

3. Why did Dr. Snow give pure oxygen for a few minutes after the cessation of anesthetic administration?

A. Isoflurane has a long duration of action, causing persistent hypoventilation and decreased oxygen uptake from the alveoli.
B. Nitrous oxide rapidly diffuses out of the blood, replacing inspired air and decreasing the alveolar (and subsequent arterial) partial pressure of oxygen.
C. Nitrous oxide rapidly diffuses out of the blood into the alveoli, causing local bronchiole irritation and cough, which is prevented by mixing with pure oxygen.
D. Isoflurane rapidly diffuses out of the blood, replacing inspired air, and decreasing the alveolar nitrogen partial pressure in favor of oxygen.
E. Nitrous oxide rapidly diffuses out of the CNS to the cardiac muscle tissue, precipitating cardiopulmonary depression, which is alleviated by mixing with a high arterial partial pressure of oxygen

- 12:45 PM: In less than 10 minutes, Matthew is breathing spontaneously and is able to respond to questions, although he is still somewhat groggy. Matthew's parents are relieved to find him awake and alert after more than 5 hours of anesthesia.

4. How does the rate of induction of anesthesia differ between children and adults?
   A. Children have a higher alveolar ventilation rate, smaller lungs, and a lower capacity of tissues for anesthetic; this shortens the time to equilibration between inspired and alveolar partial pressure, and between alveolar and tissue partial pressure.
   B. Children have a higher alveolar ventilation rate and smaller body surface area; this shortens the time to equilibration between the three tissue compartments and the inspired partial pressure.
   C. Children have a higher alveolar ventilation rate but a more rapid rate of hepatic metabolism of anesthetics, so they require a higher inspired partial pressure.
   D. Children have proportionally greater cardiac output; this decreases the time to equilibrate between alveolar and tissue partial pressure.
   E. Children have a higher alveolar ventilation rate and smaller lungs; this increases the time for inspired anesthetic to diffuse into the blood.

5. The potency of an anesthetic increases as:
   A. its solubility in cardiac muscle tissue increases
   B. its solubility in blood increases
   C. its solubility in oil increases
   D. its MAC increases
   E. its therapeutic index increases

■ CASE 2

On August 31, 1999, a 22-year-old junior physics major at Massachusetts Institute of Technology, was found dead in a campus dorm room after reportedly inhaling nitrous oxide in an attempt to get high. He was found with a plastic bag over his head and was pronounced dead at the scene. Two MIT students were charged with drug possession with intent to distribute. The nitrous oxide canister found at the scene had been stolen from a campus lab.

QUESTIONS

1. Which of the following properties of nitrous oxide predisposes to asphyxia?
   A. Nitrous oxide has a small blood/gas partition coefficient.
   B. Nitrous oxide has a low MAC.
   C. Nitrous oxide has a high analgesic index.
   D. Nitrous oxide is hepatically metabolized.
   E. Nitrous oxide has a small brain/blood partition coefficient.

2. Nitrous oxide is a "perfusion-limited anesthetic." This means that:
   A. The time constant for equilibration of alveolar and inspired partial pressures is longer than the time constant for equilibration of tissue and arterial partial pressures.
   B. It has a high blood/gas partition coefficient.
   C. It has a high rate of uptake into the bloodstream from the alveoli.
   D. The time constant for equilibration of alveolar and inspired partial pressures is similar to the time constant for equilibration of tissue and arterial partial pressures.
   E. Induction time is slow.

3. The brain is considered to be in a vessel-rich group. This means that it has:

A. a low capacity for anesthetic and low blood flow to the compartment
B. a very high capacity for anesthetic but low blood flow to the compartment
C. a low capacity for anesthetic but high blood flow to the compartment
D. a high capacity for anesthetic and high blood flow to the compartment
E. a high capacity for anesthetic but moderate blood flow to the compartment

4. Most of the general anesthetics can cause cardiopulmonary depression. Which of the following anesthetic agents increases cardiac output?
   A. isoflurane
   B. propofol
   C. ketamine
   D. thiopental
   E. diethyl ether

5. Malignant hyperthermia is a rare but potentially lethal adverse effect of halothane administration. Symptoms of malignant hyperthermia are caused by:
   A. uncontrolled influx of potassium via the sodium pump
   B. uncontrolled sequestration of calcium by the sarcoplasmic reticulum
   C. uncontrolled efflux of potassium through the sarcolemma
   D. uncontrolled influx of calcium through the sarcolemma
   E. uncontrolled efflux of calcium from the sarcoplasmic reticulum

16

Pharmacology of Analgesia

OBJECTIVES

■ Understand the mechanisms by which noxious stimuli lead to physiologic, inflammatory, neuropathic, and dysfunctional pain perception.

■ Understand the pharmacology and uses of opioid and non-opioid analgesics for the treatment of acute pain.

■ Understand the pathophysiology of, and potential pharmacologic therapies for dysfunctional pain syndromes.

■ CASE 1

J.D., a 15-year-old boy, receives severe burns while escaping from a building fire. The extensive burns include first- and second-degree burns covering much of his body and a local, full-thickness burn on his right forearm. He reaches the emergency department in severe pain and is treated with intravenous morphine in increasing quantities until he reports that the pain has subsided. This dose of morphine is then maintained. The next day, he receives a skin graft covering the region of his full-thickness burn. During the operation, an anesthesiologist provides a continuous intravenous infusion of remifentanil, with a bolus dose of morphine added 15 minutes before the end of the operation. At the end of the operation and for 4 days thereafter, J.D. receives intravenous morphine through a patient-controlled analgesia device. As the burns heal, the morphine dose is tapered and eventually replaced with an oral codeine/acetaminophen combination tablet.

QUESTIONS

1. Pain perception is the result of neuronal processing and transmission of noxious sensory stimulation, occurring in the periphery but perceived in the central nervous system. When J.D. was burned, which of the following pathways was responsible for the sequential transmission and modulation of this sensory stimulation?

   A. Intense heat stimulated ATP receptors; tissue burn injury stimulated the production of chemical activators, including glutamate; and voltage-gated calcium channels in Aδ and C fibers were activated and transmitted signals to the dorsal horn of the spinal cord, where transmitted signals were modulated by TRPV receptors.

   B. Intense heat stimulated voltage-gated sodium channels in Aδ fibers; tissue burn injury stimulated the production of chemical activators, including bradykinin and glycine; and voltage-gated sodium channels in Aδ and C fibers were activated and transmitted signals to the dorsal horn of the spinal cord, where inhibitory neurotransmitters stimulated the release of opioids.

   C. Intense heat stimulated thermosensitive TRPV receptors; tissue burn injury stimulated the production of chemical activators, including protons and kinins; and voltage-gated sodium channels in Aδ and C fibers were activated and transmitted signals to the dorsal horn of the spinal cord, where N-type voltage-gated calcium channels controlled release of neurotransmitters at the secondary projection neurons.

   D. Intense heat stimulated thermosensitive ATP receptors and tissue burn injury stimulated voltage-gated calcium channel activation in C fibers and transmitted signals to the dorsal horn of the spinal cord, where N-type sodium channels controlled the release of morphine.

   E. Intense heat stimulated thermosensitive TRPV receptors, tissue burn injury inhibited TRPM channels, which allowed voltage-gated sodium channels to be activated in Aδ and C fibers, which transmitted signals to the dorsal horn of the spinal cord, where N-type voltage-gated calcium channels controlled release of neurotransmitters at the secondary projection neurons.

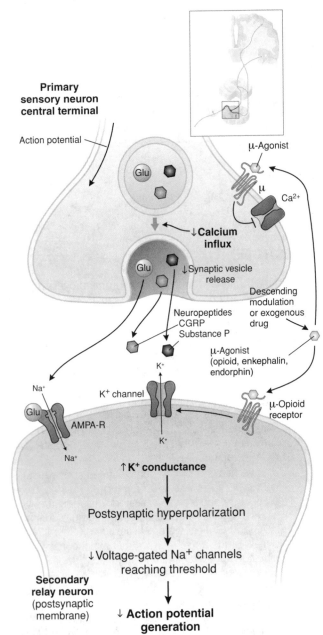

Figure 16-1. Mechanism of Action of μ-Opioid Receptor Agonists in the Spinal Cord. Activation of both presynaptic and postsynaptic μ-opioid receptors by descending and local circuit inhibitory neurons inhibits central relaying of nociceptive stimuli. In the presynaptic terminal, μ-opioid receptor activation decreases Ca^{2+} influx in response to an incoming action potential. Postsynaptic μ-opioid receptor activation increases K^+ conductance, thereby decreasing the postsynaptic response to excitatory neurotransmission. CGRP = calcitonin gene-related peptide.

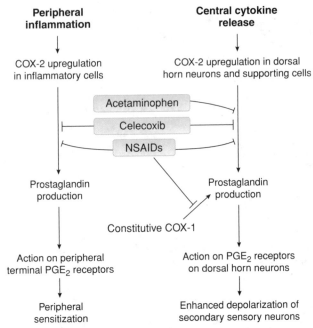

Figure 16-2. Mechanism of Analgesic Action of Cyclooxygenase (COX) Inhibitors. Inflammatory states are often associated with the production of prostaglandins, which are important mediators of both peripheral (left) and central (right) pain sensitization. In the periphery, prostaglandins produced by inflammatory cells sensitize peripheral nerve terminal prostaglandin (EP) receptors, making them more responsive to a painful stimulus. In central pain pathways, cytokines released in response to inflammation induce prostaglandin production in the dorsal horn of the spinal cord. These prostaglandins sensitize secondary nociceptive neurons, thereby increasing the perception of pain. Nonsteroidal antiinflammatory drugs (NSAIDs) block peripheral and central sensitization mediated by prostanoids that are released in inflammation; NSAIDs also reduce the extent of inflammation. PGE_2 = prostaglandin E2.

2. J.D. was treated with intravenous opioids, morphine and remifentanil, on his initial presentation and perioperatively. What is the mechanism of action through which these medications relieve pain?

   A. These μ receptor agonists inhibit calcium reuptake in postsynaptic secondary afferent neurons.

   B. These κ receptor antagonists stimulate vesicle release from primary afferents and hyperpolarize primary afferents.

   C. These μ receptor agonists block reuptake of serotonin and hyperpolarize inhibitory interneurons.

   D. These μ receptor agonists inhibit synaptic vesicle release from primary afferents and hyperpolarize postsynaptic neurons.

   E. These adrenergic receptor antagonists stimulate release of calcium from primary afferents and depolarize postsynaptic neurons.

3. As his burns began to heal, J.D.'s morphine dose was tapered and he was administered an oral codeine/acetaminophen combination tablet for pain control. What is the rationale for using this combination medication to treat pain?

A. Opioid–acetaminophen combination analgesics act through different mechanisms to reduce painful sensations, and are synergistic in their effect.

B. Opioid–acetaminophen combination analgesics enhance each other's metabolism to active metabolites, and have a longer duration of action.

C. Opioid–acetaminophen combination analgesics prevent NSAID-induced gastric upset.

D. Opioid–acetaminophen combination analgesics inhibit each other's metabolism, and have a longer duration of action.

E. Opioid–acetaminophen combinations do not cause tolerance and addiction.

Three months later, J.D. reports severe loss of sensation to touch in the area of the skin graft. He also describes a persistent tingling sensation in this area with occasional bursts of sharp, knife-like pain. After referral to a pain clinic, J.D. is prescribed oral gabapentin, which partially reduces his symptoms. However, he reports to the pain clinic again 2 months later, still in severe pain. At this time, amitriptyline is added to the gabapentin, and the pain is further relieved. Three years later, J.D.'s lingering pain has resolved, and he no longer requires medication, but the lack of forearm sensation persists.

4. Months after his injury J.D. experiences a persistent tingling sensation in the area of his skin graft with occasional bursts of severe sharp pain. He is treated with amitriptyline. What type of medication is amitriptyline, and how does it control neuropathic pain?

A. It is a specific serotonin reuptake inhibitor that blocks reuptake of serotonin in the periphery, and limits peripheral sensitization.

B. It is an antidepressant that blocks sodium channels, increases cannabinoid activity, limits peripheral sensitization, and alleviates depression associated with dysfunctional pain.

C. It is an antidepressant that blocks sodium channels, increases noradrenergic and serotonergic activity in the spinal cord, limits abnormal neurotransmission, and reduces central sensitization.

D. It is a cannabinoid receptor agonist that blocks sodium channels, increases cannabinoid and noradrenergic activity in the spinal cord, and limits abnormal neurotransmission.

E. It is an antidepressant that blocks calcium channels in the spinal cord, limits abnormal vesicle release by primary afferents, and limits central sensitization.

5. Which of the following medications is an antiinflammatory analgesic?

A. remifentanil

B. indomethacin

C. acetaminophen

D. carbamazepine

E. misoprostol

 CASE 2

Jayne S., a 51-year-old woman, is seeing her primary doctor for the fourth visit in 2 months for a recurrent but progressive pain in her face. She first noted intermittent, sharp, shooting pains in the right side of her jaw 3 months ago. Her doctor found her examination to be normal and suggested she might have inflammation of her temporomandibular joint. He prescribed a high dose of naproxen, an NSAID, to control the inflammation and pain. Ms. S. took naproxen as prescribed and sometimes took an extra dose at night in an attempt to control the painful episodes. However, after 4 weeks, she did not feel the pain was being well controlled and was starting to experience some gastric upset and heartburn.

QUESTIONS

1. How might naproxen control the pain of an inflamed temporomandibular joint?

A. Naproxen inhibits the activation of sodium channels and prevents abnormal neuronal signal transmission.

B. Naproxen non-selectively inhibits COX and prevents the formation of prostaglandins.

C. Naproxen is an agonist at the μ receptor and inhibits the release of neurotransmitters in the spinal cord.

D. Naproxen is an agonist at spinal cord cannabinoid receptors.

E. Naproxen has monoaminergic and opioid effects in the central nervous system.

One month ago during her follow-up visit with her doctor, Ms. S. complained that the pain was occurring more frequently and was unbearable. She described intense "electrical shocks" of pain shooting over the side of her cheek and nose whenever she brushed her teeth or chewed. Her doctor prescribed oxycodone for dental pain. Ms. S. took the oxycodone every 4 hours as directed, and initially felt the pain to be fairly controlled with less frequent episodes and slightly less severe intensity. However, within 1 week, the pain seemed to be more intense despite her use of oxycodone. Ms. S. felt she needed to increase her use of oxycodone to every 1 to 2 hours to control the painful episodes. She called her doctor, who refilled her oxycodone prescription and referred her to a myofascial pain specialist. One night, in disgust, Ms. S. decided to discontinue her use of oxycodone because she was sure that the medication was no longer working to control her pain. She flushed the bottle of pills down the toilet. Within 24 hours, she felt the pain was worse, but of greater concern, she felt nauseated, with diffuse muscle aches and abdominal cramping. She could not sleep.

2. What is the explanation for Ms. S.'s requirement of increasing doses of oxycodone to control her pain, and her subsequent symptoms when she discontinued oxycodone?

- **A.** central sensitization and withdrawal
- **B.** COX deficiency and prostaglandin rebound
- **C.** opioid metabolism induction and subtherapeutic drug concentration
- **D.** opioid tolerance and withdrawal
- **E.** opioid addiction and central sensitization

Ms. S. finally saw the pain specialist 1 week ago. He diagnosed her with tic douloureux (trigeminal neuralgia), a painful condition of the fifth cranial nerve characterized by abnormal impulse transmission. He prescribed another medication, which he felt would be successful in controlling this nerve ''sensitivity'' and her pain syndrome.

3. Given the pathophysiology of tic douloureux, which of the following medications is most likely to be effective in treating this condition?

- **A.** gabapentin
- **B.** anandamide
- **C.** diclofenac
- **D.** dynorphins
- **E.** naloxone

Ms. S. has now been taking the new medication for 1 week. She thinks the episodes of sharp electrical pain are slightly less frequent, but still very painful. However, she complains to her primary doctor that she is having unpleasant adverse effects, which make it difficult for her to drive and work.

4. What are common adverse effects that limit the therapeutic use of anticonvulsants in the treatment of neuropathic pain?

- **A.** COX-2 inhibitor-associated cardiovascular toxicity
- **B.** allergic reaction to acetaminophen
- **C.** flushing and nausea
- **D.** dizziness, confusion, and unsteady gait
- **E.** postural hypotension

5. Which of the following (analgesic : mechanism of action) pairs is correct?

- **A.** celecoxib : blocks calcium channels
- **B.** gabapentin : binds to voltage-dependent calcium channels
- **C.** ibuprofen : blocks voltage-gated sodium channels
- **D.** dextromethorphan : COX-2 inhibitor
- **E.** naltrexone : μ receptor agonist

17

Pharmacology of Drug Dependence and Addiction

OBJECTIVES

- Understand the neuropharmacology associated with drug dependence and addiction.

- Understand how the mechanisms of action of prescribed and non-prescribed substances are associated with the development of tolerance and potential drug dependence.

- Understand the pharmacologic actions of agents used to treat drug dependence and addiction.

■ CASE 1

Mr. B., a 25-year-old man with a history of heavy heroin use, is brought to the emergency department of a suburban Phoenix hospital with an 8-hour history of increasing nausea, vomiting, diarrhea, muscle aches, and anxiety. Mr. B. explains that he is trying to "kick the habit" and that his last "hit" was approximately 24 hours ago. He expresses an intense craving for heroin and is extremely fidgety and uncomfortable. On physical examination, he has a temperature of 103°F, enlarged pupils, a blood pressure of 170/95 mm Hg, and a heart rate of 108 bpm. He is irritable and exquisitely sensitive to touch, and his responses to painful stimuli, such as a pinprick, are out of proportion to the intensity of the stimulus. Mr. B. is given 20 mg of methadone, a long-acting opioid. He becomes slightly more comfortable and is given a second dose of 20 mg, after which he is noticeably more comfortable and the worst of his symptoms abate. Mr. B. is then admitted to an inpatient detoxification center to complete a 28-day treatment program.

QUESTIONS

1. What caused Mr. B.'s physical symptoms of nausea and vomiting and signs of fever, hypertension, and enlarged pupils on his visit to the emergency department?
   A. Mr. B. has opioid withdrawal symptoms.
   B. Mr. B. has been given an adulterated (poisoned) hit of heroin.
   C. Mr. B. has developed the symptoms of inverse tolerance.
   D. Mr. B. has the symptoms of addiction.
   E. Mr. B. has developed the symptoms of drug avoidance.

2. Why was Mr. B. treated for heroin withdrawal with methadone, another opioid?
   A. Methadone speeds the hepatic metabolism of heroin to hasten its removal from the body.
   B. Methadone has a longer duration of action than heroin and can be tapered to avoid the physical symptoms of acute withdrawal.
   C. Methadone is an oral drug that reverses the cellular mechanisms of opioid tolerance.
   D. Methadone dosages can be measured in milligram doses to precisely determine the amount of drug needed to bind to unoccupied μ opioid receptors.
   E. Methadone is a legal and cheap alternative to heroin.

Over the course of the next week, his methadone dose is decreased by approximately 20% each day. Mr. B. is enrolled in a Narcotics Anonymous (NA) program, where he tells the tale of his addiction.

A Acute administration of morphine decreases cellular activity

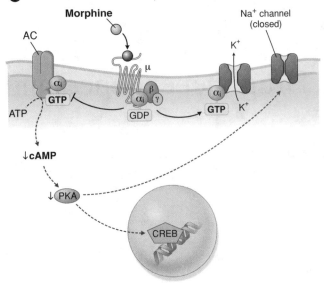

B Chronic administration of morphine induces tolerance

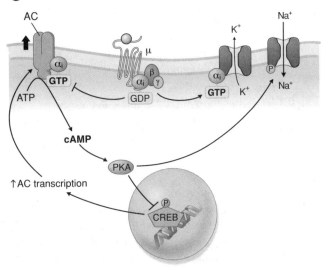

Figure 17-1.   Induction of Tolerance to Morphine. A. The μ-opioid receptor is coupled to a G protein that activates potassium channels and inhibits adenylyl cyclase (AC), resulting in membrane hyperpolarization and in decreased production of cyclic adenosine monophosphate (cAMP). Because cAMP activates protein kinase A (PKA), which in turn regulates the threshold of the voltage-gated sodium channel, the decreased cAMP levels indirectly decrease sodium channel conductance. Decreased cAMP also decreases activation of the transcription factor cAMP response element-binding protein (CREB), which regulates the level of AC expression. **B.** Chronic administration of morphine upregulates CREB, which stimulates the transcription of adenylyl cyclase, which in turn restores cAMP production toward normal levels. The increased cAMP stimulates PKA, which phosphorylates (and thereby activates) both CREB and the voltage-gated sodium channel. Therefore, upregulation of the cAMP pathway counteracts the acute effects of the drug, resulting in tolerance. GDP = guanosine diphosphate; GTP = guanosine triphosphate.

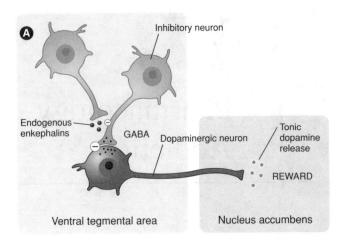

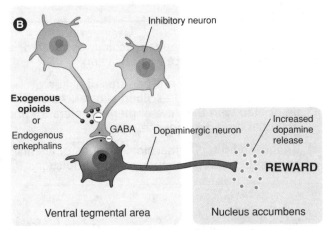

Figure 17-2.   Role of Opioids in the Brain Reward Pathway. A. GABAergic neurons tonically inhibit the dopaminergic neurons that arise in the ventral tegmental area and are responsible for reward. These GABAergic neurons can be inhibited by endogenous enkephalins, which locally modulate the release of neurotransmitter at the GABAergic nerve terminal. **B.** Administration of exogenous opioids results in decreased GABA release and disinhibition of the dopaminergic reward neurons. The increased release of dopamine in the nucleus accumbens signals a strong reward.

3. How can programs such as NA help treat addiction?
    A. These programs teach addicts about the pathophysiology of their addiction.
    B. These programs run detoxification units where drug users can return when they relapse.
    C. These programs provide a community of support and mentoring to recovering addicts.
    D. These programs provide financial support for the cost of methadone maintenance.
    E. These programs teach recovering addicts how to learn moderation management of their drug.

It had started out slowly, with only a few hits of heroin each month, ''on special occasions,'' as he puts it. Over time, however, he had found that the high he got from the drug was not as intense as it had been when he first started, and he found himself shooting (i.e., injecting intravenously) larger amounts of heroin, and injecting them more frequently. Eventually, he was shooting twice a day and felt as if he were "trapped" by the drug.

4. Why did Mr. B. find that, over time, the effect of heroin was less intense than when he first started using?
   A. Mr. B. was reusing needles, which limited the amount of drug he was injecting.
   B. Mr. B. was consciously adapting his behavior to conditioned tolerance.
   C. Mr. B. had innate tolerance to the effects of heroin.
   D. Mr. B. had acquired tolerance to the effects of heroin.
   E. Mr. B. was using less potent, adulterated heroin.

Although Mr. B. finds the sessions at NA useful, his attendance is sporadic. Over the next few weeks, he experiences cyclical changes in weight, alternating periods of insomnia and anxiety, and craving for heroin despite opioid-free urine tests. Two months later, he relapses and is again shooting heroin twice daily.

5. Why did Mr. B. experience intense cravings for heroin after his physiologic symptoms abated?
   A. Cravings and relapse are most commonly associated with heroin abstinence.
   B. Cravings and relapse can occur as a result of long-lasting molecular and cellular adaptations in the brain as a result of drug abuse.
   C. Cravings can occur as a result of drug-induced destruction of the brain's reward center neurons.
   D. Cravings can occur as a result of frequent group discussion about drug abuse.
   E. Cravings occur more commonly in men than in women.

■ CASE 2

Sam W. is a 52-year-old man who calls 911 on a Saturday night for complaints of palpitations, chest pain, and dizziness. When paramedics arrive at his apartment, he tells them that he has been sick with a bad cold for a week, with nasal congestion, sneezing, cough, and fevers. Despite taking "swigs" of a liquid over-the-counter cold medication this evening, he feels much worse! Shortly after drinking the medication, he started to feel hot and flushed and weak, with palpitations, chest pain, dizziness, nausea, and vomiting.

The paramedics apply a cardiac monitor to Mr. W.'s chest and note a sinus tachycardia with a rate of 127 bpm, a respiratory rate of 22 breaths/min., and a blood pressure of 100/65 mm Hg. Mr. W. is anxious and in moderate distress. His skin is warm and flushed. As the paramedics insert a peripheral intravenous catheter, Mr. W. relates a history of heavy tobacco and alcohol use and says, "But I'm quitting drinking! My doctor gave me that medicine to make me stop drinking, and I haven't had a drop of liquor in 2 weeks."

QUESTIONS

1. What medication did Mr. W.'s doctor give him to help him avoid drinking alcohol?
   A. topiramate
   B. naltrexone
   C. disulfiram
   D. rimonabant
   E. buprenorphine

2. Several pharmacologic therapies have been used to help patients abstain from their drug of abuse. Which of the following statements regarding the role of pharmacologic agents in the management of addiction is correct?
   A. When buprenorphine is administered in a sublingual preparation with naloxone, the partial agonist effects of buprenorphine are manifest.
   B. When heroin is injected in patients receiving methadone, the combination of opioids can cause life-threatening heroin overdose.
   C. Naltrexone is effective in treating opioid addiction but can cause withdrawal symptoms when its use is discontinued.
   D. Acamprosate modulates GABA receptors and is being studied in the treatment of alcohol dependence.
   E. Antidepressants such as desipramine are effective in preventing cocaine use based on their ability to block norepinephrine reuptake.

3. How do drugs of abuse affect the function of the brain reward system in the development of psychological dependence and potential addiction?
   A. In contrast to psychological dependence, physical dependence occurs when a drug affects the brain reward system, resulting in pleasurable sensations associated with the drug's use.
   B. Opioids enhance dopamine activity in the ventral tegmental area of the brain through their excitatory effects on GABA interneurons.
   C. Cocaine and amphetamines decrease dopamine concentrations in the synapse of dopaminergic neurons acting at the nucleus accumbens.
   D. Drugs capable of causing psychological dependence destroy the neurons in the ventral tegmental area of the brain.
   E. Drugs capable of causing psychological dependence enhance dopamine activity in the nucleus accumbens.

4. The pharmacokinetic characteristics of a drug contribute to its addictive potential. Which of the following scenarios of drug use would put a person at greatest risk for addiction?

   A. An 18-year-old man injects a very hydrophilic drug.

   B. An 18-year-old man orally ingests a long-acting opioid.

   C. An 18-year-old man applies a transdermal opioid patch.

   D. An 18-year-old man smokes a very lipophilic drug.

   E. An 18-year-old man orally ingests a short-acting drug with extensive first-pass metabolism.

5. Which of the following characteristics contribute to an individual person's increased risk of drug abuse or misuse, and potential addiction?

   A. Using a drug under unpleasant, frightening conditions

   B. Having a high sensitivity to the effects of a drug

   C. Having a high rate of metabolism of ethanol to acetaldehyde

   D. Having a high innate tolerance to the effects of a drug

   E. Using a drug covertly while at work or school

ANSWERS TO SECTION II

CHAPTER 6 ANSWERS

CASE 1

1. **The answer is C. The exchange of three sodium for two potassium ions across the cell membrane is an energy-dependent process.** This process occurs via the ATP-dependent sodium/potassium pump, which plays an important role in maintaining ion gradients. The extracellular sodium ion concentration is greater than the intracellular sodium ion concentration. This contributes to a chemical gradient for sodium entry into the cell. When sodium channels open to allow sodium flux across the cell membrane, the membrane potential becomes more positive. The permeability of the neuronal cell membrane is greatest for potassium ions. Therefore, the resting membrane potential of the cell most closely approximates the Nernst potential for potassium ions (approximately −90 mV).

2. **The answer is D. The membrane potential is unaffected by sodium channel blockade** because, at rest, there are no open sodium channels. However, membrane depolarization will be difficult or impossible in a neuron with blocked sodium channels.

3. **The answer is C. The action potential will be inhibited** by sodium channel blockade. The action potential is regulated by the balance between voltage-gated sodium and potassium channels. Voltage-gated sodium channels conduct an inward current that depolarizes the cell at the beginning of the action potential.

4. **The answer is A. Flaccid muscle paralysis** in an ascending pattern is a result of tetrodotoxin-induced sodium channel blockade at the neuromuscular junction. Death is usually the result of respiratory muscle paralysis and respiratory failure. Interestingly, although Fugu fish contain and accumulate tetrodotoxin, they have adapted point mutations in their own sodium channels that make them immune to the effects of tetrodotoxin.

5. **The answer is E. Repolarization is prolonged due to the slower opening and closing of delayed rectifier potassium channels.** These channels open in response to depolarization and contribute to the initial rapid repolarization, but because they open and close more slowly than the rapid sodium channels, they dominate the later repolarization phase of the action potential. Depolarization is caused by the rapid opening of voltage-gated sodium channels.

CASE 2

1. **The answer is B. In cardiac cells, voltage-gated calcium channels are involved in the depolarization phase of the action potential.** This is especially true in nodal cells, which lack voltage-gated sodium channels. In ventricular muscle cells, inward calcium flux contributes to the plateau phase of depolarization. The plasma membrane is least permeable to calcium ions, which may be exchanged with intracellular sodium ions through the sodium/calcium ion exchanger. Leak channels allow potassium ions to passively exit the cell, contributing to the resting membrane potential. When sodium channels are in the inactivated state, the cell cannot be stimulated to depolarize and produce an action potential. This contributes to the refractory state of the cell.

2. **The answer is D. Calcium influx triggers the exocytosis of neurotransmitter-containing synaptic vesicles.** In contrast, calcium channel blockade dampens and inhibits neurotransmission and cellular excitation. Pharmacologic calcium channel blockade has been used to treat patients with hypertension and cardiac tachy-dysrhythmias. Calcium influx causes an inward positive current and contributes to the plateau phase of depolarization in cardiac cells. The sequestration of neurotransmitters within presynaptic vesicles is an ATP-dependent process.

3. **The answer is B. Calcium influx caused massive release of neurotransmitters,** including acetylcholine and norepinephrine. Neurotransmitters activated their postsynaptic receptors, causing Mr. M.'s clinical symptoms of muscle contraction and autonomic stimulation.

4. **The answer is D.** The resting membrane potential results from three factors, including **transmembrane ion pumps, which maintain ion gradients.** These may be energy-requiring, such as the sodium/potassium pump, or passive, such as the sodium/calcium exchanger. These pumps contribute to an unequal distribution of positive and negative charges on each side of the plasma membrane. The lipid bilayer membrane is highly impermeable to ions. Therefore, a difference in the permeability of the membrane to various cations and anions through selective ion channels also contributes to the resting membrane potential. Specific ion channels open or close based on the voltage difference across the membrane.

5. **The answer is C. Voltage-gated (delayed rectifier) potassium channels are responsible for the repolarization** phase of the action potential. The voltage-independent (leak) potassium channels contribute to the resting membrane potential. The voltage-gated sodium channels are responsible for the rapid phase of depolarization. When they open, the voltage-gated calcium channels initiate the process of vesicle exocytosis.

CHAPTER 7 ANSWERS

CASE 1

1. **The answer is B. Initiation of movement** is controlled by dopaminergic neurons of the nigrostriatal tract. The nigrostriatal tract contains a dopaminergic pathway that begins in the substantia nigra and terminates in the striatum, specifically the caudate and putamen of the basal ganglia. These nuclei help initiate and control intended movement and inhibit irrelevant movements. Degeneration of these neurons prevents the basal ganglia from properly initiating motor activity. Arousal and alertness are primarily controlled by the reticular activating system and the tuberomamillary nucleus. The hypothalamus controls behaviors related to hunger, thirst, and temperature regulation. Emotions are largely controlled by the limbic system.

2. **The answer is C. An inability to get out of a deep armchair** is a clinical effect that could occur as a result of dopamine neuron degeneration. Because the dopaminergic neurons control the initiation of normal movement, their degeneration makes it difficult for patients to initiate movements. Other clinical symptoms and signs include muscle rigidity, unintended tremor, uncontrolled forward propulsion on walking, postural instability, and a flat facial affect. The combination of muscle rigidity and tremor can result in the presence of cogwheeling, which is a "catching" sensation an examiner might appreciate on testing movements of the patient's joints. Inability to move one side of the body (hemiparesis) would result from injury to the precentral gyrus of the frontal cortex on the contralateral side. Hypothalamic injury would adversely affect temperature regulation. Emotional lability might result from lesions in portions of the limbic sys-

tem. The nucleus accumbens is involved in the control of the brain reward pathway, which can be disrupted as a result of illicit drug use.

3. **The answer is D.** Levodopa is transported across the blood–brain barrier by the large amino acid transporter. After high-protein meals, **protein components compete with levodopa for transport across the blood–brain barrier**, the transporter can become overwhelmed, and its transport of levodopa ineffective.

4. **The answer is E. Levodopa is L-dopa, which is metabolized by dopamine decarboxylase to dopamine in the central nervous system.** Because levodopa can also be metabolized by dopamine decarboxylase in the periphery, it is used in combination with carbidopa. Carbidopa prevents the peripheral metabolism of levodopa to dopamine, in order to allow levodopa to cross the blood–brain barrier. In the CNS, it is metabolized to dopamine to exert its agonist effect on dopamine receptors. Dopamine β-hydroxylase converts dopamine to norepinephrine.

5. **The answer is E. Psychosis** could result from excessive dopaminergic stimulation. Dopamine receptor antagonists have been used to control the psychotic symptoms of schizophrenia, as well as vomiting (through dopamine antagonism in the vomiting center).

CASE 2

1. **The answer is A.** The clinical symptoms of strychnine poisoning are caused by competitive **inhibition of glycine activity in the spinal cord**. Strychnine inhibits the binding of glycine to its receptor in the spinal cord. Glycine is an inhibitory amino acid neurotransmitter. Its inhibition by strychnine leads to excessive stimulation of afferent motor nerve impulses, causing muscle twitching and extensor spasm (opisthotonos) and a classic facial grimace (risus sardonicus). Typically, the patient has an awake mental status between episodes of muscle spasm. The cause of death in this rare poisoning is respiratory failure. Enhanced GABA activity inhibition of histamine activity and inhibition of histamine activity cause central nervous system depression and drowsiness. Glutamate is an excitatory amino acid neurotransmitter in the central nervous system, not the peripheral muscle cells. Inhibition of acetylcholine activity at parasympathetic postganglionic neurons causes antimuscarinic effects and neuromuscular blockade.

2. **The answer is C. Benzodiazepines** enhance the effects of inhibitory GABA neurons in the cerebral cortex. Enhanced GABA activity decreases all central nervous system stimulation and would have an inhibitory effect on the excessive muscle excitability caused by strychnine. Levodopa is a dopamine agonist used in the treatment of Parkinson's disease. MAOIs inhibit the metabolism of catecholamines. Phenytoin is a sodium channel blocker used in the treatment of cerebral seizures and neuropathic pain syndromes.

3. The answer is D. Glutamate exerts its excitatory effect by **opening ligand-gated ion channels** as well as acting at metabotropic (G protein–coupled) glutamate receptors. Excessive glutamate activity is associated with neuronal cell death in the setting of ischemia. Enkephalins are opioids. Caffeine inhibits adenosine receptors, causing alertness by enhancing the release of norepinephrine from presynaptic neurons. Tricyclic antidepressants and selective serotonin reuptake inhibitors prevent the reuptake of biogenic amines (catecholamines and indoleamines).

4. The answer is B. Donepezil exerts its therapeutic effect by enhancing the activity of **acetylcholine**. Acetylcholine is a diffuse central nervous system neurotransmitter that regulates sleep and wakefulness. Donepezil is a reversible acetylcholinesterase inhibitor that prevents the breakdown of acetylcholine in the brain. This allows for an increased concentration and effect of acetylcholine at its receptors. Scopolamine is an anticholinergic drug that causes antimuscarinic effects such as drowsiness and altered sleep. Caffeine is an adenosine receptor antagonist. Serotonin is an indoleamine neurotransmitter associated with the regulation of emotions.

5. The answer is D. Lipophilic substances with high oil–water partition coefficients can generally diffuse across the blood–brain barrier most easily. Water-soluble, hydrophilic substances with low oil–water partition coefficients are excluded. Substances of high molecular weight or high polarity do not easily cross the blood-brain barrier, and may require facilitated transport to enter the central nervous system.

CHAPTER 8 ANSWERS

CASE 1

1. The answer is D. Both conditions are characterized by weakness caused by a diminished number of available postsynaptic N_M receptors. Tubocurare causes a direct, competitive blockade of N_M receptors, while autoantibodies destroy the N_M receptor and promote receptor internalization in myasthenia gravis. In both cases, the number of available receptors for ACh binding is reduced, preventing depolarization, and leading to muscle weakness. The Eaton-Lambert syndrome is characterized by weakness caused by a lack of presynaptic ACh release as a result of autoantibodies against presynaptic calcium channels. Hemicholinium blocks the presynaptic uptake of choline, inhibiting ACh synthesis. Vesamicol prevents the transport of ACh into presynaptic storage vesicles.

2. The answer is B. Physostigmine prevents the degradation of ACh. Physostigmine, a carbamic acid ester, forms a labile covalent bond with AChE, preventing its degradation. This allows for an increased concentration of endogenously released ACh within the synaptic cleft, which is then available to act at the postsynaptic N_M receptor site. ACh does not undergo reuptake at the presynaptic neuron. Rather, ACh is degraded within the synaptic cleft, and choline is recycled into the presynaptic neuron.

3. The answer is C. Organophosphate poisoning can cause muscle weakness and paralysis due to a sustained depolarization at the N_M receptors of the neuromuscular junction (depolarizing blockade). Organophosphates such as diisopropyl fluorophosphate phosphorylate and poison the AChE and prevent ACh degradation. The excessive muscle cell depolarization and weakness induced by organophosphate poisoning would be worsened by the administration of physostigmine, another AChE inhibitor. Succinylcholine causes sustained muscle cell depolarization and neuromuscular blockade. Physostigmine would also worsen muscle weakness caused by succinylcholine. In fact, all AChE inhibitors are ineffective in reversing muscle weakness when it is caused by the sustained depolarization of the N_M receptor. Physostigmine administration should improve muscle weakness caused by tubocurare and should have no significant effect on muscle weakness caused by botulism. Bethanechol is a muscarinic receptor agonist with almost complete selectivity for muscarinic receptors. Bethanechol would be expected to cause muscarinic signs, which would be worsened by physostigmine administration, but it would have little effect on muscle strength.

4. The answer is A. Scopolamine poisoning is reversed by the administration of physostigmine. Scopolamine is a direct, primarily muscarinic receptor antagonist that is able to cross the blood–brain barrier and cause significant central nervous system (CNS) effects. Physostigmine, a tertiary amine, is lipophilic and able to penetrate the CNS to reverse the anticholinergic effects of scopolamine. Muscarine and pilocarpine are direct muscarinic receptor agonists. Pralidoxime is a strong nucleophile that reverses the oxygen–phosphorous bond formed by organophosphates with AChE. Nicotine is a nAChR agonist.

5. The answer is C. Bradycardia would be a sign of ACh agonism at the muscarinic M_2 receptor within the cardiac conduction system. Antagonism of this parasympathetic innervation of the heart causes a relative tachycardia. Antagonism of ACh's effects in the bladder and salivary glands causes urinary retention and dry mucous membranes, respectively. Muscle fasciculations are a result of ACh agonism at the nicotinic N_M receptors.

CASE 2

1. The answer is E. **Botulinum toxin degrades synaptobrevin and prevents the fusion of presynaptic storage vesicles with the cell membrane.** (Synaptobrevin is one of the SNARE proteins that interacts with syntaxin to cause ACh vesicle exocytosis.) As a consequence, ACh is not released into the synaptic cleft to act at N_M receptors, resulting in muscle weakness and paralysis. Vesamicol prevents ACh transport into presynaptic storage vesicles.

2. **The answer is C. Sweating and diarrhea** could result from physostigmine administration, due to the enhanced concentration and effects of ACh at muscarinic receptors. Pupillary dilatation results from the antagonism of ACh at muscarinic receptors in the iris. Botulinum poisoning would prevent any effect of physostigmine at the neuromuscular junction.

3. **The answer is A. Atropine**, a naturally occurring alkaloid, is an antidote for muscarinic symptoms such as excessive sweating and diarrhea. Atropine is a direct muscarinic receptor antagonist. It competitively blocks the binding of ACh at muscarinic receptors, and dries secretions, reverses sweating, and limits excessive gastrointestinal motility through its parasympatholytic effects. Methacholine is a muscarinic receptor agonist that would worsen these effects. More physostigmine might also worsen symptoms by increasing the concentration of ACh at muscarinic receptors. Pralidoxime is a specific antidote for organophosphate poisoning of postsynaptic AChE. Succinylcholine causes depolarizing blockade at the neuromuscular junction.

4. **The answer is C. M_3** muscarinic ACh receptors mediate parasympathetic tone in glandular tissues and smooth muscle, contributing to sweating and diarrhea when ACh binds this receptor subtype. M_1 is expressed in the CNS and autonomic ganglia, M_4 and M_5 in the CNS, and M_2 in cardiac muscle. N_M is the nicotinic receptor at the neuromuscular junction.

5. **The answer is B. Autonomic ganglionic blockade causes vasodilation and hypotension** because sympathetic adrenergic tone normally predominates in both arterioles and veins. In contrast, parasympathetic cholinergic tone predominates in the bladder, heart, and smooth muscles of the gastrointestinal tract. As a consequence, autonomic blockade would cause urinary retention, tachycardia, and constipation, respectively.

CHAPTER 9 ANSWERS

CASE 1

1. **The answer is C. Red wine and aged cheese contain tyramine, which cannot be metabolized in the presence of MAOIs, and displaces vesicular NE.** Tyramine, a dietary amine, is the prototype indirect sympathomimetic compound. It is ordinarily metabolized in the gastrointestinal tract and liver by MAO. In patients taking MAOIs, tyramine is not metabolized in the gut and can circulate to sympathetic neurons, where it is taken up and transported by VMAT into synaptic vesicles. In this way, it displaces NE from vesicles and causes a massive release of NE through reversal of the cell membrane NE transporter. Tyramine does not act directly at the postsynaptic adrenergic receptors. Ethanol does not interact directly with MAO or with the NE transporter.

2. **The answer is A.** Phentolamine is a **nonselective α-adrenergic antagonist that blocks catecholamine-induced vasoconstriction and decreases blood pressure**. Its administration facilitates vasodilation, reduces peripheral vascular resistance, and reduces blood pressure. Tyramine-induced release of vesicular NE is via reversal of the NE transporter and is not associated with α-adrenergic receptors. Phentolamine does not interact with COMT.

3. **The answer is C. β-adrenergic receptor antagonists could block catecholamine stimulation at the heart, but allow persistent catecholamine-induced vasoconstriction at α_1-adrenergic receptors.** Catecholamines can act as agonists at both α- and β-adrenergic receptors. Blockade of their effect at β-adrenergic receptors may slow heart rate and decrease cardiac contractility, but does not prevent their effect at the peripheral vascular α-adrenergic receptors. Blood pressure may actually increase under these circumstances. Although some β-adrenergic receptor antagonists are lipophilic and can penetrate the CNS to cause sedation, they do not interact with the NE transporter and would not contribute to worsening depression or psychosis. β-adrenergic receptor antagonists are not involved in tyramine metabolism.

4. **The answer is A.** The tyramine–MAOI interaction could be prevented by **inhibition of the vesicular monoamine transporter**. This would prevent tyramine transport into presynaptic vesicles and subsequent displacement and release of NE. Inhibition of any of the steps of tyramine absorption, transport into sympathetic neurons and synaptic vesicles, or the reversal function of the NE transporter could prevent tyramine-induced non-vesicular release of NE. Induction of the aromatic L-amino acid transporter could enhance tyramine uptake into neurons. Tyrosine hydroxylase is the first step in the synthesis of dopamine from tyrosine. Induction of the NE transporter could enhance NE release. The vesicular acetylcholine transporter is expressed in cholinergic neurons.

5. **The answer is C.** Hexamethonium and mecamylamine are ganglionic blockers that block the **postsynaptic acetylcholine receptor**.

CASE 2

1. **The answer is B. Cocaine inhibits the NE transporter and prevents reuptake of synaptic catecholamines, which are thus available to act at both α- and β-adrenergic receptors.** Centrally, cocaine causes agitation and psychosis. Peripherally, it causes elevated heart rate and tachydysrhythmias, as well as peripheral vascular constriction and elevated blood pressure. Acute cocaine intoxication can result in seizures, intracerebral hemorrhage, hyperthermia, ventricular tachycardia and fibrillation, and acute myocardial infarction. Cocaine does not directly interact with adrenergic receptors or with MAO. Chronic cocaine use may cause downregulation of adrenergic receptors.

2. The answer is C. An **increase in blood pressure** could result if a β-adrenergic receptor antagonist is administered in the setting of acute cocaine intoxication. Administration of a β-adrenergic receptor antagonist would allow continued catecholamine agonist effects at peripheral α$_1$-adrenergic receptors, contributing to peripheral vasoconstriction. This is commonly referred to as an "unopposed alpha agonist effect." Blockade of β-adrenergic receptors can mask the symptoms of hypoglycemia. Blockade of β$_2$-adrenergic receptors can precipitate pulmonary smooth muscle constriction and bronchospasm, especially in asthmatic patients. Blockade of β$_1$-adrenergic receptors can cause bradycardia and decreased cardiac output.

3. The answer is C. Phentolamine is a direct acting nonselective α-adrenergic antagonist that causes arterial vasodilation, and decreases systemic vascular resistance and decreases blood pressure. This agent would decrease the patient's cocaine-induced elevated blood pressure by blocking the excessive sympathetic effects of catecholamines. Methylphenidate is an amphetamine analogue that can elevate blood pressure. Phenylephrine is a direct α$_1$-adrenergic agonist that causes arterial vasoconstriction and increased blood pressure. Yohimbine is a selective α$_2$-adrenergic antagonist that enhances NE release, and can cause tachycardia and increased blood pressure. Terbutaline is a β$_2$-adrenergic receptor agonist that causes smooth muscle relaxation and bronchodilation. Although both β$_2$ and α$_1$ receptors are present on arterial vessels, α$_1$ effects predominate in the control of arterial vascular smooth muscle tone, vascular resistance, and blood pressure.

4. The answer is C. Clonidine is a centrally acting **direct α$_2$-adrenergic receptor agonist that decreases NE release and sympathetic tone**. Its clinical adverse effects include bradycardia and sedation. These adverse effects limit its usefulness as an antihypertensive agent. Guanabenz and guanfacine, also central α$_2$-adrenergic receptor agonists, have similar effects.

5. The answer is D. If used concomitantly, **duloxetine and iproniazid** could cause a clinical serotonin syndrome because of their abilities to increase the synaptic concentration of serotonin available to act at its 5-HT$_{1A}$ receptor. The symptoms of serotonin syndrome include altered mental status with agitation, autonomic instability, often with hyperthermia, and neuromuscular abnormalities, including tremor, myoclonus, and hyperreflexia. The syndrome most commonly occurs when more than one agent is used in combination, both increasing serotonin concentrations. Agents implicated in the development of serotonin syndrome include serotonin precursors (tryptophan, lysergic acid diethylamide [LSD]), agents that enhance its presynaptic release (amphetamines), drugs that prevent serotonin reuptake (meperidine, dextromethorphan, cocaine, cyclic antidepressants such as imipramine, amitriptyline, duloxetine, and selective serotonin reuptake inhibitors), and drugs that inhibit the metabolism of serotonin (MAOIs). Complications of serotonin syndrome include hyperthermia, rhabdomyolysis, myoglobinuria, acute renal and hepatic dysfunction, and lactic acid production.

CHAPTER 10 ANSWERS

CASE 1

1. The answer is C. Lidocaine binds to an intracellular site on the voltage-gated sodium channel, inhibits its activation, and blocks the propagation of action potentials in nociceptive A- and C-fibers. Like all local anesthetics, lidocaine is a nonspecific inhibitor of peripheral sensory, motor, and autonomic pathways; its effect is related to the dose, area of administration, and the intrinsic susceptibility to blockade of different nerve fibers within the peripheral nerve (motorneurons being less susceptible than pain fibers at the same dose).

2. The answer is D. "Stinging" or sharp, highly localized pain perception is characteristic of first pain. First pain perceptions are **transmitted rapidly (5–25 m/s) by sensitive, myelinated Aδ-fibers** that are concentrated in areas such as the fingertips, face, and lips. This type of pain is in contrast to less well-localized, diffuse, dull, aching pain characteristic of second pain. Second pain perceptions are transmitted by nonmyelinated C-fibers. C-fiber impulse transmission is slower (approximately 1 m/s). Therefore, dull, second pain perception is often delayed after the initial tissue injury. When local anesthesia is administered in the area around a peripheral nerve, different fibers within the nerve are susceptible to the anesthetic's effect at different rates. This is termed **differential functional blockade**. In general, first pain is blocked first, followed by second pain, temperature, touch, proprioception, skeletal muscle tone, and voluntary tension.

3. The answer is E. Moderate hydrophobicity allows lidocaine to penetrate the neuronal cell membrane and remain near the area of administration; an amide linkage prevents its degradation by esterases. The structural groups of the local anesthetics (aromatic group, amine group, ester or amide linkage) determine the individual anesthetic's onset, duration of action, and potency. The hydrophobic aromatic group of lidocaine allows it to penetrate the neuronal cell membrane and to access the cytoplasmic side of the membrane, where it can bind at the hydrophobic site of the voltage-gated sodium channel. This accounts for its rapid onset of action and potency. This hydrophobicity also allows it to remain near the area of administration, while its amide linkage prevents its degradation by local tissue esterases. These factors account for lidocaine's medium duration of action (approximately 1 to 2 hours). Local anesthetics with low hydrophobicity are unable to easily penetrate the lipid layer of the neuronal membrane; those with high hydrophobicity penetrate well, but are unable to dissociate from the membrane on its cytoplasmic side, and are essentially "trapped" within the membrane. Local anesthetics with a relatively low pKa are primarily in a neutral form at physiologic pH and diffuse through cell membranes more easily.

4. **The answer is B. Epinephrine-induced vasoconstriction helps to maintain the concentration of lidocaine in the area of administration by slowing its rate of removal from the area.** Locally diminished blood flow in the area of administration maintains a therapeutic concentration of anesthetic near the nerve, and prevents a large concentration of anesthetic from reaching the systemic circulation.

5. **The answer is B. Amide-linked local anesthetics are primarily metabolized by hepatic microsomal cytochrome P450 enzymes.** Metabolites are produced by aromatic hydroxylation, N-dealkylation, and amide hydrolysis of the parent drug. Metabolites are then renally excreted. Ester-linked local anesthetics are metabolized by tissue and plasma esterases (pseudocholinesterases) to water-soluble metabolites, which are also renally excreted.

CASE 2

1. **The answer is D. Tetracaine is more hydrophobic than lidocaine, and therefore prolongs the duration of action and increases the potency of the topical anesthetic formulation.** Tetracaine is an ester-linked anesthetic with a butyl group attached to its aromatic group, making it highly hydrophobic. It remains in the area surrounding the nerve for a prolonged period; once it crosses the neuronal membrane, it has a prolonged interaction with the hydrophobic binding site on the intracellular side of the voltage-gated sodium channel. Both of these properties contribute to the potency and duration of action of LET. Lidocaine is moderately hydrophobic and crosses the neuronal membrane easily, but dissociates from its binding site more rapidly. Although tetracaine can be degraded by local tissue esterases, it is released slowly from its site of action, prolonging its duration of action. Lidocaine is an amide-linked anesthetic that is metabolized by hepatic enzymes.

2. **The answer is A. Local anesthetic injected into the cerebrospinal fluid penetrated the spinal cord, inhibiting the normal transmission of motor impulses.** Both epidural and spinal anesthesia are types of central nerve blockade in which local anesthetic is delivered near the spinal cord, inhibiting normal transmission in the sensory spinal roots. Because local anesthetics can cause nonspecific blockade of sensory, motor, and autonomic impulses, loss of motor function and vasodilation-induced hypotension are potential complications of central nerve blockade. Local anesthetic can also diffuse proximally and cause respiratory compromise. Other central transmitters involved in the transmission of nociceptive stimuli include the peptide, substance P, bradykinin, and the amino acid, glutamate. Receptors for these transmitters may also be inhibited by local anesthetics.

3. **The answer is B. Local anesthetics can cause cardiac toxicity by inhibiting sodium channel activation in the cardiac conduction system.** This can cause **conduction delays and blocks.** They may also contribute to reduced cardiac contractility by diminishing intracellular stores of calcium. Central nervous system stimulation and seizures may be related to excessive and selective blockade of inhibitory pathways in the cerebral cortex. Depression and coma are hypothesized to occur through inhibition of both stimulatory and inhibitory pathways in the brain by large concentrations of local anesthetic. Hypersensitivity reactions are primarily associated with ester-linked local anesthetics such as procaine.

4. **The answer is A.** The **stratum corneum** is the limiting barrier to absorption of topical local anesthetics.

5. **The answer is D. Phasic inhibition**, or use-dependent inhibition, is the phenomenon whereby action potential conduction is increasingly inhibited at higher frequencies of impulses. Rapidly arriving action potentials transmitted by nociceptors firing at high rates in areas of injury do not allow sodium channels to return to the resting state between action potentials. Progressively more channels become blocked by local anesthetic that does not have time to dissociate fully between the action potentials. The result of phasic inhibition is that administration of local anesthetic in areas of tissue injury (and rapidly firing nociceptors) will inhibit pain transmission more than other sensory or motor stimuli.

CHAPTER 11 ANSWERS

CASE 1

1. **The answer is D. Barbiturates increase the duration of chloride channel opening at the GABA$_A$ receptor**, permitting a greater influx of chloride ions and hyperpolarization of the neuron. In contrast, benzodiazepines increase the frequency of chloride channel opening at the GABA$_A$ receptor. These agents both enhance the effect of GABA, the major inhibitory neurotransmitter in the CNS. Some anesthetic barbiturates, such as pentobarbital, also directly and independently activate the GABA$_A$ receptor. Barbiturates also inhibit excitatory impulses at the AMPA receptor by decreasing glutamate activation at this receptor. Finally, at anesthetic concentrations, some barbiturates decrease the opening of voltage-gated sodium channels and inhibit neuronal firing. Because of these various mechanisms of action, and their propensity to cause profound CNS depression and coma in large doses, barbiturates have largely been replaced with safer sedatives and antiepileptic drugs.

2. **The answer is A. Both agents enhance GABA$_A$-mediated chloride influx and inhibit glutamate excitatory effects at its receptors**. Barbiturates inhibit glutamate activation of the AMPA receptor. Ethanol inhibits

glutamate activation of the NMDA receptor. Their synergistic activity can cause life-threatening CNS and respiratory depression. Benzodiazepines are positive allosteric modulators of the GABA$_A$ receptor, increasing GABA's affinity and binding to the receptor.

3. **The answer is B. Elderly patients exhibit reduced hepatic clearance of barbiturates** because of age-related decrements in hepatic metabolic function. Phenobarbital is 75% hepatically metabolized. The remainder is renally excreted in an unchanged form. Elderly patients often have reduced renal function and may accumulate drugs that are primarily dependent on renal excretion. The ratio of body fat to muscle is increased in elderly patients; this may allow for the accumulation of lipophilic drugs in these patients.

4. **The answer is C.** Because of their nonselective inhibitory effect throughout the CNS, barbiturates can cause **amnesia to recent events**, sedation, muscle relaxation, suppression of reflexes, hypnosis, coma, respiratory depression, and death. This general inhibition of excitatory neurotransmission contributes to the therapeutic efficacy of phenobarbital as a treatment for partial and tonic-clonic seizures. Etomidate, a GABA agonist and anesthetic induction agent, inhibits the synthesis of cortisol and aldosterone. Electrical (not pulmonary) shunting is the molecular basis for the inhibitory effects of GABA, which is mediated by open chloride channels that attenuate the depolarizing membrane potential caused by excitatory currents.

5. **The answer is D. The clinical effect of barbiturates in the CNS is terminated by redistribution of the drug to other highly perfused organs.** Highly lipophilic barbiturates cross the blood–brain barrier rapidly, resulting in a rapid onset of action in the CNS, but because of their lipophilicity, they also redistribute rapidly to the splanchnic circulation, muscle, and fat. Therefore, their duration of effect is shorter than less lipophilic barbiturates. Orally administered barbiturates may undergo first-pass hepatic metabolism, which limits their bioavailability and clinical effect. Barbiturates induce the hepatic P450 CYP enzymes responsible for their metabolism, and eventually enhance their own metabolism. This contributes to the development of tolerance and a reduced efficacy at the same dose. The renal elimination of barbiturates with an acidic pKa, such as phenobarbital, can be enhanced by alkalinizing the urine with bicarbonate.

CASE 2

1. **The answer is E.** Ibotenic acid exerts its effect through direct **activation of the NMDA receptor**, causing excitatory neurotransmission similar to that produced by glutamate. Ibotenic acid can also activate metabotropic glutamate receptors to some degree. The result of this toxicity is myoclonic jerking movements and seizures, seen most often in children who ingest *Amanita muscaria*.

2. **The answer is D.** Muscimol exerts its effects through direct **activation of the GABA$_A$ receptor**. Its CNS depressant effects are related to its ability to enhance GABA-mediated chloride channel opening, enhancing chloride influx, and causing hyperpolarization of neuronal cells.

3. **The answer is E. GABA agonists with more specific clinical effects show greater selectivity in their binding to GABA receptors with specific subunit compositions.** For example, the sedative, zolpidem, selectively acts at GABA$_A$ receptors containing α1 subunits. Similarly, etomidate and propofol act selectively at GABA$_A$ receptors that contain β2 and β3 subunits. Nonselective activation of GABA$_A$ receptors contributes to the numerous adverse effects of many benzodiazepines and barbiturates. Baclofen is the only clinical agonist at the GABA$_B$ receptor.

4. **The answer is B. Sodium and calcium channels open and sodium and calcium influx is enhanced** when ionotropic glutamate receptors are activated. The influx of sodium or calcium, and the efflux of potassium contribute to depolarizing membrane potentials and lead to cellular activation. Ionotropic glutamate receptors mediate fast, excitatory synaptic activity. Magnesium ions block the NMDA glutamate receptor in the resting membrane, and depolarization of the membrane concurrent with agonist binding is necessary to reverse the ion channel blockade by magnesium. Metabotropic glutamate receptors are coupled to G proteins and second messenger systems using phospholipase C or adenylyl cyclase. GABA receptor activation opens chloride channels and enhances chloride influx.

5. **The answer is C.** Excessive glutamate-mediated activation and excitation can lead to increased intracellular calcium, and cellular damage. Glutamate antagonism may be beneficial in limiting the progression of **dementia** and other neurodegenerative diseases. Glutamate antagonism has not been shown to be beneficial in preventing the sequelae of ischemic or hemorrhagic stroke; indeed, these treatments can cause schizophrenia-like effects. Glutamate antagonism may also prove to be beneficial in the treatment of hyperalgesia and central sensitization, and in antiepileptic therapy.

CHAPTER 12 ANSWERS

CASE 1

1. **The answer is D. Loss of dopaminergic neurons in the substantia nigra contributes to reduced activity of the direct pathway and movement inhibition.** In contrast, the loss of dopaminergic inhibition causes overactivity of the indirect pathway, also leading to reduced movement. Normally, dopamine stimulates the neurons of the direct pathway and inhibits neurons of the indirect pathway, resulting in purposeful movement. When these dopaminergic neurons are lost, a generalized lack of movement, or hypokinesia, results. The medium spiny neurons of the striatum release GABA, which modulates the activity and balance of the direct and indirect pathways and subsequent movement. The tubero-infundibular pathway consists of dopaminergic neurons that project within the hypothalamus. These neurons tonically inhibit the release of prolactin. The area postrema is one of the circumventricular organs, which function as blood chemoreceptors and allow communication between the blood and the CNS.

2. **The answer is C. Levodopa/carbidopa will dramatically improve Mr. S.'s symptoms.** However, levodopa will not prevent the progressive loss of dopaminergic neurons or the progression of his disease. Levodopa/carbidopa does not restore the normal function of damaged nigrostriatal dopaminergic neurons.

3. **The answer is B. He will develop tolerance to levodopa and require increasing dosages** over time to attain the same clinically significant improvement in symptoms. He will also develop sensitization to levodopa, manifesting as periods of dyskinetic movement shortly after levodopa administration. These "on" periods can be controlled by using smaller doses of levodopa but not "drug holidays". However, over time, levodopa loses it efficacy in controlling the symptoms of Parkinson's disease. The development of both tolerance and sensitization contribute to a narrowing of the drug's therapeutic index.

4. **The answer is E. Dopamine agonist therapy is an effective initial treatment for Parkinson's disease in young patients**. Monotherapy with pramipexole or ropinirole delays the onset of "off" periods and dyskinesias, although these drugs have a higher incidence of adverse effects as compared to levodopa. Levodopa therapy is very effective in the initial treatment of Parkinson's symptoms. However, because the response to its effects declines over time and it is associated with the development of "on" and "off" periods, levodopa therapy should be initiated at the point when other therapies no longer control parkinsonian symptoms. Further delay in the initiation of levodopa therapy is associated with reduced drug efficacy and increased mortality. Inhibitors of dopamine metabolism, such as selegiline, rasagiline, and entacapone, enhance the efficacy of levodopa.

5. **The answer is C. These agents modify striatal cholinergic interneurons, which regulate the direct and indirect pathways.** They are both muscarinic receptor antagonists that reduce cholinergic tone in the CNS. Amantadine blocks excitatory NMDA receptors, and is used to treat levodopa-induced dyskinesias late in the course of the disease.

CASE 2

1. **The answer is A. Amphetamines displace dopamine from presynaptic vesicles and cause CNS stimulation.** Amphetamines also directly act at postsynaptic dopaminergic receptors and have MAO inhibitory actions. The effect of these multiple actions in the mesolimbic system contributes to CNS stimulation and paranoid, schizophrenia-like behavior in patients intoxicated with amphetamines. Although ecstasy is abused in an attempt to get "high," overdose can cause a nonspecific release of many biogenic amines and resultant adrenergic and serotonergic hyperactivity. Stimulation of dopaminergic neurons in the area postrema causes nausea and vomiting, but not hallucinations.

2. **The answer is C. Excessive dopamine in the striatum** increases activity of the direct pathway and disinhibits the activity of the indirect pathway, resulting in increased motor movement. Repetitive movements such as the grinding of teeth in this patient are characteristic of amphetamine intoxication. Derangement of dopaminergic tone in the ventral tegmental area of the midbrain will affect projections to areas of the limbic system. These pathways may be involved in the development of schizophrenia.

3. **The answer is E. Seizures** may result from the use of ecstasy (or other sympathomimetic agents) while taking tranylcypromine, a MAOI. Amphetamines cause the release of dopamine and other biogenic amines from storage vesicles. These excitatory amines are unable to be metabolized in the presence of MAOIs, leading to increased dopaminergic, adrenergic, and serotonergic activity. Overstimulation of these systems can lead to CNS agitation, hallucinations, seizures, tachycardia, and elevated blood pressure.

4. **The answer is A. Shuffling gait** is an extrapyramidal effect associated with typical antipsychotic agents. These effects are caused by D2 blockade within the striatum, with resultant parkinsonian symptoms. Orthostatic hypotension and sedation are caused by α-adrenergic antagonism in the periphery and in the reticular activating system, respectively. Galactorrhea and amenorrhea can result from the disinhibition of dopaminergic effects on prolactin secretion in the pituitary.

5. **The answer is B. Haloperidol** is a butyrophenone typical antipsychotic agent with potent D2 antagonist effects. It is hypothesized that its actions at D2 receptors in the hypothalamus may contribute to its association with the development of neuroleptic malignant syn-

drome. Chlorpromazine, a phenothiazine typical antipsychotic agent, is less potent than haloperidol. Clozapine and quetiapine are atypical antipsychotic agents with even lesser affinity for D2 receptors. Clozapine is associated with a small risk of the development of agranulocytosis.

CASE 3

1. **The answer is C. Prochlorperazine acts by blocking D2 receptors in the area postrema near the fourth ventricle.** Inhibition of dopaminergic neurons in this region controls nausea. As a phenothiazine, prochlorperazine can also block peripheral muscarinic receptors, causing dry mouth, constipation, and difficulty urinating. Phenothiazines also antagonize peripheral α-adrenergic receptors, causing orthostatic hypotension. Blockade of D2 receptors in the mesolimbic system is associated with a reduction of the positive symptoms of schizophrenia. Treatments for Parkinson's disease include agents, that stimulate dopaminergic receptors in the nigrostriatal system.

2. **The answer is D.** Adverse effects of phenothiazines include "extrapyramidal effects" caused by the antagonism of D2 receptors outside of the mesolimbic and mesocortical systems. **Blockade of D2 receptors in the nigrostriatal system can cause altered muscle tone** and acute dystonic reactions. These reactions commonly manifest as muscle tightness in the face and neck region with difficulty opening the mouth (trismus), eye deviation, and neck turning. Parkinsonian symptoms and tardive dyskinesia are other extrapyramidal effects associated with long-term use of antipsychotic agents. Parkinsonian symptoms are caused by the antagonism of D2 receptors in the indirect pathway of the nigrostriatal system, and tardive dyskinesia is probably caused by receptor adaptations that result in excessive dopaminergic activity in this tract. Blockade of D2 receptors in the pituitary gland can cause prolactin secretion, which leads to amenorrhea, galactorrhea, and a false-positive pregnancy test result. A flattened affect and alogia are considered negative symptoms of schizophrenia, likely mediated by altered dopaminergic activity in the mesocortical system. Positive symptoms of schizophrenia, including delusions and disorganized speech and behavior, are thought to be mediated by excessive dopaminergic activity in the mesolimbic system.

CHAPTER 13 ANSWERS

CASE 1

1. **The answer is E.** Ms. R. is diagnosed with a major depressive disorder based on the presence of several **symptoms lasting 2 months**, including feelings of sadness, helplessness, and inadequacy, loss of appetite and weight loss, and difficulty sleeping. The presence of these symptoms for more than 2 weeks constitutes a single depressive episode. Ms. R. has symptoms of typical depression. This is in contrast to the symptoms of atypical depression, which include increased appetite, hypersomnia, and sensitivity to criticism.

2. **The answer is B. Fluoxetine prevents the reuptake of serotonin** by the serotonin transporter into presynaptic neurons. This increases the available concentration of serotonin in the synapse to act at its receptor. Fluoxetine is a selective serotonin reuptake inhibitor (SSRI). It is effective in the treatment of depression, anxiety, and obsessive-compulsive disorder. Because of its selectivity, fluoxetine (and the other SSRIs) has less toxic adverse effects than the cyclic antidepressants.

3. **The answer is D. It takes several weeks for autoreceptors to become desensitized to the increased synaptic serotonin concentrations caused by fluoxetine.** After the initiation of therapy, the increased synaptic serotonin concentrations cause presynaptic autoreceptors to downregulate serotonin synthesis and release. Chronic therapy eventually leads to downregulation of the autoreceptors and enhanced neurotransmission. This process takes several weeks and is the likely explanation for the delay in clinical efficacy of both SSRIs and norepinephrine reuptake inhibitors.

4. **The answer is E.** Patients with bipolar affective disorder can experience a rapid switch in mood from depression to mania after initiating therapy with antidepressants, such as **fluoxetine**. Even though these patients feel "good" and have an elevated mood and energy, they require treatment with mood stabilizers because they are at risk for adverse outcomes as a result of their manic behavior. In addition, patients with mixed episodes of mania and depression are at high risk for suicide.

5. **The answer is B.** Lithium has a narrow therapeutic index and can cause numerous adverse effects, including hypothyroidism and the development of a **thyroid goiter**. Other adverse effects of lithium include the development of nephrogenic diabetes insipidus, T-wave abnormalities on the ECG, and alterations in potassium balance. Acute toxicity can cause nausea, vomiting, confusion, tremors, and seizures. Psychosis can be induced by the amphetamine-like agents, which prevent vesicle storage of neurotransmitters. Sexual dysfunction is a potential adverse effect of SSRIs. Orthostatic hypotension can be an adverse effect of cyclic antidepressants.

CASE 2

1. **The answer is C. Amitriptyline** is a tricyclic antidepressant that exerts its therapeutic effect by preventing the reuptake of serotonin and norepinephrine by their respective transporters. In addition to inhibiting the effect of these transporters, cyclic antidepressants act at a number of other receptors. They can cause numerous adverse effects, including antimuscarinic (anticholinergic), antihistaminic, and antiadrenergic effects. Selegiline is an MAOI. Paroxetine is a selective serotonin reuptake inhibitor (SSRI), and less likely to cause anticholinergic adverse effects or cardiac toxicity. Bupropion is an atypical antidepressant that can cause seizures in overdose. Sumatriptan is a serotonin receptoragonist that is used in the treatment of migraine headaches.

2. **The answer is A.** In addition to their antagonist effects at muscarinic, histaminic, and adrenergic receptors, cyclic antidepressants also bind and inhibit the activity of **cardiac sodium channels**, causing slowed depolarization and conduction blocks. The treatment of cardiac sodium channel blockade is intravenous bolus therapy with sodium bicarbonate to overcome the sodium channel block. Cyclic antidepressant inhibition of α_1-adrenergic receptors contributes to hypotension, which can be profound in the setting of overdose. Lithium blocks cardiac potassium channels, causing repolarization abnormalities and abnormal T waves on the ECG.

3. **The answer is E. Mirtazapine** is an atypical antidepressant that blocks $5HT_{2A}$, $5HT_{2C}$, and α_2-adrenergic autoreceptors. Dexfenfluramine is a halogenated amphetamine derivative with both amphetamine-like effects and modest serotonergic effects. Imipramine is a cyclic antidepressant. Tyramine is the building block for catecholamine synthesis. Ondansetron is a serotonin antagonist used as an antiemetic.

4. **The answer is B.** Lithium toxicity can occur in patients who have **renal insufficiency**. As a monovalent cation, lithium is secreted and reabsorbed in the renal tubules. When renal insufficiency develops, the normal elimination of lithium is limited, and serum and central nervous system concentrations of lithium can become toxic. Hypothyroidism is a potential adverse effect of lithium therapy.

5. **The answer is B.** The rate-limiting, and first enzymatic step in serotonin synthesis is **tryptophan hydroxylase**. Tyramine hydroxylase is the first, and rate-limiting step, in the synthesis of dopamine and norepinephrine. Aromatic L-amino acid decarboxylase converts 5-hydroxytryptophan to serotonin. Catechol-O-methyltransferase metabolizes monoamines, primarily in the extracellular space of the peripheral nervous system.

CHAPTER 14 ANSWERS

CASE 1

1. **The answer is B.** Rob experienced the spread of seizure activity from the hands to the arm, and then to the leg. **This order of spread is consistent with the spread of synchronous activity across the motor homunculus**, also known as a Jacksonian march. When a local burst of neuronal activity cannot be contained by surround inhibition, the synchronized firing from a seizure focus can spread to neighboring regions of the cortex. Initially, this may manifest as an aura; in Rob's case, it manifested as a blank, fearful stare, followed by the clinical manifestations of the synchronized firing. The clinical manifestations of the seizure activity depend on the area of the brain involved.

2. **The answer is C. Loss of GABA input results in tonic activity, while an oscillation between GABA inhibitory and glutamate excitatory impulses results in clonic activity.** The initial sudden loss of GABA inhibition allows for a long train of neuronal firing to cause contraction of both agonist and antagonist muscles (i.e., tonic activity). As GABA inhibition is restored, an oscillation between GABA inhibitory effects and AMPA- and NMDA-mediated glutamate excitatory effects causes shaking movements (i.e., clonic activity).

3. **The answer is A. A focal neoplasm could alter the local neuronal environment and compromise the normally protective mechanisms, which prevent abnormal synchronous discharge.** Anything that alters the neuronal environment and compromises the normal protective mechanisms, which prevent abnormal synchronous discharge, can contribute to seizure activity. This includes ion channel abnormalities, toxins, prior brain injury (e.g., stroke, trauma), neoplasm, infection, or high fever. The *exact* mechanism by which tumors couse seizures is still unknown.

4. **The answer is E.** The antiepileptic drugs act pleiotropically. However, phenytoin, carbamazepine, valproic acid, and lamotrigine **all have sodium channel–blocking effects** in common. By enhancing sodium channel–mediated inhibition, they prolong the inactivated state of sodium channels. This prevents repetitive neuronal firing and seizure activity.

5. **The answer is A. Carbamazepine has fewer adverse effects and potential drug interactions than phenytoin** and is the drug of choice for patients with simple and complex partial seizures. Its metabolite, 10,11-epoxycarbamazepine, has similar sodium channel–blocking effects. Carbamazepine enhances its own metabolism by induction of the P450 enzyme system, so that its half-life gradually shortens with chronic therapy.

CASE 2

1. **The answer is C. Gingival hyperplasia** is a potential adverse effect of phenytoin therapy. Other adverse effects include facial coarsening, hirsutism, megaloblastic anemia, and dermatitis. Dose-related adverse effects are primarily related to the central nervous system, and include drowsiness, confusion, ataxia, incoordination, and nystagmus. Phenytoin hypersensitivity syndrome consists of rash, which can desquamate, fever, eosinophilia, and hepatitis. Rare but life-threatening pancreatitis has occurred in association with valproic acid therapy. Aplastic anemia and liver failure have been reported in association with the use of felbamate. Although they do not cause absence seizures as a potential adverse effect, barbiturates can exacerbate this type of seizure.

2. **The answer is A. Erythromycin inhibited the hepatic P450 metabolism of phenytoin** and caused an increase in its plasma concentration, and subsequent clinical toxicity. Other drugs that can inhibit this enzyme system, such as chloramphenicol, cimetidine, and isoniazid, can similarly cause phenytoin toxicity when administered concomitantly with phenytoin. Conversely, drugs that induce P450 activity, such as carbamazepine, can contribute to subtherapeutic phenytoin concentrations.

3. **The answer is D. Phenytoin blocks sodium channels in rapidly firing neurons and prevents partial and secondary generalized seizures.** Phenytoin slows the rate of sodium channel recovery from inactivation. Its effect on sodium channels is greatest in rapidly firing neurons. It prevents the paroxysmal depolarizing shift that initiates partial seizures, and prevents the spread of seizure activity associated with secondary generalized tonic-clonic seizures. Phenytoin has no effect on absence seizures, in which the rate of sodium channel opening and closing is too slow to be amenable to inhibition by use-dependent sodium channel inactivation.

4. **The answer is D. Valproic acid limits T-type calcium channel activation and enhances GABA-mediated inhibition of absence seizures.** It also slows the rate of sodium channel recovery from inactivation. Because of these many effects in limiting seizure activity, valproic acid is one of the most effective antiepileptic drugs for the treatment of epilepsy syndromes having mixed seizure types. Ethosuximide inhibits T-type calcium channel opening and is a first-line agent in the treatment of patients with absence seizures. It does not affect sodium channels. Gabapentin increases the GABA concentrations in neurons, but inhibits seizure activity primarily by inhibiting high voltage-activated calcium channel opening. Carbamazepine prolongs sodium channel inhibition and is therapeutic for partial and secondary generalized seizures, but not absence seizures.

5. **The answer is C. Benzodiazepines and barbiturates both enhance GABA-mediated inhibition, but only barbiturates are able to enhance the activity at the GABA receptor in the absence of GABA.** Both drug types bind to the GABA receptor complex. Benzodiazepines are allosteric enhancers of endogenous GABA activity, increasing GABA affinity for its receptor. In contrast, barbiturates enhance GABA effects but also act directly on the GABA channel and therefore, have broad, nonspecific activity. Barbiturate action on GABA inhibition in the thalamic relay cells enhances T-type calcium channel currents, exacerbating absence seizure activity. Benzodiazepines and barbiturates both cause sedation as an adverse effect. Both types of agents can cause acute withdrawal symptoms on withdrawal of the drug.

CHAPTER 15 ANSWERS

CASE 1

1. **The answer is E. Isoflurane allows for more potent anesthesia, while nitrous oxide facilitates more rapid induction and recovery.** This is an example of balanced anesthesia. Several anesthetic agents are used in combination to achieve the goals of rapid induction and recovery, as well as potency of anesthesia, while limiting the adverse effects of any individual agent. Isoflurane exhibits a longer induction time but is a potent, inexpensive anesthetic with a low incidence of adverse effects. Nitrous oxide exhibits fast induction and recovery times and has a high analgesic index, but lesser potency. Nitrous oxide alone is unable to provide full anesthesia, even at 80% volume.

2. **The answer is D. As the CNS partial pressure equilibrates with the higher inspired partial pressure of the anesthetic, cardiopulmonary depression can occur.** If the dose of an inhaled anesthetic is "loaded" by administering a higher inspired partial pressure, the partial pressure within the CNS will be reached more quickly. If the partial pressure within the CNS continues to rise above the anesthetic partial pressure towards the higher (loading) partial pressure of inspired anesthetic, cardiopulmonary depression can result.

3. **The answer is B. Nitrous oxide rapidly diffuses out of the blood, replacing inspired air and decreasing the alveolar (and subsequent arterial) partial pressure of oxygen.** This is an example of diffusion hypoxia. During recovery from nitrous oxide anesthesia, nitrous oxide diffuses out of the blood into the alveoli at a high rate. What distinguishes nitrous oxide from other inhalation anesthetics is the high partial pressure in the mixed venous blood returning to the lung (a consequence of its low potency). Thus, at the beginning of washout, the alveolar partial pressure of nitrous oxide will be high (>0.5atm). If the remaining partial pressure is provided by air, the PO_2 may be approximately halved at the alveoli. When the partial pressure of oxygen in the alveoli decreases, there is less oxygen available for diffusion into the blood, and hypoxia can result.

4. **The answer is A. Children have a higher alveolar ventilation rate, smaller lungs, and a lower capacity of tissues for anesthetic; this shortens the time to equilibration between inspired and alveolar partial pressure, and between alveolar and tissue partial pressure.** Higher rates of ventilation speed induction. Higher cardiac output tends to slow induction. Children have higher rates of ventilation, a proportionally greater blood flow to the vessel-rich group (brain), and a lower capacity for anesthetic in the tissues. These factors accelerate the rate at which the tissues become saturated with anesthetic in children, and more than compensate for the effect of cardiac output on slowing the rate of rise of the alveolar pressure toward the inspired partial pressure. The degree of acceleration of onset of anesthesia compared to an adult will increase with the anesthetic's blood/gas partition coefficient. Ventilation-limited anesthetics demonstrate more rapid induction in children.

5. **The answer is C.** The potency of an anesthetic increases as **its solubility in oil increases**. The Meyer Overton rule predicts that the potency of a general anesthetic can be predicted from its oil/gas partition coefficient. Anesthetic potency is inversely related to its MAC. All general anesthetics have low therapeutic indices.

CASE 2

1. **The answer is A. Nitrous oxide has a small blood/gas partition coefficient.** It equilibrates very rapidly, and diffusion of nitrous oxide out of the blood into alveoli displaces oxygen-rich air, leading to hypoxia (diffusion hypoxia.) Nitrous oxide has become a relatively common inhalant of abuse, used in an attempt to get "high". Abusers seek euphoric symptoms of lightheadedness, incoordination, hallucinations, and delusions after inhaling the gas. Symptoms of intoxication are more pronounced when nitrous oxide is inhaled in enclosed spaces. Nitrous oxide is readily available in whipped cream dispensers and is sold via the Internet. Nitrous oxide has a very high MAC, making it a less potent general anesthetic. For these reasons, it is used in combination with other inhaled anesthetics, because the high inspired partial pressure of nitrous oxide necessary to achieve full anesthesia with this agent would prevent adequate oxygenation. Nitrous oxide has a high analgesic index and is a good analgesic. Halothane is hepatically metabolized.

2. **The answer is D.** Perfusion-limited anesthetics have a **time constant for equilibration of alveolar and inspired partial pressures that is similar to the time constant for equilibration of tissue and arterial partial pressures**. Induction and recovery times are relatively short compared with those of ventilation-limited anesthetics. Ventilation-limited anesthetics have a high blood/gas partition coefficient and a high rate of uptake from the alveoli into the blood. This slows down the rate at which the alveolar partial pressure rises toward the inspired partial pressure. The time constant for equilibrium of tissue and arterial partial pressure is about the same for both groups of anesthetics.

3. **The answer is C.** Organs in the vessel-rich group (brain and visceral organs) exhibit **a low capacity for anesthetic but high blood flow to the compartment**. General anesthetics equilibrate rapidly with this compartment. The muscle group compartment has a high capacity for anesthetic and moderate blood flow, and the fat group compartment has a very high capacity for anesthetic, but low blood flow.

4. **The answer is C. Ketamine** is an unusual dissociative anesthetic agent that increases sympathetic tone and cardiac output.

5. **The answer is E.** Malignant hyperthermia is caused by an **uncontrolled efflux of calcium from the sarcoplasmic reticulum**. This rare adverse effect of halothane (and other halogenated anesthetics) is caused by an inherited mutation in the sarcoplasmic reticulum ryanodine receptor, which causes release of calcium. Symptoms include excessive muscle contraction, tetany, and heat production. Dantrolene, the treatment for malignant hyperthermia, is a muscle relaxant that blocks calcium release from the sarcoplasmic reticulum.

CHAPTER 16 ANSWERS

CASE 1

1. **The answer is C.** The initial stimulus, **intense heat, stimulated thermosensitive TRPV receptors** on primary sensory neurons. **Tissue burn injury stimulated the production of chemical activators**, including protons and kinins. (Other chemical activators associated with cell damage and inflammation include protons, ATP, cytokines, nerve growth factor, and bradykinin.) **Voltage-gated sodium channels in Aδ- and C-fibers were activated, and transmitted signals to the dorsal horn of the spinal cord, where N-type voltage-gated calcium channels controlled release of neurotransmitters at the secondary projection neurons.** ATP receptors, P2X and P2Y, are stimulated by extracellular ATP, which is usually released as a result of cell injury. TRPM receptors are stimulated by cold temperatures. The opioid peptides (dynorphins, enkephalins, and β-endorphins), norepinephrine, serotonin, glycine, and GABA are inhibitory neurotransmitters that modulate transmission in the spinal cord, and alter pain perception. Glutamate receptors in the spinal cord are altered and activated in the setting of central sensitization to pain.

2. **The answer is D.** The opioids, morphine and remifentanil, are **μ receptor agonists that inhibit synaptic transmission** in the brain, brainstem, spinal cord, and at peripheral sensory neurons. They **inhibit presynaptic vesicle release from primary afferents** by decreasing presynaptic calcium conductance. They **hyperpolarize postsynaptic neurons** by enhancing potassium conductance. In the case, remifentanil was used as a continuous infusion to maintain pain control during surgery. Because

remifentonil has a short duration of action, J.D. received bolus doses of longer-acting morphine to control pain after surgery. The opioid κ receptors are acted on by endogenous dynorphins, in contrast to enkephalins and β-endorphins, which are agonists at the μ and δ receptors.

3. **The answer is A. Opioid–acetaminophen combination analgesics act through different mechanisms to reduce painful sensations, and are synergistic in their effect.** Opioids act at μ receptors to inhibit synaptic transmission of impulses in the brain, brainstem, spinal cord, and periphery. Acetaminophen inhibits central prostaglandin synthesis. Acetaminophen is a centrally acting analgesic but is not antiinflammatory. Opioids and acetaminophen have no significant effect on each other's metabolism. Opioid tolerance and addiction can occur unrelated to the presence of acetaminophen.

4. **The answer is C.** Amitriptyline is a tricyclic **antidepressant. It increases modulating noradrenergic and serotonergic projections in the spinal cord by reducing the reuptake of these amines**. Its analgesic effect is also due to its **blockade of sodium channels** and membrane excitability. In cases of neuropathic pain, amitriptyline **limits abnormal neurotransmission and reduces central sensitization**. Specific serotonin reuptake inhibitors are not particularly effective in alleviating neuropathic pain.

5. **The answer is B. Indomethacin is an antiinflammatory analgesic.** It works by non-selectively inhibiting both COX isoenzymes, limiting the production of prostaglandins in the setting of inflammatory pain. Acetaminophen also inhibits the production of prostaglandins in the central nervous system but is not antiinflammatory. Remifentanil is an opioid analgesic. Carbamazepine is an anticonvulsant that is used to control neuropathic pain, based on its blockade of sodium channels. Misoprostol is sometimes coadministered with NSAIDs to help replace prostaglandin activity in the gastric mucosa and limit the related gastrointestinal adverse effects of NSAIDs.

CASE 2

1. **The answer is B. Naproxen is a propionic acid NSAID that non-selectively inhibits COX and prevents the formation of prostaglandins.** Naproxen inhibits both COX-1 and COX-2 and can cause adverse effects of gastric upset, gastritis, and gastrointestinal bleeding by limiting the prostaglandin protective effect on the gastric mucosa.

2. **The answer is D.** Ms. S. developed **opioid tolerance and withdrawal.** Tolerance occurs when repeatedly higher doses of drug are necessary to achieve the same therapeutic effect. The molecular basis of tolerance is related to alterations in the opioid receptor. Ms. S. also developed physical dependence such that she suffered withdrawal symptoms of nausea, abdominal cramping, and myalgias on abrupt cessation of oxycodone. This should be distinguished from addiction, which is characterized by

drug-seeking behavior in the setting of physical dependence. Central sensitization is caused by an alteration in sensory processing in the dorsal horn of the spinal cord, leading to pain hypersensitivity and allodynia.

3. **The answer is A. Gabapentin**, an anticonvulsant, has been used in the treatment of tic douloureux. Gabapentin binds to calcium channels and reduces neuronal transmission in the setting of neuropathic pain. Anticonvulsants and antidepressants block sodium channels and also limit abnormal neuronal impulse transmission. Anondomide is an endogenous cannabinoid receptor ligand. Diclofenac is a pyrrole acetic acid derivative NSAID that inhibits COX-1 and COX-2. Dynorphins are endogenous opioid peptide agonists at opioid κ receptors. Naloxone is a specific opioid receptor antagonist.

4. **The answer is D. Dizziness, confusion, and unsteady gait** are common adverse effects that limit the therapeutic usefulness of anticonvulsants in the treatment of pain. COX-2 inhibitors have been associated with cardiovascular toxicity. Postural hypotension is an adverse effect of clonidine, an adrenergic α_2-receptor agonist.

5. **The answer is B. Gabapentin binds to the α_2d** subunit of voltage-dependent calcium channels and reduces neuronal activity by an as yet unknown mechanism presumed to be a reduction in transmitter release. It has been shown to be effective in the treatment of painful diabetic neuropathy, post-herpetic neuralgia, and tic douloureux. Celecoxib is a specific COX-2 inhibitor. Ibuprofen is a nonspecific COX inhibitor. Dextromethorphan is a NMDA receptor antagonist that can cause analgesia only at very high doses, limiting its clinical usefulness as an analgesic. Naltrexone is a specific opioid receptor antagonist used in the treatment of opioid addiction and withdrawal.

CHAPTER 17 ANSWERS

CASE 1

1. **The answer is A. Mr. B. has opioid withdrawal symptoms** caused by the abrupt cessation of heroin. These adverse physical symptoms and signs result from the absence of the drug at the μ opioid receptors, consistent with a state of physiologic dependence. The clinical symptoms of irritability and hypersensitivity to painful stimuli are nearly the converse of the sedative, analgesic effects induced by the opioid. Inverse tolerance is another name for sensitization, or the mechanism by which repeated drug administration results in greater effect at a given dose compared with initial doses. Addiction is the result of long-term drug use. Its development is influenced by multiple variables, including genetic predisposition, the type of drug used, and environmental factors, all of which contribute to some degree of both physiologic and psychological dependence on the presence of drug at its effector site. Addictive behavior is related to the long-lasting adaptation and altered homeostasis of the brain, contingent on the presence of drug.

2. **The answer is B. Methadone has a longer duration of action than heroin and can be tapered to avoid the physical symptoms of acute withdrawal.** It is administered orally; has a slower onset of action; and does not cause the sudden "high" associated with heroin's rapid movement into the central nervous system. It has a long plasma half-life and can be tapered slowly to avoid acute withdrawal. Methadone has been used in heroin treatment programs since the late 1940s in the United States, and for maintenance in the treatment of heroin addiction since the mid-1960s. While difficult for some patients to discontinue, methadone is the most widely used and effective maintenance treatment for heroin addiction. Methadone is also used therapeutically to treat severe pain.

3. **The answer is C. Twelve-step programs, such as Alcoholics and Narcotics Anonymous, provide a community of support and mentoring to recovering addicts.** They emphasize positive steps in fostering sobriety, including an admission by the patient of his or her problem. The community these programs provide helps to reduce the sense of isolation felt by drug abusers. Moderation management is a strategy of managing alcohol abuse, in which the abuser is taught how to establish boundaries related to their alcohol use.

4. **The answer is D. Mr. B. had acquired tolerance to the effects of heroin.** Tolerance results when repeated administration of the drug causes less effect at the same dosage and larger amounts of drug are required to produce the same clinical effect. Acquired tolerance can occur as a result of three mechanisms: 1) an increased ability to metabolize or excrete a drug; 2) a change in the drug-receptor interaction caused by altered receptor binding affinity, inactivation of receptors or their signaling pathways, or as a result of altered regulation of gene expression of drug receptors or their signaling proteins; or 3) learned behavioral tolerance, in which the person consciously alters his or her behavior to hide the drug's effects.

    Conditioned tolerance is a type of learned behavioral tolerance in which environmental cues associated with the drug use unconsciously cause a conditioned response in the abuser. Innate tolerance refers to the differences in individuals' sensitivity to the effects of a drug before the first dose of drug is administered. Innate tolerance is determined by both genetic and environmental factors.

5. **The answer is B. Cravings and relapse can occur as a result of long-lasting molecular and cellular adaptations in the brain as a result of drug abuse.** These long-term effects may be caused by genetically modified cellular adaptations to the presence of drug. These adaptations may alter the release of neurotrophic factors and cause persistent changes in synaptic function.

CASE 2

1. **The answer is C. Disulfiram,** or tetraethylthiuram, is a sulfur-containing agent, that blocks aldehyde dehydrogenase, an enzyme in the alcohol metabolic pathway. Aldehyde dehydrogenase is responsible for the metabolism of acetaldehyde, an intermediate metabolite of ethyl alcohol. When disulfiram is present and alcohol (or an alcohol-containing substance) is ingested, acetaldehyde builds up, causing facial flushing, nausea, vomiting, headache, and palpitations. Disulfiram also inhibits the activity of dopamine beta hydroxylase. This may lead to an increase in brain dopamine, and relative depletion of norepinephrine synthesis, contributing to orthostatic hypotension. Many over-the-counter cold preparations contain ethanol as a diluent, which can cause the disulfiram-ethanol interaction. Topiramate is an antiepileptic drug that inhibits AMPA/kainate glutamate receptors. It is under study for the treatment of alcohol abuse. Naltrexone is a long-acting opioid antagonist that competitively blocks the binding of opioid agonists to the μ opioid receptor and prevents the "high" associated with opioid agonist use. Rimonabant is a CB1 cannabinoid receptor antagonist that blocks the effects of exogenous cannabinoids. Buprenorphine is a partial opioid agonist that alleviates cravings for opioids and opioid withdrawal symptoms, while antagonizing the "high" associated with the use of full opioid agonists.

2. **The answer is A. When buprenorphine is administered in a sublingual preparation with naloxone, the partial agonist effects of buprenorphine are manifest,** while the naloxone is inactivated. This combination, suboxone, is intended to reduce the abuse potential of buprenorphine. If it is administered parenterally as a drug of abuse, the naloxone antagonizes the opioid agonist effect of buprenorphine. Methadone produces cross-tolerance to other opioids and blunts the opioid agonist effects of injected heroin in patients taking methadone. Naltrexone antagonizes the "high" associated with opioid use but may not alleviate cravings. Naltrexone does not produce withdrawal effects by itself. Acamprosate modulates glutamate receptors. Antidepressants, such as desipramine and fluoxetine, reduce cocaine cravings but have not been shown to prevent cocaine use.

3. **The answer is E. Drugs capable of causing psychological dependence enhance dopamine activity in the nucleus accumbens.** Normally, GABA interneurons in the ventral tegmental area of the brain tonically inhibit dopaminergic neurons, which activate the brain reward pathway in the nucleus accumbens. Opioids enhance dopamine activity in the ventral tegmental area through their inhibitory effects on GABA interneurons. Cocaine and amphetamines increase the dopamine concentration in the synapse of dopaminergic neurons acting at the nucleus accumbens. Psychological dependence occurs when a drug affects the brain reward system, resulting in pleasurable sensations associated with the drug's use.

4. **The answer is D. An 18-year-old man smokes a very lipophilic drug.** The pharmacokinetics of this method of drug use are associated with potential abuse and addiction. Rapid absorption and entry into the central nervous system of lipophilic (or hydrophobic) drugs with rapid clinical onset and short duration of action is associated with potential drug abuse and addiction. In contrast, drugs that have a slower rate of absorption and slower entry into the central nervous system, with long durations of action that slowly resolve, are less likely to cause abrupt withdrawal symptoms and abuse.

5. **The answer is D. Having a high innate tolerance to the effects of a drug** places a person at greater risk of abuse and addiction. This relative insensitivity to the drug's effects makes it more likely that a person will require greater amounts of drug to achieve the intended effect. Using a drug under pleasurable circumstances is also associated with repeat drug use. Genetic variability in drug metabolism is also associated with a relative risk of drug dependence and abuse. For example, genetic variations in ethanol metabolism are associated with a variable risk of ethanol abuse and addiction.

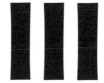

Principles of Cardiovascular Pharmacology

18

Pharmacology of Cardiac Rhythm

OBJECTIVES

■ Understand the molecular basis for the electrical physiology of the cardiac conduction system.

■ Understand the pharmacology, therapeutic uses, and adverse effects of the various classes of antiarrhythmic agents in the setting of cardiac electrical dysfunction.

■ CASE 1

One winter morning, Dr. J., a 56-year-old professor, is lecturing on the treatment of cardiomyopathies to the second-year medical school class. He feels his heart beating irregularly and becomes nauseated. He is able to finish his lecture but continues to feel significantly short of breath throughout the morning. His persistent symptoms prompt him to walk down the street to the local emergency department.

Physical examination reveals an irregular heartbeat ranging from 120 to 140 bpm. Dr. J.'s blood pressure is stable (132/76 mm Hg), and his oxygen saturation is 100% on room air. An electrocardiogram (ECG) confirms that Dr. J. has atrial fibrillation, without any evidence of ischemia. Several intravenous boluses of diltiazem are administered, and his heart rate decreases to a range of 80 to 100 bpm but remains irregular. Further laboratory studies and a chest X-ray do not reveal any underlying cause for Dr. J.'s atrial fibrillation.

QUESTIONS

1. Why did diltiazem slow Dr. J.'s heart rate without affecting his underlying heart arrhythmia, atrial fibrillation?

   A. Diltiazem slowed AV nodal conduction, but accelerated bypass tract conduction from the ventricles to the atria.

   B. Diltiazem slowed atrial impulse conduction, but contributed to atrial irritability and ectopic impulse formation.

   C. Diltiazem slowed sinoatrial (SA) nodal depolarization, but accelerated the atrial reentry circuit.

   D. Diltiazem slowed atrioventricular (AV) nodal conduction, but had no effect on the atrial reentry circuit.

   E. Diltiazem slowed Purkinje fiber conduction, but accelerated SA nodal depolarization.

During observation over the next 12 hours, Dr. J. remains in atrial fibrillation, and he continues to feel palpitations despite his pulse rate being under better control. Under continuous ECG monitoring, a cardiologist administers an intravenous infusion of ibutilide. Twenty minutes after receiving ibutilide, Dr. J.'s heart returns to a normal sinus rhythm. Based on his age and generally good health, Dr. J. is sent home with a prescription for aspirin. He is instructed to call his doctor if he develops further symptoms of atrial fibrillation.

2. What is the mechanism of action of ibutilide, and why does it potentially cause a clinical effect that requires that it be administered only under carefully monitored circumstances?

   A. Ibutilide inhibits delayed rectifier K^+ channels and prolongs repolarization, which can predispose to a prolonged QT interval and *torsades de pointes*.

   B. Ibutilide inhibits delayed rectifier K^+ channels and delays phase 0 depolarization, which can predispose to complete conduction block.

   C. Ibutilide inhibits delayed rectifier K^+ channels in a use-dependent manner such that repolarization will be greatly prolonged when the rate of depolarization is fast.

   D. Ibutilide inhibits delayed rectifier K^+ channels as well as slow inward Na^+ channels, which slows conduction velocity and contributes to conduction block.

   E. Ibutilide inhibits fast inward Na^+ channels and prolongs depolarization, which can predispose to reentry and ventricular tachyarrhythmias.

Dr. Johnson initially feels fine, but he develops recurrent palpitations within 3 weeks of his initial event. After discus-

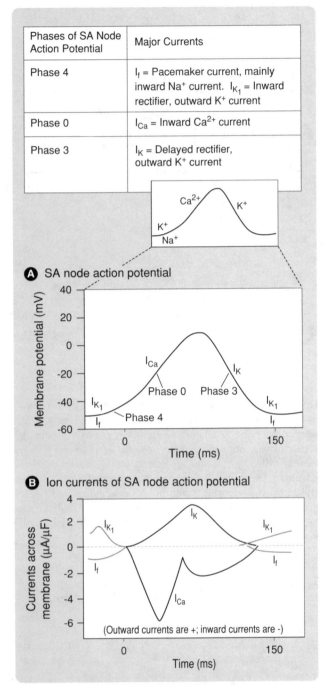

Phases of SA Node Action Potential	Major Currents
Phase 4	I_f = Pacemaker current, mainly inward Na+ current. I_{K_1} = Inward rectifier, outward K+ current
Phase 0	I_{Ca} = Inward Ca^{2+} current
Phase 3	I_K = Delayed rectifier, outward K+ current

A SA node action potential

B Ion currents of SA node action potential

(Outward currents are +; inward currents are -)

Figure 18-1. Sinoatrial (SA) Node Action Potential and Ion Currents. A. SA nodal cells are depolarized slowly by the pacemaker current (I_f) (phase 4), which consists of an inward flow of sodium (mostly) and calcium ions. Depolarization to the threshold potential opens highly selective voltage-gated calcium channels, which drive the membrane potential toward E_{Ca} (phase 0). As the calcium channels close and potassium channels open (phase 3), the membrane potential repolarizes. **B.** The flux of each ion species correlates roughly with each phase of the action potential. Positive currents indicate an outward flow of ions, and negative currents are inward. Adapted from Ackerman M, Clapham DE. Normal cardiac electrophysiology. In: Chien KR, Breslow JL, Leiden JM, Rosenberg RD, Seidman CE, eds. Molecular Basis of Cardiovascular Disease: A Companion to Braunwald's Heart Disease, Figure 12-2, page 284. Philadelphia: WB Saunders, 1999. With permission from Elsevier.

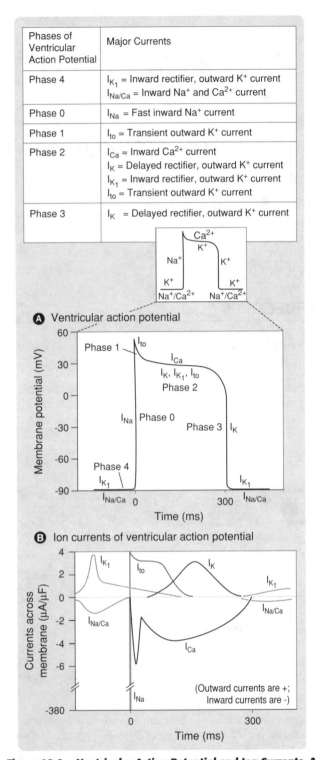

Phases of Ventricular Action Potential	Major Currents
Phase 4	I_{K_1} = Inward rectifier, outward K+ current $I_{Na/Ca}$ = Inward Na+ and Ca^{2+} current
Phase 0	I_{Na} = Fast inward Na+ current
Phase 1	I_{to} = Transient outward K+ current
Phase 2	I_{Ca} = Inward Ca^{2+} current I_K = Delayed rectifier, outward K+ current I_{K_1} = Inward rectifier, outward K+ current I_{to} = Transient outward K+ current
Phase 3	I_K = Delayed rectifier, outward K+ current

A Ventricular action potential

B Ion currents of ventricular action potential

(Outward currents are +; Inward currents are -)

Figure 18-2. Ventricular Action Potential and Ion Currents. A. At the resting membrane potential (phase 4), the inward and outward currents are equal and the membrane potential approaches the K+ equilibrium potential (E_K). During the action potential upstroke (phase 0), there is a large transient increase in Na+ conductance. This is followed by a brief period of initial repolarization (phase 1), which is mediated by a transient outward K+ current. The plateau of the action potential (phase 2) results from the opposition of an inward Ca^{2+} current and an outward K+ current. The membrane repolarizes (phase 3) when the inward Ca^{2+} current decreases and the outward K+ current predominates. **B.** The ion fluxes that give rise to the ventricular action potential consist of a complex pattern of changing ion permeabilities that are separated in time. Note especially that the Na+ current in phase 0 is very large but extremely

sion with his cardiologist, he elects to start amiodarone at a maintenance dose of 200 mg/day in addition to continuing his aspirin. Dr. J. tolerates the amiodarone well and reports no difficulty breathing. He remains symptom free during the rest of his cardiology lectures.

3. Which of the following is a potential adverse effect of amiodarone when it is used in high daily dosages?

   A. lupus-like syndrome
   B. pulmonary fibrosis
   C. renal insufficiency
   D. urinary retention
   E. bronchospasm and impotence

4. Quinidine is a prototypical class IA antiarrhythmic that was often used in the past to treat atrial flutter. However, its anticholinergic adverse effects can convert an atrial:ventricular rate from 2:1 to 1:1, with subsequent cardiac decompensation. What is the mechanism responsible for this effect?

   A. Sodium channel blockade slows atrial conduction, while potassium channel blockade enhances ventricular conduction.
   B. Sodium channel blockade slows atrial conduction, while anticholinergic effects increase AV nodal conduction velocity.
   C. Sodium channel blockade slows AV nodal conduction, while anticholinergic effects allow rapid bypass tract conduction velocity.
   D. Sodium channel blockade slows atrial conduction, while anticholinergic effects increase the frequency of SA nodal firing.
   E. Sodium channel blockade is overcome by anticholinergic release of sodium from the sarcoplasmic reticulum.

5. Dihydropyridine calcium channel blockers have a preferential effect on calcium channels in:

   A. skeletal muscle
   B. vascular smooth muscle
   C. the AV node
   D. the myocyte
   E. the Purkinje fibers

Figure 18-2. brief. Adapted from Ackerman M, Clapham DE. Normal cardiac electrophysiology. In: Chien KR, Breslow JL, Leiden JM, Rosenberg RD, Seidman CE, eds. Molecular Basis of Cardiovascular Disease: A Companion to Braunwald's Heart Disease, Figure 12-1 and Figure 12-2, pages 282 and 284. Philadelphia: WB Saunders, 1999. With permission from Elsevier.

 CASE 2

Paramedics bring a 68-year-old man with a history of coronary artery disease and hypertension to the emergency department after he had a witnessed seizure at home. On arrival, the patient is lethargic. His examination is remarkable for a heart rate of 42 bpm and a blood pressure of 62/55 mm Hg. His temperature and respiratory rate are normal. The patient is placed on a cardiac monitor and administered supplemental oxygen. An ECG is performed and shows a rate of approximately 40 bpm and a narrow QRS complex. No P waves are apparent on the ECG. The patient's fingerstick glucose is 100 mg/dL. Despite intravenous fluid boluses, the patient's blood pressure does not improve. The resident administers 1 mg of atropine (an antimuscarinic drug) with only a transient increase in the heart rate but no improvement in the hypotension. The medical student asks, ''Do you want to see his medication list?''

QUESTIONS

1. Which of the following medications could cause this patient's bradycardia?

   A. nifedipine
   B. atropine
   C. propranolol
   D. nitroglycerine
   E. epinephrine

2. What is the mechanism of action of atropine in transiently increasing the heart rate in this case?

   A. Atropine inhibits the parasympathetic effects of the vagus nerve, enhances calcium entry into ventricular myocytes, and enhances the firing of ectopic ventricular pacemakers.
   B. Atropine reduces calcium channel opening in pacemaker cells and increases the rate of rise of phase 0 depolarization.
   C. Atropine has a direct agonist effect at sympathetic β_1-adrenergic receptors in the SA node and increases the frequency of pacemaker cell firing.
   D. Atropine enhances ventricular myocyte potassium conductance through the delayed rectifier K+ channels, shortens repolarization, and allows ectopic ventricular pacemakers to fire more frequently.
   E. Atropine decreases parasympathetic tone by inhibiting the release of acetylcholin from the vagus nerve, enhances pacemaker current, facilitates depolarization, and increases the rate of pacemaker cell firing.

This patient is taking propranolol. The family arrives in the emergency department and reports that he has been very depressed since the death of his wife earlier this year. They have been concerned that he has been feeling hopeless and suspect that he may have been considering suicide. An empty bottle of propranolol was subsequently found at the patient's home. In the emergency department, the patient is orally intubated and mechanically ventilated. An orogastric tube is inserted, and the patient is administered activated charcoal in an attempt to prevent further gastrointestinal absorption of the propranolol. He is subsequently admitted to the cardiac care unit for antidotal therapy of this overdose.

3. What is the mechanism of action of the class II antiarrhythmic agents, β-adrenergic receptor antagonists?
   A. β-adrenergic receptor antagonists decrease the rate of phase 0 depolarization and prolong repolarization.
   B. β-adrenergic receptor antagonists increase the rate of phase 3 repolarization and shorten conduction time.
   C. β-adrenergic receptor antagonists decrease the rate of calcium entry during the plateau phase 2 and shorten the refractory period.
   D. β-adrenergic receptor antagonists decrease the rate of phase 4 depolarization and prolong repolarization.
   E. β-adrenergic receptor antagonists decrease the rate of phase 4 depolarization and shorten repolarization.

4. Which of the following is an example of "state-dependent" ion channel block that is useful in the treatment of arrhythmia?
   A. Amiodarone has a high affinity for potassium channels when the heart rate is slow.
   B. Lidocaine has a high affinity for inactivated sodium channels in ischemic tissue.
   C. Lidocaine has a high affinity for closed sodium channels during intense exercise.
   D. Lidocaine blocks sodium channels independent of action potential firing rates.
   E. Flecainide has a high affinity for sodium channels in the resting state.

5. Adenosine is used as first line therapy for which of the following arrhythmias?
   A. narrow-complex supraventricular tachycardias
   B. atrial fibrillation
   C. junctional bradycardia after propranolol overdose
   D. ventricular ectopic pacemakers
   E. ventricular fibrillation

19

Pharmacology of Cardiac Contractility

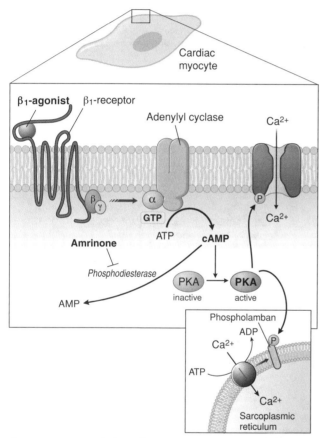

Figure 19-1. Regulation of Cardiac Contractility by β-Adrenergic Receptors. β-Adrenergic receptors increase cardiac myocyte contractility but also enhance relaxation. Binding of an endogenous or exogenous agonist to β₁-adrenergic receptors on the surface of cardiac myocytes causes Gα proteins to activate adenylyl cyclase, which in turn catalyzes the conversion of ATP to cAMP. cAMP activates multiple protein kinases, including protein kinase A (PKA). PKA phosphorylates and activates sarcolemmal Ca^{2+} channels and thereby increases cardiac myocyte contractility. PKA also phosphorylates phospholamban. The SERCA pump becomes disinhibited and pumps Ca^{2+} into the sarcoplasmic reticulum; the increased rate of Ca^{2+} sequestration enhances cardiac myocyte relaxation. cAMP is converted to AMP by phosphodiesterase, resulting in termination of β₁-adrenergic receptor-mediated actions. The phosphodiesterase is inhibited by amrinone, a drug that can be used in the treatment of heart failure.

OBJECTIVES

■ Understand the molecular basis for cardiac contraction.

■ Understand the pharmacology, therapeutic uses, and adverse effects of the various agents used for the treatment of cardiac contractile dysfunction.

■ CASE 1

G.W., a 68–year-old man with known systolic dysfunction and heart failure, is admitted to the hospital with shortness of breath and nausea. The patient's cardiac history is notable for two prior myocardial infarctions, the more recent occurring about 2 years ago. Since the second infarction, the patient has had significant limitation of his exercise capacity. A two-dimensional echocardiogram is notable for a left ventricular ejection fraction of 25% (normal, > 55%) and moderate mitral valve regurgitation. G.W. has been treated with aspirin, carvedilol (a β-receptor antagonist), captopril (an angiotensin-converting enzyme inhibitor), digoxin (a cardiac glycoside), furosemide (a loop diuretic), and spironolactone (an aldosterone receptor antagonist). He has also had an automatic internal cardioverter/defibrillator (AICD) placed to prevent sustained ventricular arrhythmia and sudden cardiac death.

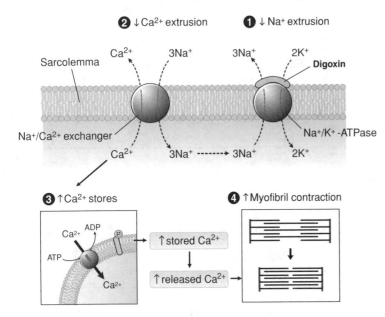

Figure 19-2. Positive Inotropic Mechanism of Digoxin. 1. Digoxin selectively binds to and inhibits the Na^+/K^+-ATPase. Decreased Na^+ extrusion *(dashed arrows)* leads to an increased concentration of cytosolic Na^+. 2. The increased intracellular Na^+ decreases the driving force for the Na^+/Ca^{2+} exchanger *(dashed arrows)*, leading to decreased extrusion of Ca^{2+} from the cardiac myocyte into the extracellular space and to increased cytosolic Ca^{2+}. 3. An increased amount of Ca^{2+} is then pumped by the SERCA Ca^{2+}-ATPase *(large arrow)* into the sarcoplasmic reticulum, creating a net increase in Ca^{2+} that is available for release during subsequent contractions. 4. During each contraction, the increased Ca^{2+} release from the sarcoplasmic reticulum leads to increased myofibril contraction, and therefore increased cardiac inotropy.

QUESTIONS

1. Why is G.W., a patient with heart failure, being treated with a β-receptor antagonist and a positive inotrope (digoxin) at the same time?
   A. This combination of agents allows for both drugs to be dosed in a nontoxic range.
   B. This combination of agents prevents recurrent myocardial infarction in ischemia-induced heart failure patients.
   C. This combination of agents reduces mortality and improves the functional status of heart failure patients.
   D. This combination of agents negates the need for diuretic therapy in chronic heart failure patients.
   E. This combination of agents causes cardiac remodeling and return of normal left ventricular ejection fraction, curing heart failure.

Physical examination in the emergency department is notable for a blood pressure of 90/50 mm Hg and a heart rate of 120 bpm. An electrocardiogram indicates that the underlying cardiac rhythm is atrial fibrillation. He is started on amiodarone (a class III antiarrhythmic), and his heart rate decreases to approximately 80 bpm. Laboratory tests show serum Na^+ of 148 mEq/L (normal, 135–145), BUN of 56 mg/dl (normal, 7–19), K^+ of 2.9 mEq/L (normal, 3.5–5.1), and creatinine of 4.8 mg/dL (normal, 0.6–1.2). The serum digoxin level is 3.2 ng/mL (therapeutic concentration, typically ~1 ng/mL).

2. What is the mechanism of action of digoxin?
   A. Digoxin inhibits the plasma membrane sodium pump, leading to an increase in the intracellular calcium concentration.
   B. Digoxin stimulates G protein–coupled receptors, leading to an increased formation of cyclic adenosine monophosphate (cAMP) and an increase in the intracellular calcium concentration.

C. Digoxin binds to neuronal sodium pumps, leading to an increase in sympathetic stimulation of the myocytes.
   D. Digoxin inhibits the reuptake of calcium by sarcoplasmic reticulum ATPase (SERCA) into the sarcoplasmic reticulum, maintaining a uniform concentration of intracellular calcium.
   E. Digoxin inhibits the plasma membrane sodium pump, causing $β_1$-adrenergic receptors to be more sensitive to the effect of circulating epinephrine.

3. Supratherapeutic digoxin can cause several adverse effects and toxicities. What is G.W.'s major clinical manifestation of digoxin toxicity?
   A. hyperkalemia
   B. atrial fibrillation
   C. renal failure
   D. yellow-green halos in the visual fields
   E. dehydration

4. Which of the following factors contributed to digoxin toxicity in this patient, and how?
   A. hypokalemia; alters the sodium-calcium exchanger such that it preferentially exchanges potassium
   B. hypokalemia; prevents renal excretion of digoxin
   C. hypernatremia; enhances the normal function of the sodium pump
   D. hypokalemia; makes the sodium pump more sensitive to digoxin
   E. hypernatremia; causes the sodium pump to preferentially exchange digoxin for potassium

Based on these findings, G.W. is admitted to the cardiology intensive care unit. His oral digoxin dose is held, and he is given intravenous K^+ to increase his serum potassium concentration. Based on the severity of his clinical decompensation, a pulmonary artery (PA) catheter is placed to monitor cardiac pressures, G.W. is also started on dobutamine and his carvedilol is held. After initiation of intravenous dobutamine, G.W. has increased urine output and begins to feel symptomatically improved. He is monitored for 7 days, and his digoxin level decreases to the therapeutic range.

5. What is the mechanism of action of dobutamine?
- **A.** Dobutamine is an agonist at the β_2-adrenergic receptor that increases intracellular potassium sequestration in the sarcoplasmic reticulum.
- **B.** Dobutamine is an antagonist at the α_1-adrenergic receptor that decreases afterload.
- **C.** Dobutamine is an agonist at the β_1-adrenergic receptor that increases the effectiveness of digoxin at the sodium pump.
- **D.** Dobutamine is an agonist at the β_1-adrenergic receptor that increases intracellular cAMP and calcium.
- **E.** Dobutamine increases norepinephrine release from sympathetic nerve terminals and enhances norepinephrine agonist effect at all adrenergic receptors.

 CASE 2

Carola L. is a 32-year-old woman, 2 weeks postpartum after a normal spontaneous vaginal delivery of a full-term infant daughter. She presents to her obstetrician for an urgent evaluation of severe fatigue and difficulty breathing. She states that she is feeling very tired and has had no energy for the past 10 days. She attributed her symptoms to lack of sleep, but for the past 5 days, she has felt very short of breath. She initially noted difficulty catching her breath when she was walking up a flight stairs with the laundry, but she now has shortness of breath with minimal exertion (getting up to nurse and change the baby) and is especially short of breath when she lies down in bed. Today she noted some substernal chest tightness associated with her shortness of breath, and ankle swelling, which has increased since her delivery. She wonders if she is anemic.

On physical examination, Mrs. L. is well developed but tachypneic. Her vital signs are remarkable for a heart rate of 127 bpm, a respiratory rate of 24 breaths/min, and a blood pressure of 78/50 mm Hg. Her doctor examines her lungs and hears bilateral crackles and wheezing. He suspects that she may have had a pulmonary embolus and calls an advanced cardiac life support ambulance to take her to the hospital for further evaluation. The paramedics place Mrs. L. on a cardiac monitor, establish an intravenous line, and administer intravenous fluids of normal saline in an attempt to increase her blood pressure. In route to the hospital Mrs. L. complains of feeling much more short of breath, and the paramedics note a narrow complex supraventricular tachyarrhythmia on the monitor. They administer a small dose of intravenous diltiazem, a calcium channel blocker, to convert this rhythm. Unfortunately, Mrs. L. remains hypotensive and her shortness of breath worsens. On arrival at the hospital, her heart rate is 116 bpm, her respiratory rate is 40 breaths/min, her systolic blood pressure is 60 mm Hg, and her oxygen saturation is 86% on room air.

QUESTIONS

1. What is the role of calcium in the cardiac myocyte contraction cycle?
- **A.** Intracellular calcium binds to troponin C, which allows it to cross link with actin and shorten the sarcomere.
- **B.** Intracellular calcium binds to tropomyosin, which allows it to "walk up" the actin filament and shorten the sarcomere.
- **C.** Intracellular calcium binds to troponin C, which allows the release of troponin I so that myosin and actin can interact to shorten the sarcomere.
- **D.** Intracellular calcium binds to the calmodulin–SERCA complex and forces the sequestration of more calcium in the sarcoplasmic reticulum.
- **E.** Intracellular calcium facilitates the formation of ATP, which binds to the actin–myosin crossbridges and causes them to release calcium during diastolic relaxation.

In the hospital, Mrs. L. is placed on a cardiac monitor and administered 10 L of oxygen by face mask. Her examination is remarkable for bilateral crackles in all lung fields, a tachycardia with a heart rate of 120 bpm and a S3 gallup, elevated jugular venous pressure to 14 cm above the sternal angle, and bilateral pitting edema of her ankles. An ECG shows a sinus tachycardia with nonspecific changes. A chest X-ray is performed and shows a large heart silhouette and alveolar pulmonary edema. A tentative diagnosis of peripartum cardiomyopathy is made and confirmed by emergency echocardiography, which shows a dilated left ventricle with an estimated ejection fraction of 35% with normal valvular function. Mrs. L. is treated with dobutamine for inotropic support, dopamine for blood pressure support, and furosemide (a loop diuretic), and is admitted to the cardiac stepdown unit.

2. Dopamine has various clinical effects at different doses. Which of the following statements regarding the effects of dopamine is true?
- **A.** Dopamine administered at low rates acts primarily as an agonist at α_1-adrenergic receptors, decreasing systemic vascular resistance.
- **B.** Dopamine administered at low rates acts as an agonist at both α_1- and β_1-adrenergic receptors, increasing heart rate and blood pressure.
- **C.** Dopamine administered at low rates acts primarily as an antagonist at β_1-adrenergic receptors, decreasing heart rate.
- **D.** Dopamine administered at high rates acts primarily as an agonist at β_2-adrenergic receptors, increasing bronchial smooth muscle tone.
- **E.** Dopamine administered at high rates acts primarily as an agonist at α_1-adrenergic receptors, increasing peripheral vascular resistance.

Mrs. L. diureses a large amount of dilute urine over the next several hours. Her blood pressure stabilizes, and she is weaned off of the dopamine infusion. She is started on oral therapy of digoxin and an angiotensin-converting enzyme inhibitor. On the second day of admission, she is weaned off of the dobutamine infusion. On the fourth hospital day, she no longer requires oxygen supplementation, her ankle edema is improved, and she is able to ambulate in the hallway. Six days after being admitted, she is able to be discharged on oral medications. She is counseled against heavy exertion and scheduled for a follow-up echocardiogram in 2 months.

3. Beta-receptor antagonists are sometimes used in heart failure patients. What is the potential disadvantage of using a β-adrenergic receptor antagonist in this patient?

   A. Beta-receptor antagonists may limit the binding of digoxin to the sodium pump.

   B. Beta-receptor antagonists may limit the beneficial effects of sympathetic tone in maintaining renal blood flow.

   C. Beta-receptor antagonists may further decrease cardiac output and cause pulmonary edema.

   D. Beta-receptor antagonists may depress heart rate and contribute to postpartum depression.

   E. Beta-receptor antagonists may prevent remodeling of the left ventricle during recovery from peripartum cardiomyopathy.

4. Which of the following agents is a phosphodiesterase inhibitor?

   A. low-dose dopamine

   B. milrinone

   C. carvedilol

   D. isoproterenol

   E. digitoxin

5. Beta-receptor agonists and phosphodiesterase inhibitors both increase cardiac contractility but through different mechanisms. What is the end effect of these agents responsible for their desired effect?

   A. Both agents increase cardiac contractility by increasing intracellular cAMP levels.

   B. Both agents increase cardiac contractility by increasing β_1-adrenergic receptor sensitivity.

   C. Both agents increase cardiac contractility by increasing the number of actin–myosin crossbridges.

   D. Both agents increase cardiac contractility by reducing peripheral vascular resistance.

   E. Both agents increase cardiac contractility by binding to an enzyme and inhibiting its action.

20

Pharmacology of Volume Regulation

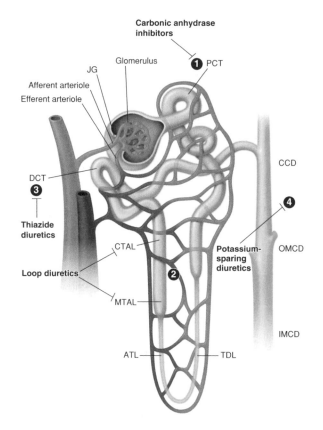

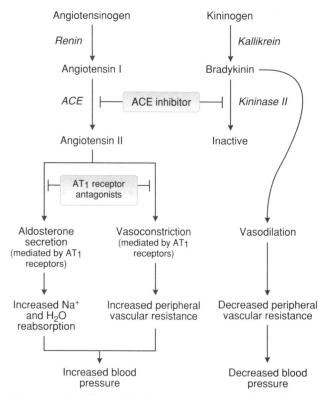

Figure 20-1. Nephron Anatomy and Sites of Action of Diuretics. Nephron fluid filtration begins at the glomerulus, where an ultrafiltrate of the plasma enters the renal epithelial (urinary) space. This ultrafiltrate then flows through four sequential segments of the nephron (1–4). **1.** From the glomerulus, ultrafiltrate travels to the proximal convoluted tubule (PCT), then to the **2.** loop of Henle, which includes the thin descending limb (TDL), ascending thin limb (ATL), medullary thick ascending limb (MTAL), and cortical thick ascending limb (CTAL) of Henle. **3.** The distal convoluted tubule (DCT) includes the macula densa and juxtaglomerular (JG) apparatus. **4.** The collecting duct consists of the cortical collecting duct (CCD), outer medullary collecting duct (OMCD), and inner medullary collecting duct (IMCD). Pharmacologic agents inhibit specific solute transporters within each segment of the nephron. Carbonic anhydrase inhibitors act at the proximal convoluted tubule, loop diuretics act at the medullary and cortical thick ascending limbs, thiazide diuretics inhibit solute transport in the distal convoluted tubule, and potassium-sparing diuretics inhibit collecting duct Na^+ reabsorption.

Figure 20-2. Effects of Renin–Angiotensin System Inhibitors on Blood Pressure. Angiotensin-converting enzyme (ACE) inhibitors prevent the conversion of angiotensin I to angiotensin II (both in the lung and locally in blood vessels and tissues) and inhibit the inactivation of bradykinin. Both actions of ACE inhibitors lead to vasodilation. The inhibition of angiotensin I conversion decreases AT_1-mediated vasoconstriction and decreases aldosterone secretion; both of these effects act to decrease blood pressure. The inhibition of kininase II activity results in higher bradykinin levels, which promote vasodilation. The increased vasodilation decreases peripheral vascular resistance, which decreases blood pressure. In contrast, AT_1 antagonists (also known as angiotensin receptor blockers [ARBs]) decrease aldosterone synthesis and interrupt AT_1-mediated vasoconstriction but do not alter bradykinin levels. Note that bradykinin-induced cough is a major side effect of ACE inhibitors but not of AT_1 antagonists. Adapted with permission from Katzung BG, ed. Basic & Clinical Pharmacology, 8th Ed, Figure 11-6, page 173. New York: Lange Medical Books/The McGraw-Hill Companies, Inc., 2001.

OBJECTIVES

▪ Understand the physiology and pathophysiology of extracellular volume regulation.

▪ Understand the pharmacology of, indications for, and adverse effects of agents that modify the neurohormonal signals controlling volume regulation.

▪ Understand the pharmacology of, indications for, and adverse effects of agents that alter renal sodium and water reabsorption.

▪ CASE 1

Seventy-year-old Mr. R. is taken by ambulance to the emergency department at 1:00 AM after waking up with shortness of breath for the fourth night in a row. Each time he "felt tight in the chest" and "couldn't get a breath"; this discomfort was relieved somewhat by sitting up in bed. He also recalls previous episodes of shortness of breath while climbing stairs.

Physical examination reveals tachycardia, mild hypertension, pedal edema (edema of the feet and lower legs), and bilateral pulmonary crackles on inspiration. Serum chemistries show no elevation of troponin T (a marker of cardiomyocte injury) but mildly elevated creatinine and blood urea nitrogen (BUN). The electrocardiogram shows evidence of an old myocardial infarction. Echocardiography reveals diminished left ventricular ejection fraction (the fraction of blood in the ventricle at the end of diastole that is ejected when the ventricle contracts) without ventricular dilatation.

Based on the clinical findings of decreased cardiac output, pulmonary congestion, and peripheral edema, Mr. R. is diagnosed with acute heart failure. His increased creatinine and BUN also indicate an element of renal insufficiency.

QUESTIONS

1. What mechanisms led to Mr. R.'s pulmonary congestion and pedal edema?
   A. Acute renal failure caused sodium and water reabsorption, volume overload, and increased pulmonary congestion and pedal edema.
   B. Acute myocardial infarction diminished left ventricular function and caused increased pulmonary congestion and pedal edema.
   C. Compromised cardiac function caused renal sodium and water reabsorption, leading to pulmonary congestion and pedal edema.
   D. Acute lung injury caused transudation of fluid into the pulmonary interstitium and pulmonary congestion.
   E. Compromised cardiac function caused pedal edema, which progressed to pulmonary congestion according to the overflow model of volume regulation.

Pharmacologic therapy is started, including a positive inotrope, a coronary vasodilator, an antihypertensive angiotensin-converting enzyme (ACE) inhibitor, and a loop diuretic. After Mr. R.'s condition stabilizes over the course of 3 days, the dose of the loop diuretic is decreased and then discontinued.

2. Why was Mr. R. given a loop diuretic?
   A. Loop diuretics inhibit sodium reabsorption in the distal convoluted tubule, while causing a direct vasodilatory effect, which is beneficial in patients with heart failure.
   B. Loop diuretics inhibit the high capacity for sodium reabsorption in the thick ascending loop of Henle and cause a rapid diuresis and reduction in intravascular volume.
   C. Loop diuretics inhibit sodium reabsorption in the collecting duct where the highest intralumenal sodium concentration is delivered in the setting of heart failure.
   D. Loop diuretics inhibit sodium, calcium, and potassium reabsorption throughout the nephron, reducing intravascular volume and enhancing the secretion of dangerously elevated electrolytes.
   E. Loop diuretics inhibit sodium reabsorption in the thick ascending loop of Henle while reversing the pathologic cardiac contractile dysfunction associated with heart failure.

3. Diuretic drugs decrease renal sodium reabsorption along four segments of the nephron, regulating urinary volume and composition. Which of the following statements regarding diuretic agents is correct?
   A. Carbonic anhydrase inhibitors can precipitate acute glaucoma.
   B. Thiazide diuretics can exacerbate nephrolithiasis.
   C. Loop diuretics rapidly reduce cerebral intravascular volume in the setting of closed head trauma.
   D. Potassium-sparing diuretics inhibit the action of aldosterone at the mineralocorticoid receptor.
   E. Mannitol is associated with ototoxicity.

Elective coronary angiography reveals significant stenosis of the left anterior descending coronary artery. Mr. R. undergoes balloon angioplasty and stent placement and remains stable as an outpatient. His discharge drug regimen is accompanied by a low-salt, low-fat diet.

4. How do ACE inhibitors improve cardiovascular hemodynamics?
   A. ACE inhibitors prevent pregnancy-associated cardiomyopathy.
   B. ACE inhibitors increase bradykinin levels to inhibit tachyarrhythmias.

C. ACE inhibitors antagonize the vasoconstrictive effects of angiotensin at its receptors.

D. ACE inhibitors inhibit antidiuretic hormone synthesis and reduce water reabsorption and intravascular volume.

E. ACE inhibitors cause arterial vasodilation and limit the development of post–myocardial infarction cardiomyopathy.

5. Sodium reabsorption is greatest in the:
A. proximal tubule
B. sinusoids
C. thick ascending limb of the loop of Henle
D. distal convoluted tubule
E. collecting duct

 CASE 2

Kathy M. is a 42-year-old woman with a long history of alcohol abuse, drinking up to 2 pints of vodka on a daily basis for 10 to 15 years. She last saw her primary doctor, Dr. Binney, for a routine visit 5 years ago. He counseled her regarding her alcohol use and urged her to consider joining Alcoholics Anonymous. He warned her that she was risking many long-term complications if she did not stop drinking.

Ms. M. returns to Dr. Binney today with fears that she may be ill. She has gained approximately 12 pounds in the past 2 weeks and notes that her feet and ankles are swollen. Her sneakers are tight and her socks leave a mark around her ankles. She feels generally fatigued.

On his examination, Dr. Binney notes that Ms. M. looks rather pale, but has palmar erythema and scattered spider angiomata over her chest. Her abdomen is somewhat protuberant, and he notes a nontender nodular liver edge extending 3 cm below the right costal margin. He also notes shifting dullness on percussion of her abdomen when he moves her from a supine to a decubitus position. Her ankles and feet are swollen with pitting edema. He orders an ultrasound, which shows a small, nodular liver, but no focal masses, consistent with cirrhosis..

QUESTIONS

1. What is the relationship between hepatic cirrhosis and the development of ascites and edema?
A. The underfill theory proposes that increased intrahepatic hydrostatic pressure causes ascites, diminishes intravascular volume, and promotes renal sodium reabsorption.
B. Hepatic synthetic function is diminished, including the production of peptide hormones, which are responsible for maintaining vascular endothelial cell tight junctions.
C. The overflow model of ascites proposes that renal failure leads to excessive sodium retention, volume overload, and increased intrahepatic hydrostatic pressure.

D. Hepatic damage allows albumin to cross the hepatic sinusoids into the interstitial tissues, reversing oncotic pressures and causing ascites and interstitial edema.
E. Hepatic cirrhosis obstructs flow in the portal vein, shunting blood to the lower extremities.

Dr. Binney orders laboratory studies, including complete blood count with platelet count; electrolytes, including potassium; and tests of synthetic liver function and renal function. After reviewing the results, he warns Ms. M. that she has significant damage to her liver, probably caused by her chronic alcohol use. He gives her instructions for strict sodium restriction and a prescription for spironolactone, a potassium-sparing diuretic. She is to weigh herself daily until he sees her in 3 weeks. Lastly, he again urges her to get help with alcohol abstinence.

2. What is the role of spironolactone in the treatment of cirrhosis-induced edema?
A. Spironolactone retards the progression of hepatic cirrhosis by inhibiting growth factor–mediated fibrosis.
B. Spironolactone is a potent diuretic that rapidly reduces the extent of ascites and peripheral edema.
C. Spironolactone promotes the retention of potassium, which is lost from the intravascular space through transudation into ascitic fluid.
D. Spironolactone inhibits the androgen receptor and the development of gynecomastia in chronic alcohol use with cirrhosis.
E. Spironolactone antagonizes the effects of hyperaldosteronism in cirrhosis with edema.

Ms. M. takes the spironolactone and restricts her sodium intake. She loses approximately 8 pounds, and although her feet are swollen by the end of the day, her sneakers are less tight when she puts them on in the morning. Two weeks after her visit to Dr. Binney, she gets a phone call in the middle of the night with the tragic news that her son has been killed in a motorcycle crash. In the midst of her grief, she neglects taking her medication, and within a week, she is again drinking heavily on a daily basis. She misses her follow-up appointment with Dr. Binney, and despite a phone call and reminder letters from his office, she does not return to primary care.

3. Potential adverse effects of potassium-sparing diuretics include:
A. hypokalemic metabolic alkalosis
B. hirsutism
C. hyperkalemic contraction alkalosis
D. hyperkalemic metabolic acidosis
E. diabetes insipidus

Six months later, Dr. Binney receives a call from an urgent care clinic. Ms. M. has arrived there complaining of severe shortness of breath and abdominal "tightness." She is transported by ambulance to the local emergency department, where Dr. Binney meets her. She is disheveled and in moderate respiratory distress. Her vital signs reveal a normal temperature, heart rate of 132 bpm, respiratory rate of 24 breaths/min., and blood pressure of 96/52 mm Hg. When Dr. Binney examines her, he notes scleral icterus, bilateral basilar pulmonary crackles, and a firm, distended abdomen with a fluid wave, consistent with grade 3 severe ascites. He also notes that Ms. M. has edema of her lower extremities, which starts at her feet and reaches to the inguinal ligament. She is admitted to the hospital.

4. After the resident physician performs a paracentesis to remove approximately 5 L of thin, yellowish ascitic fluid from Ms. M.'s abdomen, Dr. Binney asks the nurse to administer intravenous fluids. Which of the following intravenous agents will act as a volume expander by increasing the intravascular oncotic pressure, and promoting the movement of interstitial fluid back into the intravascular space?
    A. mannitol
    B. potassium
    C. desmopressin
    D. albumin
    E. water

5. Which of the following is elevated in response to volume overload?
    A. kininase II
    B. renin
    C. B-type natriuretic peptide
    D. vasopressin
    E. albumin

21

Pharmacology of Vascular Tone

Figure 21-1. Mechanism of Vascular Smooth Muscle Cell Contraction and Relaxation. Vascular smooth muscle cell contraction and relaxation are controlled by the coordinated action of several intracellular signaling mediators. Ca^{2+} entry through L-type voltage-gated Ca^{2+} channels (left panel) is the initial stimulus for contraction. Ca^{2+} entry into the cell activates calmodulin (CaM). The Ca^{2+}–CaM complex activates myosin light chain kinase (MLCK) to phosphorylate myosin light chain (Myosin-LC). The phosphorylated myosin-LC interacts with actin to form actin–myosin crossbridges, a process that initiates vascular smooth muscle cell contraction. Relaxation (right panel) is a coordinated series of steps that act to dephosphorylate (and hence inactivate) myosin-LC. Nitric oxide (NO) diffuses into the cell and activates guanylyl cyclase. The activated guanylyl cyclase catalyzes the conversion of guanosine triphosphate (GTP) to guanosine 3',5'-cyclic monophosphate (cGMP). cGMP activates myosin-LC phosphatase, which dephosphorylates myosin light chain, preventing actin–myosin crossbridge formation. As a result, the vascular smooth muscle cell relaxes. The active form of each enzyme is italicized.

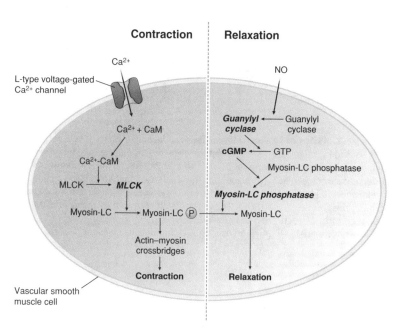

OBJECTIVES

- Understand the molecular basis for the control of vascular tone.
- Understand the pharmacology, therapeutic uses, and adverse effects of various classes of vasodilators.

■ CASE 1

G.F., a 63-year-old man with a history of hypertension, diabetes, and hypercholesterolemia, begins to develop episodes of chest pain on exertion. One week after his first episode, a bout of chest pain occurs while he is mowing the lawn. Twenty minutes after the onset of this pain, G.F. takes two of his wife's sublingual nitroglycerin tablets. Within a few minutes, he feels much better.

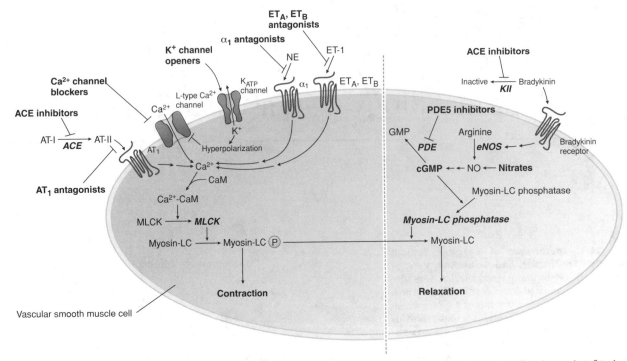

Figure 21-2. Sites of Action of Vasodilators. Vasodilators act at several sites in the vascular smooth muscle cell. Left panel: Ca^{2+} channel blockers and K^{+} channel openers inhibit the entry of Ca^{2+} into vascular smooth muscle cells by decreasing activation of L-type Ca^{2+} channels. Angiotensin-converting enzyme (ACE) inhibitors, angiotensin I (AT$_1$) antagonists, α_1-antagonists, and endothelin receptor (ET$_A$, ET$_B$) antagonists all decrease intracellular Ca^{2+} signaling. The decreased cytosolic Ca^{2+} results in less vascular smooth muscle cell contraction, and, hence, in relaxation. Right panel: ACE inhibitors inhibit kininase II (KII), leading to increased levels of bradykinin. Nitrates release NO. Sildenafil inhibits phosphodiesterase (PDE). These agents all cause an increase in cGMP, an effect that promotes vascular smooth muscle relaxation. The active form of each enzyme is italicized. α_1 = α_1-adrenergic receptor; CaM = calmodulin; eNOS = endothelial nitric oxide synthase; ET-1 = endothelin-1; MLCK = myosin light chain kinase; Myosin-LC = myosin light chain; PDE = phosphodiesterase.

QUESTIONS

1. What is the mechanism by which sublingual nitroglycerin acts so quickly to relieve chest pain?

    A. Sublingual nitroglycerin is rapidly absorbed and metabolized to nitric oxide, which increases intracellular concentrations of peroxynitrite and inhibits guanylyl cyclase-associated vasoconstriction of epicardial arteries, and increases myocardial oxygen supply.

    B. Sublingual nitroglycerin is rapidly absorbed and activated by a first-pass metabolism in the coronary artery epithelial cells to inhibit nitric oxide breakdown and increase nitric oxide–associated epicardial arterial dilation and myocardial oxygen supply.

    C. Sublingual nitroglycerin is rapidly absorbed and metabolized to nitric oxide, which dilates the pulmonary vasculature, relieving pulmonary hypertension and increasing myocardial oxygen supply.

    D. Sublingual nitroglycerin is rapidly absorbed and metabolized to nitric oxide, which dilates systemic veins and epicardial arteries, decreasing myocardial oxygen demand and increasing myocardial oxygen supply.

    E. Sublingual nitroglycerin is rapidly absorbed and metabolized to nitric oxide, which dilates systemic arterioles, decreasing systemic vascular resistance and reducing myocardial oxygen demand.

2. Which of the following is a common adverse effect of nitroglycerin administration?

    A. hepatitis
    B. transient vision loss
    C. bradycardia
    D. nausea
    E. headache

G.F. feels so well that he decides to take one of the sildenafil (Viagra) pills that a friend had previously offered to him. A few minutes after taking sildenafil, he feels flushed, develops a throbbing headache, and feels his heart racing. Upon standing, G.F. feels lightheaded and faints. He is taken immediately to the emergency department, where he is found to have severe hypotension.

3. How do sildenafil and organic nitrates interact to precipitate severe hypotension?

    A. Both agents promote vasodilation.
    B. Both agents reduce myocardial contractility.
    C. Both agents divert systemic blood flow to the corpus cavernosum.
    D. Both agents decrease the normal sympathetic tone of the systemic vasculature.
    E. Both agents promote transudation of fluid from the systemic vasculature and reduce the circulating intravascular volume.

G.F. is quickly placed in a supine position with his legs raised, and monitored until he regains consciousness. The physician considers administering an α-adrenergic agonist, such as phenylephrine, but the rapid amelioration of G.F.'s hypotension after he is placed in a supine position suggests that pharmacologic intervention is unnecessary. After G.F. recovers, his physician discusses with him the dangers of taking medications without a prescription and, specifically, the risk of concurrent administration of organic nitrates and sildenafil.

4. How would phenylephrine be effective in treating G.F.'s hypotension?

- **A.** Stimulation of α_1-adrenergic receptors in vascular smooth muscle would promote arterial vasoconstriction, and increase systemic vascular resistance and blood pressure.
- **B.** Stimulation of α_1-adrenergic receptors in the cardiac conduction system would increase heart rate and contractility, and increase cardiac output and blood pressure.
- **C.** Stimulation of α_1-adrenergic receptors in the vascular smooth muscle would promote venous constriction, decrease venous capacitance, and increase preload, cardiac output, and blood pressure.
- **D.** Stimulation of α_2-adrenergic receptors in the central nervous system would increase general sympathetic tone and increase cardiac output, systemic vascular resistance, and blood pressure.
- **E.** Stimulation of α_2-adrenergic receptors in the vascular smooth muscle would promote negative feedback of norepinephrine release and increase blood pressure.

5. Which of the following is the mechanism of action of minoxidil?

- **A.** It opens potassium channels, hyperpolarizes the cell, and promotes calcium release from the sarcoplasmic reticulum.
- **B.** It opens potassium channels and prevents binding of endothelin receptor agonists.
- **C.** It opens potassium channels and prevents depolarization and calcium influx.
- **D.** It opens calcium channels and promotes calcium influx.
- **E.** It blocks calcium channels and prevents depolarization and calcium influx.

■ CASE 2

Jack, a 15-year-old high school student, has a history of severe allergic reactions to bee stings. He carries an epinephrine auto-injector (EpiPen®) with him in case he is stung by a bee while outside at lacrosse practice. Jack is showing his teammates how it works when one of his friends accidentally discharges the injector and injects the palmar surface of the

base of his left index finger with 0.3 mg of a 1:1000 epinephrine solution. Within several minutes, his index finger looks pale and feels cold.

QUESTIONS

1. Under normal physiologic conditions, what is the control of epinephrine?

- **A.** Epinephrine is released at preganglionic receptors, which subsequently control norepinephrine release at the postsynaptic α- and β-adrenergic receptors.
- **B.** Epinephrine is released from the adrenal gland into the systemic circulation, where it provides negative feedback for the presynaptic release of norepinephrine.
- **C.** Epinephrine is released from presynaptic adrenergic nerve terminals on to postsynaptic α- and β-adrenergic receptors.
- **D.** Epinephrine is released from the adrenal gland directly on to postganglionic α- and β-adrenergic receptors.
- **E.** Epinephrine is released from the adrenal gland into the systemic circulation, where it can act at both α- and β-adrenergic receptors.

Jack's friend goes to the school nurse who soaks his finger in a hot water bath for 30 minutes. However, there is no change in the appearance of the finger. The lacrosse coach takes him to the nearest emergency department for evaluation. On arrival, his examination is remarkable for a heart rate of 68 bpm and blood pressure of 118/72 mm Hg. His finger is pale and cool. The capillary refill when the fingertip is compressed is delayed, approximately 5 seconds. The intern is concerned that the fingertip may become ischemic and initiates treatment with topical nitroglycerin paste.

2. What is the mechanism by which topical nitroglycerin paste might treat this patient's finger?

- **A.** Topical nitroglycerin is absorbed transdermally and inhibits phosphodiesterase type 3 to cause vasodilation.
- **B.** Topical nitroglycerin is absorbed transdermally and inhibits calcium influx to cause vasodilation.
- **C.** Topical nitroglycerin is absorbed transdermally and stimulates β_2-adrenergic receptors to cause vasodilation.
- **D.** Topical nitroglycerin is absorbed transdermally and releases nitric oxide to cause vasodilation.
- **E.** Topical nitroglycerin warms the skin locally to enhance the metabolism of epinephrine.

After 20 minutes, there is minimal improvement in the patient's finger. The attending physician uses a small-gauge needle to locally infiltrate phentolamine around the autoinjector site. Within 5 minutes, the finger is normal in color.

3. How did phentolamine treat this patient's pale, cool finger?

  A. Phentolamine stimulated calcium influx into the digital arteries.

  B. Phentolamine blocked α_1-adrenergic vasoconstriction of the digital arteries.

  C. Phentolamine released NO from endothelial cells of the digital arteries.

  D. Phentolamine enhanced the metabolism of epinephrine.

  E. Phentolamine enhanced β_2-adrenergic vasodilation of the digital arteries.

4. Which of the following statements regarding calcium channel blockers is true?

  A. Nifedipine can be administered once daily to control tachyarrhythmias.

  B. Diltiazem has high bioavailability because of its first-pass hepatic metabolism.

  C. Nifedipine can cause atrioventricular nodal block in overdose.

  D. Verapamil can cause a reflex tachycardia.

  E. Amlodipine has a delayed onset but a long duration of action.

5. Sodium nitroprusside non-enzymatically liberates nitric oxide to dilate both arteries and veins. What other compound is released during sodium nitroprusside metabolism, and what is the resultant toxicity?

  A. endothelin: pulmonary artery constriction and hypertension

  B. thiocyanate: metabolic acidosis, ventricular arrhythmias

  C. cyanide: acute renal failure

  D. cyanide: metabolic acidosis, ventricular arrhythmias

  E. cyanide: cyanosis, peripheral edema

22

Pharmacology of Hemostasis and Thrombosis

OBJECTIVES

- Understand the physiology of hemostasis and the pathogenesis of thrombosis.

- Understand the pharmacology of, indications for, and adverse of antiplatelet, anticoagulant, and thrombolytic agents.

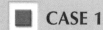 CASE 1

Mr. S., a 55-year-old man with a history of hypertension and cigarette smoking, is awakened in the middle of the night with substernal chest pressure, sweating, and shortness of breath. He calls 911 and is taken to the emergency department. An electrocardiogram shows deep T-wave inversions in leads V2–V5. A cardiac biomarker panel shows a creatine kinase level of 800 IU/L (normal, 600–400 IU/L) with 10% MB fraction (the heart-specific isoform), suggesting myocardial infarction. He is treated with intravenous nitroglycerin, aspirin, unfractionated heparin, and eptifibatide, but his chest pain persists. He is taken to the cardiac catheterization laboratory, where he is found to have a 90% mid-LAD (left anterior descending artery) thrombus with sluggish distal flow.

QUESTIONS

1. Which of the following factors could have contributed to a blood clot arising in Mr. S.'s coronary artery?
   A. aspirin use
   B. turbulent blood flow in the right atrium
   C. high blood pressure
   D. asthma
   E. neutropenia

Mr. S. undergoes successful angioplasty and stent placement. At the time of stent placement, an intravenous loading dose of clopidogrel is administered. The heparin is stopped, the eptifibatide is continued for 18 more hours, and he is transferred to the telemetry ward.

2. If low-molecular-weight heparin had been used instead of unfractionated heparin, how could the patient's coagulation status have been monitored?
   A. The prothombin time (PT) would accurately measure the anticoagulant effect of low-molecular-weight heparin.
   B. The activated partial thromboplastin time (aPTT) would accurately measure the anticoagulant effect of low-molecular-weight heparin.
   C. Measurement of antithrombin activity would reflect the anticoagulant effect of low-molecular-weight heparin.
   D. Accurate measurement of the anticoagulant effect of low-molecular-weight heparin would depend on the measurement of anti-factor Xa activity.
   E. Measurement of the anticoagulant effect of low-molecular-weight heparin would be inaccurate if Mr. S. had renal insufficiency.

Six hours later, Mr. S. is noted to have an expanding hematoma (an area of localized hemorrhage) in his right thigh below the arterial access site. The eptifibatide is stopped and pressure is applied to the access site. The hematoma ceases to expand.

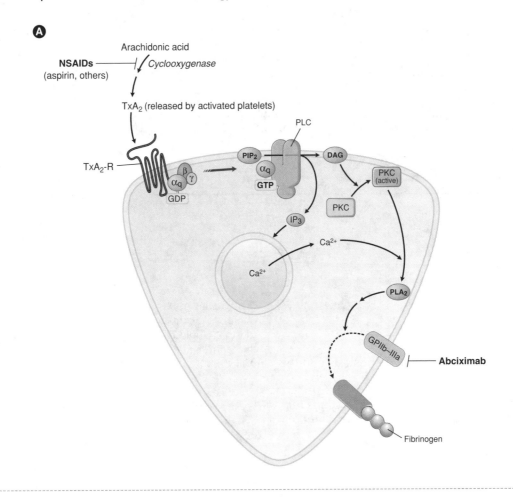

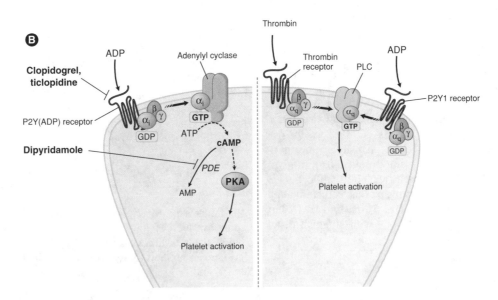

Figure 22-1.   Mechanism of Action of Antiplatelet Agents. A. Nonsteroidal anti-inflammatory drugs (NSAIDs) and glycoprotein IIB–IIIa (GPIIb–IIIa) antagonists inhibit steps in thromboxane A_2 (TxA$_2$)–mediated platelet activation. Aspirin inhibits cyclooxygenase by covalent acetylation of the enzyme near its active site, leading to decreased TxA$_2$ production. The effect is profound because platelets lack the ability to synthesize new enzyme molecules. GPIIb–IIIa antagonists, such as the monoclonal antibody abciximab and the small-molecule antagonists eptifibatide and tirofiban (not shown), inhibit platelet aggregation by preventing activation of GPIIb–IIIa (dashed line), leading to decreased platelet crosslinking by fibrinogen. **B.** Clopidogrel, ticlopidine, and dipyridamole inhibit steps in adenosine diphosphate (ADP)–mediated platelet activation. Clopidogrel and ticlopidine are antagonists of the P2Y(ADP) receptor. Dipyridamole inhibits phosphodiesterase (PDE), thereby preventing the breakdown of cyclic adenosine monophosphate (cAMP) and increasing cytoplasmic cAMP concentration.

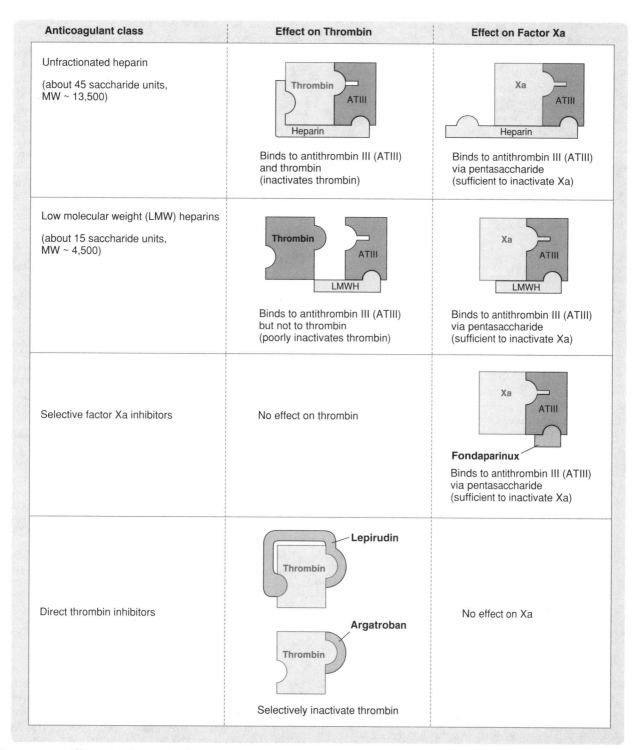

Figure 22-2. Differential Effects of Unfractionated Heparin and Low Molecular Weight Heparin on Coagulation Factor Inactivation.
Effect on thrombin: To catalyze the inactivation of thrombin, heparin must bind both to antithrombin III via a high-affinity pentasaccharide unit and to thrombin via an additional 13-saccharide unit. Low molecular weight heparin (LMWH) does not contain a sufficient number of saccharide units to bind thrombin, and therefore is a poor catalyst for thrombin inactivation. Selective factor Xa inhibitors do not inactivate thrombin, while direct thrombin inhibitors selectively inactivate thrombin. *Effect on factor Xa:* Inactivation of factor Xa requires only the binding of antithrombin III to the high-affinity pentasaccharide unit. Since unfractionated heparin, low molecular weight heparin, and fondaparinux all contain this pentasaccharide, these agents are all able to catalyze the inactivation of factor Xa. Direct thrombin inhibitors have no effect on factor Xa.

3. What accounts for the efficacy of eptifibatide in inhibiting platelet aggregation?
  A. Eptifibatide enhances endothelial cell production of prostacyclin, which inhibits platelet aggregation.
  B. Eptifibatide is an antagonist at the platelet GPIIb–IIIa receptor, preventing fibrinogen binding to platelets.
  C. Eptifibatide is a mouse–human monoclonal antibody directed against platelet-derived thromboxane, preventing its activation of platelet aggregation.
  D. Eptifibatide catalyzes the degradation of fibrinogen, preventing its binding to activated platelets.
  E. Eptifibatide inhibits adenylyl cyclase and reduces intracellular cyclic adenosine monophosphate (cAMP) levels and subsequent platelet activation and aggregation.

4. When the expanding hematoma was observed, could any measure other than stopping the eptifibatide have been used to reverse the effect of this agent?
  A. Infuse vitamin K to reverse the effect of this agent.
  B. Infuse washed and irradiated platelets to reverse the effect of this agent.
  C. Infuse protamine to reverse the effect of this agent.
  D. Infuse fresh-frozen plasma to reverse the effect of this agent.
  E. There is no measure to reverse the effect of this agent other than stopping the eptifibatide.

Mr. S. is discharged 2 days later with prescriptions for clopidogrel and aspirin, which are administered to prevent subacute thrombosis of the stent.

5. Aspirin, heparin, clopidogrel, and eptifibatide all have actions that limit thrombus formation. Which of the following statements correctly describes how these agents will treat Mr. S.'s blood clot and prevent recurrent thrombus formation?
  A. Clopidogrel modifies and inactivates the platelet ADP receptor and inhibits adenylyl cyclase production of cAMP, preventing platelet aggregation.
  B. Heparin prevents the generation of reduced vitamin K, which is necessary for the hepatic production of activated clotting factors.
  C. Aspirin inhibits endothelial cell COX-2 generation of platelet-activating thromboxane.
  D. Eptifibatide enhances the normal activity of anti-thrombin III.
  E. Clopidogrel antagonizes fibrinogen binding to the ADP receptor and inhibits platelet aggregation.

■ CASE 2

Ms. Eliza S. is a 32-year-old business consultant for an information technology start-up firm. She has just returned from a 5-day business trip to Tokyo. Despite flying business class in both directions, she notes some discomfort in her left calf on the return trip and cannot get comfortable. The following day, the discomfort is more pronounced and painful in the thick part of her calf and behind her knee. It hurts when she walks, especially in high heels. She calls her family practitioner for a checkup.

Ms. S.'s doctor examines her and notes normal vital signs. Her examination is unremarkable except for some swelling and tenderness in her left calf. When she measures the circumference of Ms. S.'s calves 8 cm below the inferior edge of the patella, the left calf measures 2 cm greater in circumference than the right. She sends Ms. S. to the local hospital vascular diagnostic lab for a lower extremity noninvasive ultrasound of her calf. The test reveals lack of compressibility in Ms. S.'s left popliteal vein, consistent with a deep venous thrombosis.

QUESTIONS

1. What is the major cause of venous thrombus formation?
  A. turbulent blood flow associated with valves in lower extremity veins
  B. stasis of blood flow
  C. cigarette smoking
  D. atrial fibrillation
  E. aneurysm formation in lower extremity veins

Ms. S.'s doctor explains the diagnosis to her. On further questioning, she learns that Ms. S.'s older sister had a "blood clot in her lung" several years ago. Her doctor questions her further regarding her personal and family history and reviews her medication list with her.

2. Which of the following is a *primary* cause of hypercoagulability?
  A. oral contraceptive use
  B. postpartum state
  C. antiphospholipid syndrome
  D. transcontinental plane flights
  E. factor V Leiden mutation

Ms. S.'s doctor explains that she will need to begin anticoagulation therapy while the workup for hypercoagulability is begun. She is started on subcutaneous low-molecular-weight heparin and oral warfarin therapy. She is instructed to return to the office in 3 days to have blood drawn for laboratory studies to measure the degree of anticoagulation achieved with warfarin therapy.

3. Why does Ms. Smith need to be treated with low molecular weight heparin in addition to warfarin?
  A. It takes several days for warfarin to reach a steady-state plasma concentration.
  B. Warfarin's degradation of clotting factors begins to affect coagulation after 3 to 4 drug half-lives.
  C. Warfarin's pharmacologic effect on the inhibition of

clotting factor activation is not manifested for 3 to 4 clotting factor half-lives.

D. Warfarin's destruction of reduced vitamin K takes several days to affect the synthesis of activated clotting factors.

E. It takes several days for warfarin to build up toxic levels in the liver.

Three months pass, and Ms. S. continues her warfarin as directed while her prothrombin time is monitored intermittently. Four months after the initiation of warfarin therapy, Ms. S. and her partner are surprised and pleased to find that she is pregnant! She calls her family practitioner to arrange an obstetric visit. Her doctor tells her she must discontinue her warfarin and come in for an evaluation of her pregnancy and her need for further anticoagulation.

4. What is a pregnancy-associated adverse effect of warfarin therapy?

A. Warfarin can induce the P450 enzyme system, and hasten the metabolism of prenatal vitamins.

B. Prenatal vitamins can enhance the gastrointestinal absorption of warfarin.

C. Warfarin can cause congenital malformations in the fetus.

D. Warfarin can cause microvascular thromboses as a result of its effects on the synthesis of activated protein C and S.

E. Warfarin can inhibit the formation of vitamin K, which is necessary for fetal heart development.

5. Which of the following statements regarding thrombolytic agents is correct?

A. The administration of streptokinase can elicit an antigenic response.

B. The administration of orgatroban can elicit an antigenic response.

C. Tenecteplase has a longer half-life than tissue plasminogen activator (t-PA) and must be administered as a slow, continuous infusion.

D. Recombinant tissue plasminogen activator (t-PA) activates plasminogen only at the site of newly formed thrombi.

E. Aprotinin activates plasmin, but its use has been associated with postoperative acute renal failure.

23

Pharmacology of Cholesterol and Lipoprotein Metabolism

OBJECTIVES

■ Understand the biochemistry and physiology of cholesterol and lipoprotein metabolism.

■ Understand the pharmacology of, indications for, and adverse effects of agents used in the modification of lipid metabolism.

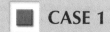

CASE 1

In June 1998, Jake P., a 29-year-old construction worker, makes an appointment to see Dr. Cush. Mr. P. complains of hard, elevated swellings around his Achilles tendon that seem to rub constantly against his construction boots. He had been hesitant to see the doctor (his last appointment was 10 years ago), but he remembers that his dad, who died at age 42 of a heart attack, had similar swellings. On examination, Dr. Cush recognizes the Achilles swellings as xanthomas (lipid deposits); the physical examination is otherwise within normal limits. Mr. P. comments that his daily diet is quite ''fatty,'' including three to four doughnuts each day and frequent hamburgers. Dr. Cush explains that the xanthomas on Mr. P.'s feet are the result of cholesteryl ester deposition, probably from high cholesterol levels in his blood. Dr. Cush orders a fasting plasma cholesterol level and recommends that he reduce his intake of foods high in saturated fat and cholesterol, and increase his intake of poultry, fish, whole cereal grains, fruits, and vegetables. Mr. P. has gained about 15 pounds since he was 19 and has a small ''paunch.'' Dr. Cush recommends regular exercise and weight loss.

Results of the blood test reveal a total plasma cholesterol concentration of 300 mg/dL (normal, < 200), with elevated low-density lipoprotein (LDL) cholesterol of 250 mg/dL (desirable, <100), low high-density lipoprotein HDL of 35 mg/dL (normal, 35–100), and normal concentrations of triglycerides and very low-density lipoprotein (VLDL). Based on these test results, his age, the Achilles heel xanthomas, and a family history for an early myocardial infarction, Dr. Cush tells Mr. P. that he likely has an inherited disorder of cholesterol metabolism, probably heterozygous familial hypercholesterolemia. This disease puts him at high risk for early atherosclerosis and myocardial infarction, but aggressive lowering of cholesterol levels can ameliorate many of the disease sequelae. The low HDL cholesterol level also contributes to his increased risk of cardiovascular disease.

QUESTIONS

1. What is the etiology of familial hypercholesterolemia?
A. an autosomal dominant disease causing an excess of LDL receptors
B. an autosomal dominant disease causing defective LDL receptor formation
C. an autosomal dominant disease causing decreased affinity of LDL for its receptor
D. an autosomal recessive disease causing absence of LPL (lipoprotein lipase)
E. an autosomal dominant disease causing increased hepatic triglyceride synthesis

2. How do high cholesterol levels predispose to cardiovascular disease?
A. Excess LDL cholesterol damages the cap over atherosclerotic lesions.
B. Excess LDL cholesterol upregulates LDL receptor expression and LDL uptake by macrophages.
C. Excess LDL cholesterol downregulates LDL receptor expression and LDL uptake by hepatocytes.
D. Excess LDL cholesterol accumulates in macrophages in atherosclerotic lesions.
E. Excess LDL cholesterol downregulates HMG CoA reductase activity.

In addition to the dietary changes, Dr. Cush prescribes a statin to help reduce Mr. P.'s cholesterol. A starting dose of a statin reduces his LDL by 30% to 175 mg/dL, while his

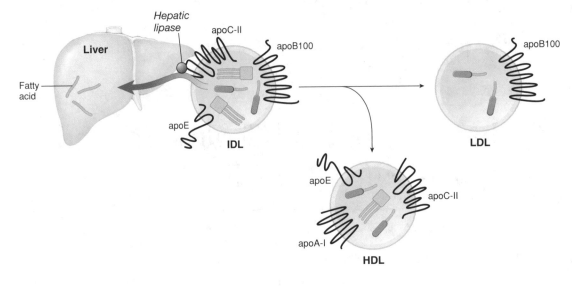

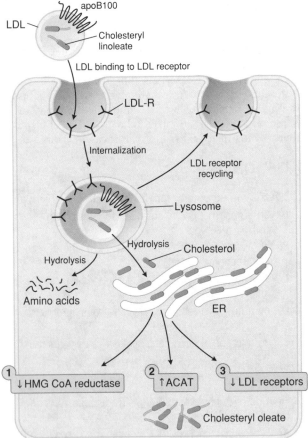

Figure 23-1. Formation and Clearance of Low-Density Lipoprotein (LDL) Particles. Top. Formation of LDL occurs when IDL particles interact with hepatic lipase to become denser and cholesteryl ester enriched. As a result, both apoE and apoCII lose affinity for the particle and are transferred to high-density lipoprotein (HDL), leaving only apoB100. **Bottom.** Binding of apolipoprotein B100 to LDL receptors on hepatocytes or other cell types promotes LDL internalization into endocytic vesicles and fusion of the vesicles with lysosomes. Whereas LDL receptors are recycled to the cell surface, lipoprotein particles are hydrolyzed into amino acids, releasing free cholesterol. Intracellular cholesterol has three regulatory effects on the cell. First, cholesterol decreases the activity of HMG-CoA reductase, the rate-limiting enzyme in cholesterol biosynthesis. Second, cholesterol activates acetyl CoA: cholesterol acyltransferase (ACAT), an enzyme that esterifies free cholesterol into cholesteryl esters for intracellular storage or export. Third, cholesterol inhibits the transcription of the gene encoding the LDL receptor, thereby decreasing further uptake of cholesterol by the cell. ER, endoplasmic reticulum.

Figure 23-2. Reverse Cholesterol Transport. A. The process of reverse cholesterol transport begins when apoAI is secreted from the liver. ApoAI in plasma interacts with ATP binding cassette protein AI (ABCA1), which incorporates a small amount of phospholipid and unesterified cholesterol from hepatocyte plasma membranes to form a discoidal-shaped pre-β-HDL particle. Due to the activity of lecithin cholesterol: acyltransferase (LCAT) in plasma, pre-β-HDL particles mature to form spherical α-HDL. Spherical α-HDL particles function to accept excess unesterified cholesterol from the plasma membranes of cells in a wide variety of tissues. The unesterified cholesterol is transferred from the cell to nearby HDL particles by diffusion through the plasma. As explained in Panel B, LCAT and phospholipid transfer protein (PLTP) increase the capacity of HDL to accept unesterified cholesterol molecules from cells by allowing for expansion of the core and the surface coat of the particle. Cholesteryl ester transfer protein (CETP) removes cholesteryl ester molecules from HDL and replaces them with triglycerides from remnant particles. HDL particles interact with scavenger receptor, class B type I (SR-BI), which mediates selective hepatic uptake of cholesteryl esters, but not apoAI. This process is facilitated when hepatic lipase hydrolyzes triglycerides from the core of the particle. The remaining apoAI

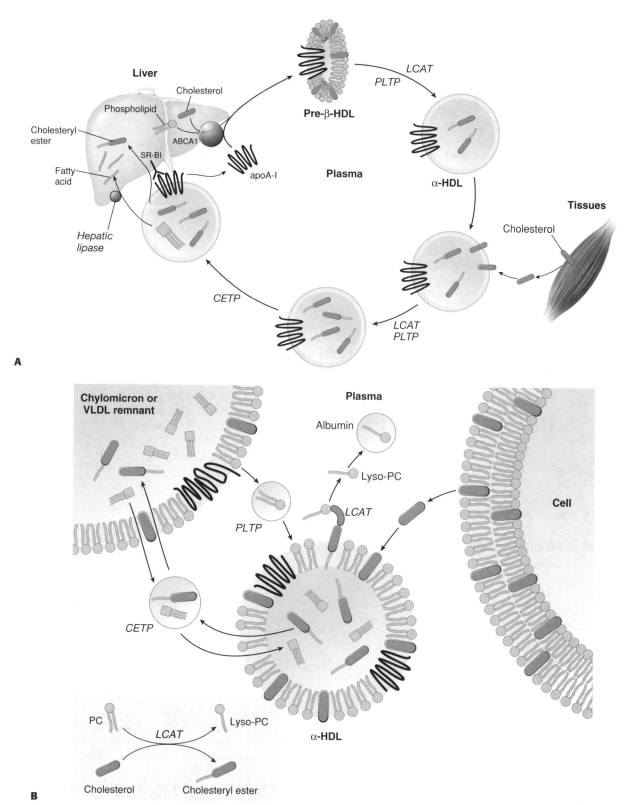

Figure 23-2. molecules may begin the cycle of reverse cholesterol transport again. **B.** LCAT, PLTP, and CETP promote the removal of excess cholesterol from the plasma membranes of cells. LCAT removes a fatty acid from a phosphatidylcholine molecule in the surface coat of α- (or pre-β-) HDL and esterifies an unesterified cholesterol molecule on the surface of the particle. The resulting lysophosphatidylcholine (lyso-PC) becomes bound to albumin in the plasma, whereas the cholesteryl ester migrates spontaneously into the core of the lipoprotein particle. The unesterified cholesterol molecules that are consumed by LCAT are replaced by unesterified cholesterol from cells. HDL phospholipids that are consumed by LCAT action are replaced with excess phospholipids from remnant particles by the activity of PLTP. As described in Panel A, CETP increases the efficiency of cholesterol movement to the liver by transporting cholesteryl ester molecules from α-HDL to VLDL remnants in exchange for triglycerides. Unlike phospholipids, triglycerides, and cholesteryl esters, unesterified cholesterol and lyso-PC move by diffusion through the plasma. Adapted with permission from Scapa Ef, Kanno K, Cohen DE. Lipoprotein Metabolism. In: Benhamou JP, Rizzetto M, Reichen J, Rodés J, Blei A, eds. The Textbook of Hepatology: From Basic Science to Clinical Practice. 3rd Ed, Figure 6B, Oxford, UK: Blackwell, 2006.

HDL slightly increases. Dr. Cush then increases the statin dose, and this produces an additional 12% reduction in LDL.

3. Which of the following statements regarding statins is correct?
   A. Statins upregulate the activity of LPL.
   B. Statins competitively inhibit the activity of the LDL receptor.
   C. Statins competitively inhibit the activity of HMG CoA reductase.
   D. Statins begin to reduce cardiovascular mortality once coronary artery disease becomes clinically apparent.
   E. Statins reduce LDL cholesterol, such that the higher the drug dose, the greater the reduction in LDL.

Because Mr. P.'s LDL has still not reached <100 mg/dL and his HDL remains low, Dr. Cush adds the cholesterol absorption inhibitor ezetimibe, as well as extended-release niacin. After these modifications, Mr. P.'s LDL drops below 100 mg/dL, and his HDL increases to 45 mg/dL. He experiences cutaneous flushing during the first few months of niacin treatment, but after that period, he has only occasional flushing episodes.

4. What is the mechanism of action of ezetimibe in lowering cholesterol?
   A. Ezetimibe inhibits cholesterol incorporation into VLDL by the liver.
   B. Ezetimibe displaces cholesterol from chylomicrons and facilitates its transport to the liver.
   C. Ezetimibe binds to, and interrupts, bile acid and cholesterol enterohepatic circulation.
   D. Ezetimibe displaces dietary cholesterol from micelles and enhances its loss in the feces.
   E. Ezetimibe inhibits cholesterol uptake through a brush border protein on enterocytes.

5. Niacin is nicotinic acid, vitamin B_3. How does it lower cholesterol and triglycerides?
   A. Niacin enhances hepatic triglyceride uptake and decreases hepatic VLDL synthesis.
   B. Niacin enhances peripheral triglyceride uptake and decreases hepatic VLDL synthesis.
   C. Niacin decreases peripheral triglyceride breakdown and decreases hepatic triglyceride synthesis.
   D. Niacin enhances prostaglandin-mediated cholesterol uptake by foam cells.
   E. Niacin promotes the formation of HDL and limits cholesterol circulation.

■ CASE 2

In 1998, Jenny J., a 42-year-old woman with familial hypercholesterolemia, was being treated with cerivastatin and gemfibrozil for her elevated lipids. She knew that a reduction in her LDL and cholesterol would protect her heart.

QUESTIONS

1. In addition to reducing LDL cholesterol concentrations, statins have also been demonstrated to have other pharmacologic effects, which may ameliorate the underlying pathophysiologic states associated with the development of atherosclerotic cardiovascular disease. These pleiotropic effects include:
   A. enhanced fibrinogen expression
   B. decreased nitric oxide production
   C. decreased inflammation
   D. induction of foam cell apoptosis
   E. enhanced smooth muscle remodeling

Within 1 month of initiating therapy, Ms. J. complained to her doctor that she felt an aching in her legs when she walked up the stairs. Sometimes the leg pain and weakness were so severe that she would limit her usual daily exercise. Her doctor ordered a serum creatine kinase level, which returned within normal limits. He suggested that she increase her fluid intake because it was an especially hot summer. When she went on vacation for 2 weeks, Ms. J. forgot to bring her medications. Remarkably, her leg pain and weakness did not bother her, and she had a wonderful time playing tennis at a resort in the Caribbean.

2. Statin-associated myositis and rhabdomyolysis is associated with:
   A. fenofibrate therapy
   B. concomitant administration of drugs, which induce the P450 enzymes
   C. elevated plasma creatine kinase screening levels in patients
   D. high dosages of more potent statins
   E. low dosages of less potent statins

When she returned home and resumed her medications, Ms. J. noted recurrent leg aches and difficulty walking upstairs within 2 days of restarting her medicines. Within 1 week, she noted that her urine was dark, and one night she was admitted to the hospital with severe weakness, nausea, muscle cramps, and shortness of breath when walking. Her vital signs revealed a temperature of 99°F, heart rate of 123 bpm, respiratory rate of 32 breaths/min., and blood pressure of 148/90 mm Hg. After laboratory testing, she was diagnosed with acute renal failure caused by rhabdomyolysis.

In August, 2001 Bayer Pharmaceutical Division voluntarily withdrew its HMG CoA reductase inhibitor Baycol (cerivastatin) from the U.S. market after reports of fatal rhabdomyolysis. The rare muscle disorder had been reported in patients using cerivastatin in combination with gemfibrozil, as well as those taking cerivastatin monotherapy. A review of Food and Drug Administration adverse event reports noted that the rate of fatal rhabdomyolysis was very rare but was 10 to 50 times as high in patients taking cerivastatin, compared with other statins.

3. What is a major adverse effect of concomitant statin and niacin therapy?
   A. facial flushing
   B. P450 enzyme inhibition
   C. abdominal bloating
   D. rhabdomyolysis
   E. vitamin B$_3$ wasting

4. Gemfibrozil and fenofibrate bind and activate receptors, which promote gene transcription associated with the expression of specific proteins involved in lipid metabolism. The clinical laboratory result of their action includes:

   A. increase in plasma HDL concentrations
   B. decrease in plasma total cholesterol levels
   C. increase in plasma VLDL concentrations
   D. decrease in plasma HDL concentrations
   E. increase in plasma LDL concentrations

5. Secondary factors that can lead to hyperlipidemia include:
   A. excessive ethanol intake
   B. niacin deficiency
   C. hyperthyroidism
   D. prolonged fasting
   E. excessive weight loss

24

Integrative Cardiovascular Pharmacology: Hypertension, Ischemic Heart Disease, and Heart Failure

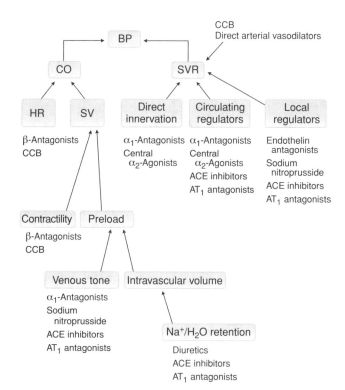

Figure 24-1. Pharmacologic Effects of Commonly Used Antihypertensive Agents. Antihypertensive agents modulate blood pressure by interfering with the determinants of blood pressure. Many of these antihypertensive drugs have multiple actions. For example, renin–angiotensin system blockers, such as angiotensin-converting enzyme (ACE) inhibitors and angiotensin II type 1 (AT_1) antagonists, alter the levels of local regulators and circulating regulators, and affect renal Na^+ retention and venous tone. BP = blood pressure; CCB = Ca^{2+} channel blocker; CO = cardiac output; HR = heart rate; SV = stroke volume; SVR = systemic vascular resistance. Adapted with permission from Deshmukh R, Smith A, Lilly LS. Hypertension. In: Lilly LS, ed. Pathophysiology of Heart Disease, 2nd Ed, Figure 13.10, page 286. Baltimore: Williams & Wilkins, 1998.

OBJECTIVES

▪ Understand the pharmacology, indications for, and adverse effects of agents used in the treatment of patients with hypertension, ischemic heart disease, and heart failure.

▪ CASE 1

Thomas N., a 45-year-old manager at a telecommunications company, presents to the cardiology clinic for evaluation of exertional shortness of breath. Mr. N. had always been zealous in maintaining aerobic fitness, but about 6 months before his cardiology clinic visit, he began to note severe breathlessness as he approached the completion of his daily run, which concludes with a long but gentle uphill climb. During the intervening 6 months, the patient reports a progression in his symptoms to the point that, now he rarely completes the first half of his daily run without resting. He denies chest discomfort at rest or with exercise. His family history is notable for hypertension and premature atherosclerosis. Mr. N. has never used tobacco products.

On examination, the patient is hypertensive (blood pressure, 160/102 mm Hg), and a prominent presystolic S4 is heard at the left ventricular apex. The examination is otherwise unremarkable. The chest X-ray is reported as normal. The 12-lead electrocardiogram (ECG) reveals normal sinus rhythm with voltage criteria for left ventricular hypertrophy. Mr. N. is referred for noninvasive cardiac evaluation, including a treadmill exercise test and a transthoracic echocardiogram. He reaches a peak heart rate of 170 bpm during exercise and has to terminate the test because of severe dyspnea at a workload of 7 METS. (METS are metabolic equivalents, a measure of energy consumption; a value of 7 METS is below normal for this patient's age.) There is no evidence of myocardial ischemia by ECG criteria. The two-dimensional

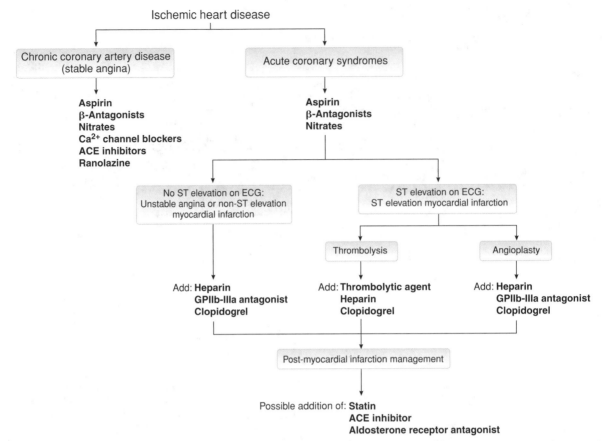

Figure 24-2. Pharmacologic Management of Acute Coronary Syndromes. All patients with chronic coronary artery disease are given aspirin unless a life-threatening contraindication is present. β-Antagonists, nitrates, calcium channel blockers, ACE inhibitors, and ranolazine are primarily used to reduce myocardial oxygen demand. All patients with symptoms that raise concerns about a possible acute coronary syndrome are given aspirin and, if tolerated, a β-antagonist. Sublingual or intravenous nitrates can also be given to relieve chest discomfort and minimize ischemia. Electrocardiographic (ECG) findings of ST elevation should prompt emergency measures to open the occluded artery, either with a thrombolytic agent (thrombolysis) or mechanical revascularization (angioplasty). Additional adjunctive pharmacologic therapies for ST elevation myocardial infarction may include aspirin, β-antagonists, nitrates, heparin, GPIIb–IIIa antagonists, and clopidogrel. For patients with acute coronary syndrome but no ST elevation on the electrocardiogram, laboratory assays of myocyte damage (e.g., troponin I or troponin T) determine whether the patient is classified as experiencing unstable angina or non-ST elevation myocardial infarction. In either case, management generally includes administration of aspirin, β-antagonists, nitrates, heparin, GPIIb–IIIa antagonists, and clopidogrel. For all patients with acute coronary syndrome, post-myocardial infarction management should include modification of risk factors, and possible addition of lipid-lowering agents (statins), ACE inhibitors, and aldosterone receptor antagonists. Adapted with permission from Libby P. Current concepts of the pathogenesis of acute coronary syndromes. Circulation. 2001;104:365–372.

echocardiogram reveals concentric-pattern left ventricular hypertrophy, an enlarged left atrium, and normal aortic and mitral valves. Left ventricular diastolic filling is abnormal with a reduced rate of early rapid filling and a significant increase in the extent of filling during atrial systole.

QUESTIONS

1. Given the severity of hypertension in this case, Mr. N. will likely require at least two drugs to achieve adequate control of his blood pressure. Which of the following statements concerning current recommendations for the initiation of drug therapy and therapeutic goals is correct?

   A. Initiate drug therapy for a diastolic blood pressure greater than 99 mm Hg; reduce diastolic blood pressure to less than 80 mm Hg.

   B. Initiate drug therapy for a systolic blood pressure greater than 140 mm Hg and diastolic blood pressure greater than 90 mm Hg; reduce blood pressure by 25%.

   C. Initiate drug therapy for a systolic blood pressure greater than 120 mm Hg; reduce systolic blood pressure to less than 120 mm Hg and diastolic blood pressure to less than 80 mm Hg.

   D. Initiate drug therapy for a systolic blood pressure greater than 150 mm Hg; reduce systolic blood pressure to less than 120 mm Hg.

   E. Initiate drug therapy for a systolic blood pressure greater than 160 mm Hg and diastolic blood pressure greater than 100 mm Hg; reduce systolic blood pressure to less than 120 mm Hg and diastolic blood pressure to less than 80 mm Hg.

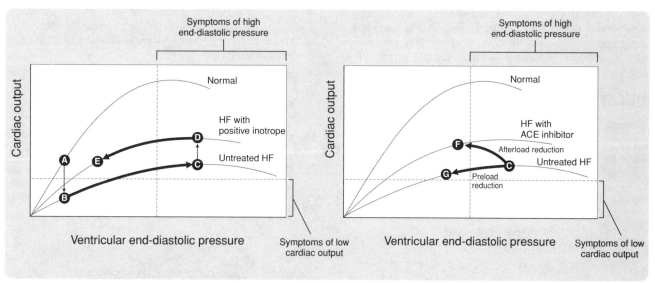

Figure 24-3. The Frank–Starling Relationship in Heart Failure. Left panel: The normal Frank–Starling relationship shows a steep increase in cardiac output with increasing ventricular end-diastolic pressure (preload). Point A describes the end-diastolic pressure and cardiac output of a normal heart under resting conditions. With contractile dysfunction (untreated heart failure [HF]), cardiac output falls (**B**) and the Frank–Starling curve flattens, so that increasing preload translates to only a modest increase in cardiac output (**C**). This increase in cardiac output is accompanied by symptoms of high end-diastolic pressure, such as dyspnea. Treatment with a positive inotrope, such as digitalis, shifts the Frank–Starling curve upward, and cardiac output increases (**D**). The improvement in myocardial contractility supports a sufficient reduction in preload that the venous congestion is relieved (**E**). **Right panel:** Two of the principal pharmacologic treatments of HF are afterload reduction (e.g., angiotensin-converting enzyme [ACE] inhibitors) and preload reduction (e.g., diuretics). Afterload reduction (**F**) increases cardiac output at any given preload, thereby elevating the Frank–Starling relationship. Preload reduction (**G**) alleviates congestive symptoms by decreasing ventricular end-diastolic pressure along the same Frank–Starling curve. Adapted with permission from Harvey RA, Champe PC, eds. Lippincott's Illustrated Reviews: Pharmacology, Figure 16-6, page 157. Philadelphia: Lippincott Williams & Wilkins, 1992.

2. Thiazide diuretics have been used for many years as "first-line" therapy in patients with hypertension. What is a potential adverse effect of monotherapy with a thiazide diuretic?
   A. hyperkalemia
   B. elevated triglycerides and hyperkalemia
   C. compensatory volume depletion and hypokalemia
   D. volume depletion and renal failure
   E. compensatory volume retention and hypokalemia

3. "High-output" hypertension may be caused by an increased sensitivity of the heart to basal levels of neurohumoral regulators. The hemodynamic pattern of increased cardiac output with normal systemic vascular resistance is often seen in younger patients, such as Mr. N., who have essential hypertension. An appropriate initial therapy for blood pressure control in these patients might include:
   A. metoprolol, a β-receptor antagonist
   B. prazosin, an α-receptor antagonist
   C. furosemide, a loop diuretic
   D. trimethaphan, a ganglionic blocker
   E. dietary salt restriction

4. Angiotensin-converting enzyme (ACE) inhibitors prevent the ACE-mediated conversion of angiotensin I to the vasoconstrictor angiotensin II. The effects of ACE inhibitors also include:

   A. decreased aldosterone release, promoting natriuresis
   B. increased bradykinin metabolism, contributing to the development of a chronic cough
   C. prevention of renin release and protection of the glomerular filtration rate
   D. inhibition of angiotensin II binding to its receptors, facilitating vasodilation
   E. development of a lupus-like syndrome, resulting in acute renal failure

5. Causes of secondary hypertension include:
   A. genetic predisposition
   B. oral contraceptive use
   C. excessive dietary salt intake
   D. elevated triglycerides
   E. excessive ethanol intake

■ CASE 2

Mr. N. is treated for hypertension with a β-blocker and an ACE inhibitor. He returns for follow-up visits at 1 month and 6 months and reports that he is doing well. He has faithfully adhered to his prescribed medical regimen and has noted a definite improvement in exercise capacity. His regular blood pressure measurements now show readings of 130–150/ 86–90 mm Hg. A serum lipid profile is notable for increased total cholesterol, with a moderately elevated low-density lipoprotein (LDL). Low-dose aspirin is added to his regimen. Treatment with a lipid-lowering agent is also advised, but Mr. N. declines, instead requesting that his profile be re-checked after a period of diet and lifestyle modifications.

QUESTIONS

1. Clinical studies indicate that drugs that lower serum LDL cholesterol decrease the risk of ischemic cardiovascular events in patients with known coronary artery disease. HMG CoA reductase inhibitors are the most frequently used and well-studied lipid-lowering agents. They reduce hepatic cholesterol synthesis. For which of the following patients is an HMG CoA reductase inhibitor the most appropriate lipid-lowering agent?
   A. a 45-year-old man with hepatic cirrhosis
   B. a 39-year-old woman who is 3 months' pregnant
   C. a 37-year-old woman who is breastfeeding
   D. a 45-year-old man who has pure variant angina
   E. a 52-year-old man who has exertional angina

An exercise tolerance test 1 year after his initial visit is notable for improved exercise capacity (10 MET workload), with blunting of the heart rate and blood pressure at peak exercise (120 bpm and 190/90 mm Hg, respectively); there is no evidence of myocardial ischemia by ECG criteria. A repeat LDL cholesterol determination is within the normal range. His medications (aspirin, β-receptor antagonist, and ACE inhibitor) are continued, and routine follow-up is established.

One week later, Mr. N. experiences the abrupt onset of severe retrosternal chest pressure. He is visibly diaphoretic and dyspneic. He calls 911 and is transported to the local emergency department, where an ECG shows sinus tachycardia and ST segment elevation in the inferior leads.

2. Mr. N.'s ECG shows regional ST segment elevation consistent with a transmural myocardial infarction. The treatment of ST-elevation myocardial infarction is aimed at expeditious reperfusion of the occluded epicardial coronary artery. Which of the following listed agents is emergently indicated while preparing the patient for emergency cardiac catheterization?
   A. aspirin, heparin, and alteplase
   B. clopidogrel, a GPIIb/IIIa inhibitor, and alteplase
   C. aspirin, clopidogrel, and streptokinase
   D. aspirin, clopidogrel, and a GPIIb/IIIa inhibitor
   E. acetaminophen, heparin, and clopidogrel

3. Which of the following agents would reduce myocardial oxygen demand and the risk of cardiac death in the setting of acute myocardial ischemia?
   A. aspirin
   B. a β-receptor antagonist
   C. a calcium channel blocker
   D. tenecteplase
   E. an HMG CoA reductase inhibitor

4. Organic nitrates are useful antianginal agents, as well as therapy for acute and chronic left ventricular failure. Which of the following statements regarding nitrate therapy is correct?
   A. Nitrates improve exercise tolerance in the setting of non–ST-elevation myocardial infarction (NSTEMI).
   B. Tolerance to the vasodilatory effect of nitrates complicates their long-term use.
   C. Sublingual nitrates reduce preload, while intravenous nitrates induce coronary arterial vasodilation.
   D. Nitrates are the primary therapy in the management of acute left ventricular heart failure by causing systemic arterial dilation and reducing afterload.
   E. Impotence is the most common adverse effect of nitrate therapy.

Emergent cardiac catheterization is performed, confirming total occlusion of a dominant right coronary artery, and percutaneous transluminal coronary angioplasty (PTCA) with stent placement is performed. The procedure is successful, and Mr. N. remains free of chest pain and is hemodynamically stable. Electrocardiographic and enzymatic changes (peak creatine kinase [CK], 2400 IU/L [normal, 60–400 IU/L]; cardiac isoform [MB] fraction, positive) are consistent with an evolving myocardial infarction. A repeat echocardiogram immediately before Mr. N.'s discharge from the hospital demonstrates concentric left ventricular hypertrophy with a left ventricular ejection fraction of 35% (normal, > 55%); the inferior wall from the base to the apex is akinetic, with thinning of the myocardium in this akinetic region.

5. Mr. N.'s discharge echocardiogram demonstrates a reduced left ventricular ejection fraction of 35%. Which of the following agents is a critical drug component of a postmyocardial infarction treatment regimen in the setting of left ventricular dysfunction?
   A. calcium channel blockers
   B. long-acting oral nitrates
   C. ACE inhibitors
   D. reteplase
   E. clopidogrel

 CASE 3

Mr. N. is discharged from the hospital on a multi-drug regimen that includes aspirin, clopidogrel, metoprolol, atorvastatin, captopril, and eplerenone. He does well as he increases his activity level during the first 4 to 6 weeks after the infarction. At that point, however, he again experiences breathlessness at moderate levels of exertion. He initially attributes this to deconditioning but becomes concerned when he wakes from sleep with severe breathlessness in the early morning hours. He schedules an appointment with his physician for later that day.

On examination in the physician's office, Mr. N. appears comfortable seated in the upright position. His heart rate is

64 bpm, and his blood pressure is 168/100 mm Hg. The pulmonic component of S2 is prominent (representing a change from his previous examinations), and the apical S4 is again noted; there is a grade III/VI apical holosystolic murmur with radiation to the left axilla. An echocardiogram reveals akinesis of the basal segment of the inferior wall of the left ventricle, with more prominent thinning and aneurysmal remodeling of the segment. The left ventricular ejection fraction is 35%. Although the mitral valve leaflets and the supporting structures of the valve appear structurally normal, there is a degree of posterior leaflet prolapse (LV → LA) during ventricular systole. A Doppler study confirms the presence of mitral regurgitation that is at least moderate in severity. The right ventricle is dilated and hypertrophic, with relative preservation of systolic function.

QUESTIONS

1. Mr. N.'s echocardiogram demonstrates biventricular heart failure. Which of the following pharmacologic agents would be an effective initial treatment of right heart failure?
   A. hydralazine
   B. dobutamine
   C. furosemide
   D. aspirin
   E. clopidogrel

Repeat catheterization is performed to assess the cause of the patient's new biventricular heart failure. Angiography shows wide patency of the right coronary artery at the site of the previous PTCA/stent intervention, and the left coronary system is free of obstruction. Hemodynamic data demonstrate increased pulmonary artery and right ventricular pressures.

2. If digoxin is added to Mr. N.'s medication regimen, what potential drug interactions should he be aware of?
   A. Captopril and digoxin may cause renal insufficiency.
   B. Metoprolol and digoxin may cause symptomatic bradycardia.
   C. Aspirin may inhibit digoxin metabolism.
   D. Metoprolol and digoxin may precipitate atrial fibrillation.
   E. Clopidogrel and digoxin may increase the risk of bleeding.

3. Mr. N.'s blood pressure remains elevated on this visit (168/100 mm Hg). This persistently increased afterload impedes left ventricular output from his weakened left ventricle. Which of the following statements regarding vasodilator drugs is correct?
   A. Milrinone dilates both arterial and venous vessels, but long-term use is associated with an increased incidence of mortality.
   B. Nitrates primarily dilate the venous system and do not affect arterial blood pressure.
   C. Calcium channel blockers prevent calcium entry into smooth muscle and venodilate, reducing preload.
   D. ACE inhibitors cause vasodilation by preventing renin release and the resulting neurohumoral vasoactive cascade.
   E. β_2-receptor antagonists promote arterial smooth muscle relaxation and vasodilation.

4. Which of the following inotropic agents can be administered parenterally to treat acute decompensated heart failure?
   A. digoxin-specific antibodies
   B. minoxidil
   C. hydralazine
   D. metoprolol
   E. dobutamine

5. Acute exacerbations of heart failure are often multifactorial in their etiology. Which of the following would be likely to contribute to an acute exacerbation of heart failure?
   A. getting a sunburn
   B. daily exercise
   C. dieting
   D. enjoying a big holiday meal
   E. sleep disturbances

ANSWERS TO SECTION III

CHAPTER 18 ANSWERS

CASE 1

1. **The answer is D. Diltiazem, a calcium channel blocker, slowed AV nodal conduction** by inhibiting inward calcium current during phase 0 depolarization. The calcium channel blockers (Class IV antiarrhythmics) act preferentially on the SA and AV nodal tissues, but do not have a significant effect on atrial conduction. Dr. J.'s atrial fibrillation was caused by a reentrant circuit within the atria above the AV node. **Diltiazem had no effect on the atrial reentry circuit.** If SA or AV nodal rates are pathologically slow, ectopic foci with more rapid rates of automaticity can take over as ectopic pacemakers.

2. **The answer is A. Ibutilide inhibits delayed rectifier K^+ channels and prolongs repolarization, which can predispose to a prolonged QT interval and *torsades de pointes.*** Ibutilide also enhances slow inward Na^+ conduction, further prolonging repolarization. The Class III antiarrhythmics, with the exception of amiodarone, exhibit "reverse-use dependency." Their prolongation of the action potential is greatest at slow rates and least pronounced at fast rates. Ibutilide does not have any effect on phase 0 depolarization or conduction velocity.

3. **The answer is B. Pulmonary fibrosis,** as well as hypotension, hyper- and hypothyroidism, elevated liver enzymes, and peripheral neuropathy and tremors, are all potential complications of high-dose amiodarone. A lupus-like syndrome with positive antinuclear antibodies can develop in association with procainamide use. Urinary retention is a potential anticholinergic adverse effect of quinidine and disopyramide. Bronchospasm and impotence are potential adverse effects of β_2 antagonists.

4. **The answer is B. Sodium channel blockade slows atrial conduction, while anticholinergic effects increase AV nodal conduction velocity.** In this setting, the atrial rate can decrease while impulse conduction through the AV node can be facilitated, causing a 1:1

atrial:ventricular conduction at rapid rates of 200/min. Quinidine does not have any effect on potassium channels. Calcium, not sodium, is sequestered in the sarcoplasmic reticulum.

5. **The answer is B.** Dihydropyridine calcium channel blockers such as nifedipine act preferentially on **vascular smooth muscle.** Verapamil and diltiazem act preferentially at calcium channels in cardiac tissues.

CASE 2

1. **The answer is C. Propranolol,** a prototypical first generation β-adrenergic receptor antagonist, nonselectively antagonizes normal sympathetic stimulation at both β_1 and β_2 receptors. Although β-adrenergic receptor antagonists are useful in the treatment of supraventricular and ventricular tachyarrhythmias and are cardioprotective after myocardial infarction, in overdose, they can cause profound bradycardia and conduction blocks. Nifedipine, a dihydropyridine calcium channel blocker, preferentially antagonizes calcium channels on vascular smooth muscle cells, causing vasodilation, hypotension, and a reflex tachycardia. Atropine inhibits the parasympathetic effects of the vagus nerve at the SA and AV nodes, enhancing pacemaker current and facilitating depolarization and increasing the rate of pacemaker cell firing. Nitroglycerin relaxes smooth muscles, vasodilates and causes hypotension, usually accompanied by a reflex tachycardia. Epinephrine is an adrenergic receptor agonist that increases sympathetic tone and the rate of pacemaker firing through activation of the β_1-adrenergic receptor, and increases peripheral vascular resistance at high doses through its activation of the α_1-adrenergic receptor.

2. **The answer is E. Atropine decreases the parasympathetic tone by inhibiting the release of acetylcholine from of the vagus nerve, enhances pacemaker current, facilitates depolarization, and increases the rate of pacemaker cell firing.** The vagus nerve, part of the parasympathetic nervous system, releases acetylcholine primarily onto the atria, SA and AV nodes. Atropine is a competitive antagonist of muscorinic acetylcholine receptors. Atropine has no effect on β_1-adrenergic receptors or the ventricular myocytes. Muscarinic receptors activate inward rectifier potassium channels, which hyperpolarize myocytes and slow

pacemaker depolarization. In addition, muscarinic receptors inhibit voltage-dependent calcium channels, which decreases the rate of phase O depolarization. Both effects slow heart rate. Phase O depolarization of pacemaker cells is dependent on intracellular calcium entry. Reduced calcium entry slows the rate of increase of phase O depolarization and slows heart rate.

3. **The answer is D. β-adrenergic receptor antagonists decrease the rate of phase 4 depolarization and prolong repolarization.** These drugs block the sympathetic stimulation of β_1-adrenergic receptors in the SA and AV nodes, slowing heart rate. Beta$_1$-adrenergic receptors have the opposite of muscarinic acetylcholine receptors; they speed pacemaker and phase O depolarization rates. Therefore, blockade of these receptors abrogates sympathetic effects, resulting in reduced heart rate. They also increase the effective refractory period (by enhancing voltage-gated potassium channels governing the plateau duration), thus decreasing the incidence of reentry.

4. **The answer is B. Lidocaine has a high affinity for inactivated sodium channels in ischemic tissue.** This is an example of state-dependent ion channel blockade. Lidocaine, a (Class IB antiarrhythmic sodium channel blocker, has a higher affinity for the open and inactivated states of the sodium channel (like most sodium channel blockers). When myocardial tissue is ischemic, the length of myocyte depolarization is prolonged and sodium channels spend more time in the inactivated state. As a consequence, lidocaine binds to the sodium channels of ischemic myocytes. This is a desirable effect such that lidocaine acts preferentially to inhibit arrhythmogenic foci in ischemic tissues. Class III potassium channel blockers (except amiodarone) exhibit "reverse-use dependency" such that their effect on action potential prolongation is most pronounced at slow heart rates and least pronounced at fast heart rates. This is not a desirable property of these agents.

5. **The answer is A.** Adenosine acts on purinergic receptors to activate the same intracellular pathways as muscarinic acetylcholine repectors. Adenosine opens inward rectifier potassium channels and inhibits voltage-dependent calcium channels, inhibiting SA nodal, atrial and AV nodal conduction. The AV node is particularly sensitive to the effects of adenosine, which is used to convert reentrant **narrow-complex supraventricular tachycardias.**

CHAPTER 19 ANSWERS

CASE 1

1. **The answer is C. The combination of a β-adrenergic receptor antagonist and digoxin reduces mortality and improves the functional status of heart failure patients**. β-receptor antagonists reduce mortality by 30%, perhaps by counteracting the effects of chronic sympathetic stimulation on the heart and effect-

ing ventricular remodeling. Although digoxin itself does not reduce mortality in patients with heart failure, it may have a positive effect on contractile function, as well as neurohumoral effects, and improves the functional status of patients with systolic dysfunction.

2. **The answer is A. Digoxin inhibits the plasma membrane sodium pump, leading to an increase in the intracellular calcium concentration.** Inhibition of the sodium pump causes an increase in the intracellular sodium concentration, which alters the equilibrium of the plasma membrane sodium–calcium exchanger. This results in an increase in intracellular calcium. The intracellular calcium binds to troponin C, increasing contractile tension and contractility. Digoxin also binds to the plasma membrane sodium pump of neuronal cells, inhibiting sympathetic tone and increasing parasympathetic tone. It also decreases the automaticity of the AV node and prolongs conduction through the AV node. β-receptor agonists act through G protein–coupled receptors to increase intracellular cAMP and subsequent recycling of intracellular calcium in and out of the sarcoplasmic reticulum.

3. **The answer is B. Atrial fibrillation** is a characteristic electrical rhythm in digoxin toxic patients. This is caused by digoxin's effects of decreased automaticity at the AV node but enhanced automaticity of the His-Purkinje fibers. These divergent effects can contribute to complete heart block with an accelerated junctional or idioventricular escape rhythm. Other symptoms of digoxin toxicity include nausea and visual halos (of which G.W. does not complain). Because digoxin is approximately 70% renally excreted, acute renal failure and dehydration with altered glomerular filtration rate can predispose patients to digoxin toxicity. Serum hyperkalemia (caused by poisoning of the sodium pump) can occur in the setting of acute digoxin toxicity or digoxin overdose, and is an ominous prognostic sign.

4. **The answer is D. Hypokalemia makes the sodium pump more sensitive to digoxin.** A low extracellular potassium concentration increases the phosphorylation of the sodium pump. Digoxin has a higher affinity for the phosphorylated form of the pump. Many factors predispose patients to digoxin toxicity. They include preexisting cardiopulmonary disease, renal insufficiency, electrolyte abnormalities, and antibiotic use (which alters gastrointestinal bacterial flora and affects the amount of digoxin absorbed from the gut).

5. **The answer is D. Dobutamine is an agonist at the β_1-adrenergic receptor that increases intracellular cAMP and calcium** available affect to the myocyte contraction cycle. Dobutamine is a synthetic sympathomimetic amine that exists in a racemic mixture of (+) and (−) enantiomers. Both enantiomers stimulate β_1-adrenergic receptors (and β_2-adrenergic receptors to a lesser degree). They have opposite effects at the α_1-receptor. The end result of this formulation mixture is predominantly an agonist effect at β_1-adrenergic receptors, making dobutamine a titratable intravenous inotrope for acute cardiogenic failure.

CASE 2

1. **The answer is C. Intracellular calcium binds to troponin C, which allows the release of troponin I so that myosin and actin can interact to shorten the sarcomere.** In this way, intracellular calcium is the link between myocyte excitation and contraction. The cycling of calcium within the cell is controlled by several mechanisms. When calcium levels are high, calcium–calmodulin complexes inhibit further release of calcium into the cytosol. Intracellular calcium stimulates SERCA to pump calcium back into the sarcoplasmic reticulum, replenishing calcium stores and facilitating diastolic relaxation of the sarcomeres. Adequate intracellular ATP concentrations are also necessary to allow actin–myosin interaction and relaxation, as well as SERCA function.

2. **The answer is E. Dopamine administered at high rates acts primarily as an agonist at α_1-adrenergic receptors, increasing peripheral vascular resistance.** At low infusion rates, dopamine increases contractility (β_1-adrenergic agonist) and decreases systemic vascular resistance (β_2-adrenergic agonist.)

3. **The answer is C. β-receptor antagonists may further decrease cardiac output and cause pulmonary edema.** The initial treatment of patients with peripartum cardiomyopathy includes digoxin and an angiotensin-converting enzyme inhibitor. β-receptor antagonists may be added to the patient's treatment regimen if this initial drug combination fails to improve symptoms; however, beta-receptor antagonists should be avoided in patients with decompensated heart failure. Peripartum cardiomyopathy is rare, occurring any time from the last month of pregnancy up to 6 months postpartum.

4. **The answer is B. Milrinone** is a relatively selective PDE3 inhibitor, as is inamrinone. Dopamine is an adrenergic agonist, carvedilol is a β-adrenergic antagonist, isoproterenol is a β-adrenergic agonist, and digitoxin is a cardiac glycoside.

5. **The answer is A.** Both β-receptor agonists and phosphodiesterase inhibitors **increase cardiac contractility by increasing intracellular cAMP levels**. β-receptor agonists act through a G protein–coupled system to increase cAMP formation, while phosphodiesterase inhibitors prevent the enzymatic hydrolysis and breakdown of cAMP.

CHAPTER 20 ANSWERS

CASE 1

1. **The answer is C. Compromised cardiac function caused renal sodium and water reabsorption, and decreased cardiac output caused pulmonary congestion and pedal edema.** The diminished cardiac output is perceived as inadequate intravascular volume by the high-pressure volume receptors, including the juxtaglomerular apparatus. This induces enhanced renal sodium absorption through the renin–angiotensin–aldosterone neurohumoral mediators. Unfortunately, the compromised left ventricle is unable to adequately pump the existing intravascular volume, leading to pulmonary venous congestion and pedal edema. Although acute renal failure can lead to volume overload, Mr. R. has only renal insufficiency, which may be a reflection of inadequate renal arterial blood flow in the setting of chronic heart failure. Cardiac biomarkers do not indicate that Mr. R. has had an acute myocardial infarction. The overflow model is one hypothesis for ascites formation in hepatic cirrhosis, due to primary renal sodium retention.

2. **The answer is B. Loop diuretics inhibit the high capacity for sodium reabsorption in the thick ascending loop of Henle and cause a rapid diuresis and reduction in intravascular volume.** This reduces filling pressures in the compromised left ventricle and alleviates high pulmonary venous pressures. Loop diuretics are therefore first-line therapy for the relief of pulmonary and peripheral edema in heart failure. Long-term therapy with loop diuretics can predispose patients to hypocalcemia, hypokalemia, and hypomagnesemia. Thiazide diuretics inhibit sodium reabsorption in the distal convoluted tubule, while causing a direct vasodilatory effect. They are an important component of antihypertensive therapy. Potassium-sparing diuretics inhibit sodium reabsorption in the collecting duct. In addition to their effects in volume regulation and blood pressure control, ACE inhibitors retard the pathologic cardiac contractile dysfunction associated with heart failure after myocardial infarction.

3. **The answer is D. Potassium-sparing diuretics, specifically spironolactone and eplerenone, inhibit the action of aldosterone at the mineralocorticoid receptor.** This leads to a reduction in the number of epithelial sodium channels in the collecting duct's principal cells, and reduced sodium reabsorption. The potassium-sparing diuretics, amiloride and triamterene, inhibit the activity of principal cell apical membrane sodium channels. Potassium-sparing diuretics are mild diuretics that enhance potassium reabsorption and can cause hyperkalemic metabolic acidosis. Carbonic anhydrase inhibitors inhibit sodium reabsorption in the proximal convoluted tubule and are used in the treatment of acute glaucoma for their reduction in aqueous humor production by the ciliary process. Thiazide diuretics diminish hypercalciuria and the risk of calcium nephrolithiasis. Mannitol, an osmotic diuretic, rapidly reduces cerebral intravascular volume in the setting of closed head trauma. Loop diuretics are associated with dose-dependent ototoxicity, especially when used with aminoglycoside antibiotics.

4. **The answer is E. ACE inhibitors cause arterial vasodilation and limit the development of postmyocardial infarction cardiomyopathy.** They prevent the conversion of angiotensin I to angiotensin II, limiting the vasoconstricting effects of angiotensin II. ACE inhibitors retard the progression of cardiac contractile dysfunction after myocardial infarction, possibly through an inhibitory effect on growth factors and hormones, which pathologically stimulate tissue hypertrophy and fibrosis. Because of these effects, ACE inhibitors are a first-line therapy as antihypertensives, and are commonly prescribed after myocardial infarction for their protective effect on the remodeling of the heart. ACE inhibitors increase the levels of bradykinin, a smooth muscle relaxer and vasodilator. ACE inhibitors inhibit aldosterone synthesis and reduce potassium excretion. They reduce the release of ADH. ACE inhibitors are contraindicated in pregnancy because of their association with fetal malformations. Angiotensin receptor antagonists antagonize the vasoconstrictive effects of angiotensin at its receptors.

5. **The answer is A.** Sodium reabsorption is greatest in the **proximal tubule**, where approximately two thirds of sodium reabsorption occurs, along with most bicarbonate reabsorption and 60% of chloride absorption. Solute absorption in the proximal tubule is iso-osmotic: water is also absorbed along with ions to maintain osmotic balance. The thick ascending limb of the loop of Henle reabsorbs between 25% and 35% of filtered sodium, without accompanying water, diluting the tubular fluid. The distal convoluted tubule reabsorbs only 2% to 10% of sodium, but also mediates the reabsorption of calcium and magnesium. The collecting duct principal cells reabsorb only 1% to 5% of filtered sodium and secrete potassium under the control of aldosterone. ADH promotes water reabsorption in the collecting duct. The intercalated cells of the collecting duct secrete bicarbonate and protons, and regulate chloride and potassium absorption.

CASE 2

1. **The answer is A. The underfill theory proposes that increased intrahepatic hydrostatic pressure causes ascites, diminishes intravascular volume, and promotes renal sodium reabsorption.** The fluid filtered across the hepatic sinusoids is a transudate. The increased volume of transudate overwhelms the ability of the lymphatic system to return it to the systemic circulation, resulting in ascites and edema. Hepatic synthetic function is diminished in patients with cirrhosis, causing a decreased production of albumin, clotting factors, and peptide hormones, and eventually, disruption of metabolic functions such as gluconeogenesis. The overflow model of ascites proposes that the postsinusoidal obstruction in patients with cirrhosis stimulates a hepatorenal reflex. This autonomic response leads to primary renal sodium reabsorption. The resulting sodium retention, volume overload, and increased intrahepatic hydrostatic pressure cause ascites.

2. **The answer is E. Spironolactone antagonizes the effects of hyperaldosteronism in cirrhosis with edema.** Mineralocorticoid excess can occur in patients with cirrhosis and heart failure as a result of diminished aldosterone metabolism. Spironolactone is a mild diuretic that is unlikely to cause excessive and rapid diuresis. In the setting of diminished plasma oncotic pressure (as in cirrhosis), the ability to rapidly mobilize extravascular fluid into the vasculature is limited, so that rapid or extensive diuresis might compromise cardiovascular stability. This risk is lessened with use of spironolactone. Spironolactone promotes potassium retention. It inhibits the androgen receptor, contributing to the adverse effects of impotence and gynecomastia in men. Spironolactone and eplerenone may preserve cardiac function and slow the development of heart failure in patients with myocardial infarction, possibly related to an inhibition of cardiac fibrosis.

3. **The answer is D. Hyperkalemic metabolic acidosis** can result from the use of potassium-sparing diuretics, which are used in the treatment of hypokalemic metabolic alkalosis.

4. **The answer is D. Albumin**, globulins, and other large plasma proteins are normally confined to the intravascular space. As osmotically active agents, they contribute to the vascular oncotic pressure gradient and promote movement of transudate (water) into the intravascular space from the interstitial space. Mannitol is an osmotic diuretic that is filtered at the glomerulus and increases the intraluminal osmotic force within the nephron tubule, limiting water reabsorption. Desmopressin is an exogenous vasopressin agonist used in the treatment of patients with central diabetes insipidus. Although water can be infused directly into veins, it is able to cross into the interstitial tissue, depending on changes in hydrostatic and oncotic pressure gradients.

5. **The answer is C. B-type natriuretic peptide** is elevated in response to volume overload. The natriuretic peptides are released by the atria (A type), ventricles (B type), and vascular endothelium (C type) in response to increased intravascular volume, probably because of increased stretch in the natriuretic peptide-secreting cells. The natriuretic peptides promote vasodilation, transudation of fluid from the intravascular space into the interstitium, and natriuresis, as well as diminished thirst, decreased release of ADH, and decreased sympathetic tone. Nesiritide is a recombinant human sequence B-type natriuretic peptide approved for the acute management of decompensated heart failure.

Kininase II is another name for ACE. Renin is secreted by the juxtaglomerular apparatus in response to signals indicating low intravascular volume. Vasopressin is ADH, secreted by the posterior pituitary in response to increased plasma osmolality or hypovolemia. Albumin concentrations may be diluted in the setting of intravascular volume overload.

CHAPTER 21 ANSWERS

CASE 1

1. **The answer is D. Sublingual nitroglycerin is rapidly absorbed and metabolized to nitric oxide (NO), which dilates systemic veins and epicardial arteries, decreasing myocardial oxygen demand and increasing myocardial oxygen supply.** Enzymatic release of NO from organic nitrates occurs in specific vascular tissues, targeting the systemic veins (increasing venous capacitance, decreasing venous return to the heart, and decreasing myocardial work and oxygen demand) and the epicardial coronary arteries (vasodilating and increasing oxygen supply to the myocardium). Nitroglycerin doses sufficient to cause excessive peripheral arterial vasodilation can lead to profound hypotension. Orally administered organic nitrates have a more prolonged but delayed onset of action because of gastrointestinal absorption and some degree of first-pass hepatic metabolism. NO metabolism to peroxynitrite is one hypothesis for the development of cellular tolerance to the effects of organic nitrates. Inhaled NO has been used to treat primary pulmonary hypertension of the newborn.

2. **The answer is E. Headache** is a very common adverse effect of nitroglycerin administration caused by vasodilation of cerebral arteries. Other adverse effects of organic nitrates associated with vasodilation include hypotension, with reflex tachycardia, and facial flushing. Bradycardia occurring after nitroglycerin administration has been reported, but is rare. Transient visual loss caused by nonarteritic ischemic optic neuropathy has been reported in association with the PDE5 inhibitors, such as sildenafil. Hepatic transaminase elevation is a major adverse effect of bosentan, a competitive endothelin receptor antagonist used in the treatment of pulmonary artery hypertension.

3. **The answer is A. Both sildenafil and organic nitrates promote vasodilation.** Sildenafil is a guanosine 3',5'-cyclic monophosphate (cGMP) phosphodiesterase type V (PDE5) inhibitor. It prevents the breakdown of cGMP, which promotes smooth muscle relaxation. Although PDE5 is primarily expressed in the smooth muscle of the corpus cavernosum, it is also expressed in small amounts on vascular smooth muscle cells. Organic nitrates are metabolized to NO, which stimulates the production of intracellular cGMP. When these agents are used in combination, their vasodilatory effect is amplified, and profound hypotension can result. Although concomitant use of sildenafil and calcium channel blockers has not been proven to cause the same effect, patients taking vasodilatory antihypertensive agents with sildenafil are considered to be at risk for dangerous hypotension.

4. **The answer is A. Stimulation of α_1-adrenergic receptors in vascular smooth muscle would pro-** mote arterial vasoconstriction and increase systemic vascular resistance and blood pressure. Adrenergic innervation of the heart is primarily through β_1-receptors. α_2-adrenergic receptors are primarily located on presynaptic nerve terminals, where they are involved in negative feedback, decreasing sympathetic tone in the central nervous system, and inhibiting the release of norepinephrine from peripheral adrenergic neurons.

5. **The answer is C. Minoxidil opens potassium channels and hyperpolarizes the cell. This prevents normal depolarization and calcium influx.** The result is relaxation and vasodilation of vascular smooth muscle cells. Minoxidil does not interact with calcium channels or effect calcium release from the sarcoplasmic reticulum. Endothelin is a potent endogenous vasoconstrictor peptide.

CASE 2

1. **The answer is E. Epinephrine is released from the adrenal gland into the systemic circulation, where it can act at both α- and β-adrenergic receptors.** Norepinephrine is released from adrenergic postganglionic neurons. Both epinephrine and norepinephrine are agonists at vascular smooth muscle α_1- and β_2-adrenergic receptors. Sympathetic stimulation, particularly constriction mediated through α_1-adrenergic receptors, predominates in the autonomic control of vascular tone.

2. **The answer is D. Topical nitroglycerin is absorbed transdermally, where it releases NO to cause vasodilation** through the formation of cGMP. Phosphodiesterase inhibitors prevent the breakdown of cGMP. Calcium channel blockers prevent calcium influx. β_2-adrenergic agonists increase intracellular cAMP. All of these actions reduce smooth muscle contraction and facilitate vasodilation.

3. **The answer is B. Phentolamine blocked α_1-adrenergic vasoconstriction of the digital arteries.** Phentolamine is a nonselective α-adrenergic antagonist, which is able to reverse epinephrine-induced vasoconstriction of the digital arteries.

4. **The answer is E. Amlodipine has a delayed onset but long duration of action.** Amlodipine is a third-generation dihydropyridine agent that is positively charged at physiologic pH. This facilitates its binding to cell membranes with high affinity, accounting for a late peak plasma concentration and slow hepatic metabolism. In contrast, nifedipine is renally excreted and has a short half-life compared with amlodipine. Diltiazem undergoes significant first-pass hepatic metabolism, resulting in a low bioavailability. Both diltiazem and verapamil are cardioselective, acting as negative inotropes, as well as decreasing automaticity and conduction velocity.

5. The answer is D. Cyanide is liberated during the metabolism of sodium nitroprusside. Cyanide inhibits normal electron transfer by cytochromes and **causes metabolic acidosis and ventricular arrhythmias**. Cyanide is normally metabolized in the liver to thiocyanate, which is renally excreted. Thiocyanate can accumulate in patients with renal insufficiency, causing altered mental status and seizures. Endothelin is an endogenous vasoconstrictor peptide.

CHAPTER 22 ANSWERS

CASE 1

1. The answer is C. Three factors predispose patients to thrombus formation: endothelial injury, abnormal blood flow, and hypercoagulability (Virchow's triad). Endothelial injury is the most important factor associated with cardiac and arterial thrombus formation. Mr. S.'s **high blood pressure** and cigarette use predisposed him to coronary artery endothelial injury and thrombus formation. Turbulent blood flow at the sites of atherosclerotic plaques and blood vessel bifurcations also predisposes patients to endothelial injury. Areas of local blood stasis, such as at aneurysmal dilatations and in the venous system, contribute to thrombus formation. Genetic and acquired hypercoagulable states, such as heparin-induced thrombocytopenia, can predispose to thrombosis. Low-dose aspirin use has an antiplatelet effect that is protective against arterial thrombus formation.

2. The answer is D. Accurate measurement of the anticoagulant effect of low-molecular-weight heparin would depend on the measurement of anti-factor Xa activity. This is because low-molecular-weight heparin is more selective in catalyzing the inactivation of factor Xa than the inactivation of thrombin by antithrombin III. In contrast, unfractionated heparin nonselectively catalyzes the inactivation of both factor Xa and thrombin by antithrombin III. The activated partial thromboplastin time (aPTT) is a measure of the anticoagulant effect of unfractionated heparin. Low-molecular-weight heparins are renally excreted, and care should be taken to avoid excessive anticoagulation in patients with renal insufficiency. The prothombin time (PT) measures the anticoagulant effect of warfarin.

3. The answer is B. Eptifibatide is an antagonist at the platelet GPIIb–IIIa receptor, preventing fibrinogen binding to platelets. Functional GPIIb–IIIa is expressed on the platelet surface as a result of a number of stimuli, including thromboxane, ADP, epinephrine, collagen, and thrombin. Eptifibatide is a powerful inhibitor of platelet aggregation because it prevents the final common pathway in platelet binding of fibrinogen through its effect on the GPIIb–IIIa receptor. Abciximab, not en-

tifibotide; is a mouse–human monoclonal antibody directed against the GPIIb–IIIa receptor.

4. The answer is E. There is no measure to reverse the effect of this agent other than stopping the eptifibatide. Unlike abciximab, the effects of which can be reversed by infusing fresh platelets, eptifibatide and tirofiban are administered in such dosages that there is still a large excess of drug available to bind to platelet receptor sites. Therefore, infusion of fresh platelets is impractical in reversing the antiplatelet effect of these agents. Vitamin K repletion facilitates the hepatic synthesis of vitamin K–dependent clotting factors, which is inhibited by warfarin. Fresh-frozen plasma infusion provides clotting factors. Protamine antagonizes the anticoagulant effect of heparin.

5. The answer is A. Clopidogrel inactivates the platelet ADP receptor and inhibits adenylyl cyclase production of cAMP, preventing platelet aggregation. It is used in combination with aspirin to inhibit platelet activation and is approved for secondary prevention in patients with recent myocardial infarction and after percutaneous coronary intervention or coronary artery bypass grafting. Aspirin irreversibly inhibits both COX-1 and COX-2, and prevents the formation of platelet-derived thromboxane. Heparins enhance the normal activity of antithrombin III. Warfarin prevents the generation of reduced vitamin K, which is necessary for the hepatic production of activated clotting factors.

CASE 2

1. The answer is B. Stasis of blood flow is the major cause of venous thrombus formation. Stasis inhibits the continuous flow of fresh blood through a vascular bed, so that activated coagulation factors in the vessels are not removed or diluted. The development of venous thrombosis associated with long plane flights has been called the "economy class syndrome," or flight-related deep venous thrombosis (DVT). Local pockets of stasis can also occur as a result of dysrhythmias such as atrial fibrillation, and aneurysm formation in blood vessels or cardiac chambers. Turbulent flow at atherosclerotic plaques or bifurcations of blood vessels can cause endothelial injury, the most dominant influence on thrombus formation in the heart and the arterial circulation. Cigarette smoking also causes endothelial injury.

2. The answer is E. Factor V Leiden mutation is the most common genetic cause of hypercoagulability. The mutant factor V Leiden is resistant to proteolytic cleavage by activated protein C, and accumulates promoting coagulation. Other primary genetic causes of hypercoagulability include the prothrombin G20210A mutation, (causing increased prothrombin levels) protein C or S deficiencies, and antithrombin deficiency. Secondary, or disease or drug-induced, hypercoagulabilities include those caused by oral contraceptive use, the postpartum state, antiphospholipid syndrome, surgery or trauma, and active malignancy.

3. **The answer is C. Warfarin's pharmacologic effect on the inhibition of clotting factor activation is not manifested for three to four clotting factor half-lives.** Its onset of action parallels the half-life of the vitamin K–dependent clotting factors II, VII, IX, and X. Factor VII has the shortest half-life (6 hours), so the effect of warfarin takes approximately 18 to 24 hours (or three to four factor VII half-lives) to become manifested. This delay in action distinguishes warfarin from the other anticoagulants. Warfarin is often administered to complete a long-term course of anticoagulation that has been initiated with heparin. In this case, subcutaneous low-molecular-weight heparin would be discontinued when the anticoagulant effect of warfarin is therapeutic, as measured by the prothrombin time.

4. **The answer is C. Warfarin can cause congenital malformations in the fetus,** particularly craniofacial bone abnormalities, and is contraindicated for anticoagulation in pregnant patients. It can also cause hemorrhagic disorders in fetuses. Heparin is the anticoagulant of choice in pregnancy. Warfarin is metabolized by the P450 enzyme system in the liver to inactive metabolites. It is susceptible to numerous drug–drug interactions, which can cause P450 induction or inhibition, and to alterations in albumin binding. Warfarin can cause microvascular thromboses and skin necrosis as a result of its effects on the synthesis of activated protein C and S. The latter effect is not limited to the pregnant state.

5. **The answer is A. The administration of streptokinase can elicit an antigenic response,** which can result in anaphylaxis on subsequent administration of the drug. This is because it is a foreign protein, produced by β-hemolytic streptococci. Tenecteplase has a longer half-life than tissue plasminogen activator (t-PA) and can be administered as a single weight-based bolus. Recombinant t-PA (alteplase) activates plasminogen but can generate a systemic lytic state and cause unwanted bleeding. Argatroban is a small molecule direct thrombin inhibitor, not athrombolytic. Aprotinin inhibits plasmin, t-PA, and thrombin. Its use has been associated with postoperative acute renal failure.

CHAPTER 23 ANSWERS

CASE 1

1. **The answer is B.** Familial hypercholesterolemia is **an autosomal dominant disease causing defective LDL receptor formation.** This mutation leads to a lack of receptor synthesis, failure of receptor to reach the plasma membrane, defective LDL binding, or failure to internalize LDL particles. Heterozygotes have elevated total plasma cholesterol concentrations and LDL, but normal triglyceride levels. Homozygotes have an absence of functional LDL receptors. Familial defective apoB100 is an autosomal dominant disease causing decreased affinity of LDL for its receptor. Total cholesterol concentrations are similarly elevated, as compared to patients with familial hypercholesterolemia. Familial LPL deficiency is an autosomal recessive disease causing absence of LPL, and hypertriglyceridemia. Familial hypertriglyceridemia is an autosomal dominant disease that causes increased hepatic triglyceride synthesis, but normal LDL concentrations.

2. **The answer is D. Excess LDL cholesterol accumulates in macrophages in atherosclerotic lesions**, leading to the formation of foam cells. Foam cell death contributes to the local inflammatory response associated with plaque destabilization and rupture. In addition, oxidized LDL also upregulates the inflammatory response through promotion of cytokine production, and impairs normal endothelial function. Although excess LDL cholesterol downregulates LDL receptor expression and LDL uptake by hepatocytes, this regulation does not occur on mononuclear phagocytic cells as they begin to accumulate cholesterol. Excess LDL cholesterol downregulates HMG CoA reductase activity in the liver, one method of maintaining normal cholesterol homeostasis.

3. **The answer is C. Statins competitively inhibit the activity of HMG CoA reductase**, the rate limiting enzyme in cholesterol synthesis. This results in a decrease in cellular cholesterol concentrations and subsequent upregulation of LDL receptor expression, which further increases the cellular uptake of cholesterol. Statins have been shown to reduce cardiovascular mortality both after myocardial infarction and in patients without overt cardiovascular disease. The dose–response relationship of statins is nonlinear, referred to as the "rule of sixes". The greatest effect on LDL lowering occurs with the starting dose.

4. **The answer is E. Ezetimibe inhibits cholesterol uptake through a brush border protein on enterocytes.** This inhibition of cholesterol absorption decreases the cholesterol content of intestinal chylomicrons, cholesterol delivery to the liver, and subsequent incorporation in VLDL. Plant sterols and stanols in fruits and vegetables displace dietary cholesterol from micelles and enhance its loss in the feces. Bile acid sequestrants such as cholestyramine, colesevalam, and colestipol bind to, and interrupt, bile acid and cholesterol enterohepatic circulation.

5. **The answer is C. Niacin decreases peripheral triglyceride breakdown and decreases hepatic triglyceride synthesis.** It decreases adipose tissue lipase activity and adipose release of free fatty acids to the liver. This decreases subsequent hepatic triglyceride and VLDL synthesis. Niacin also increases plasma HDL concentrations by increasing the half-life of apoAI, the major apolipoprotein present in HDL. This may enhance reverse cholesterol transport to the liver. Flushing is a major adverse effect of niacin administration, caused by the release of cutaneous prostaglandins.

CASE 2

1. **The answer is C.** Pleiotropic effects of statin therapy include **decreased inflammation**, as evidenced by a reduced concentration of acute-phase reactants during statin therapy. Other pleitropic effects associated with statins include a reversal of endothelial dysfunction, as evidenced by enhanced nitric oxide–induced vasodilation, decreased coagulation associated with decreased prothrombin activation, and improved stability of atherosclerotic plaques. Many of these effects have been demonstrated in vitro and in animal models.

2. **The answer is D. High dosages of more potent statins** are more often associated with the development of myositis and rhabdomyolysis. Concomitant administration of drugs that inhibit P450 enzyme activity will decrease statin clearance and may increase the risk of rhabdomyolysis. Statin-associated rhabdomyolysis has been associated with concomitant gemfibrozil, but not fenofibrate therapy. Plasma creatine kinase levels are not useful for routine screening of myositis in patients treated with statins. In fact, some patients with muscle aching and myositis associated with statin use have been found to have normal creatine kinase levels.

3. **The answer is D.** A major adverse effect of concomitant statin and niacin therapy is the development of **rhabdomyolysis**. Facial flushing is an adverse effect of niacin (vitamin B_3) therapy.

4. **The answer is A.** The clinical laboratory result of fibrate therapy is an **increase in plasma HDL concentrations**, a decrease in plasma triglyceride levels, and a modest decrease in plasma LDL concentrations. Fibrates increase the expression of LPL and increase the uptake of triglycerides. They enhance hepatic fatty acid oxidation and decrease hepatic triglyceride and VLDL production.

5. **The answer is A.** Secondary factors that can lead to hyperlipidemia include excessive **ethanol intake**, insulin resistance, and hypothyroidism. In contrast, moderate ethanol consumption may increase HDL and have a cardioprotective effect.

CHAPTER 24 ANSWERS

CASE: PART 1

1. **The answer is C.** Current guidelines for the treatment of hypertension recommend the **initiation of drug therapy in the presence of elevated systolic blood pressure greater than 120 mm Hg** (isolated systolic hypertension), especially in elderly patients. This is in contrast to prior indications for drug therapy, such as isolated elevated diastolic blood pressure. The principal goal of treatment is to **reduce systolic blood pressure to 120 mm Hg and diastolic blood pressure to less than 80 mm Hg**. Blood pressures greater than 140/90 mm Hg are classified as moderate hypertension (stage 1), and blood pressures greater than 160/100 mm Hg (as in Mr. N.'s case) are classified as severe hypertension (stage 2). Because of the adverse effects associated with most antihypertensive agents and the physiologic compensatory response to their effects, multidrug therapy at submaximum doses is often necessary to achieve blood pressure control.

2. **The answer is E. Compensatory volume retention and hypokalemia** are potential adverse effects of thiazide therapy. Thiazides reduce blood pressure by decreasing intravascular volume. They increase renal excretion of sodium and water, as well as potassium. The resulting decrease in intravascular volume decreases cardiac output and blood pressure. The compensatory stimulation of the renin–angiotensin system promotes volume retention. However, the long-term antihypertensive effect of thiazides may also be caused by a vasodilatory effect. Hyperkalemia can result from the use of potassium-sparing diuretics such as spironolactone, triamterene, and amiloride. Elevated triglycerides and high-density-lipoprotein levels have been associated with β-receptor antagonists.

3. **The answer is A. Metoprolol, a β-receptor antagonist**, is an effective antihypertensive choice in younger patients with "high-output" hypertension. β-receptor antagonists work by downregulating sympathetic tone, specifically by reducing cardiac output. Over time, these agents also reduce vasomotor tone through their β_1 inhibition of renin release and subsequent inhibition of angiotensin II production. Currently, there is a move away from β-receptor antagonists as first-line therapy for hypertension because they have not shown a consistent mortality benefit. α-receptor antagonists reduce vasoconstriction and systemic vascular resistance. Loop diuretics reduce intravascular volume and are occasionally used for the treatment of patients with mild to moderate hypertension. Trimethaphan and other ganglionic blockers, such as hexamethonium, inhibit activity at sympathetic ganglia but have significant adverse effects due to both parasympathetic and sympathetic blockade. Salt restriction limits renal water absorption and intravascular volume.

4. **The answer is A.** ACE inhibitors decrease angiotensin II production, decreasing systemic vascular resistance. They also **decrease aldosterone levels, promoting natriuresis,** and reducing intravascular volume. Another effect of ACE inhibitors is a decrease in bradykinin breakdown; the increased circulating bradykinin contributes to vasodilation (as well as bradykinin-associated cough). Patients with intravascular volume depletion are at risk for developing acute renal insufficiency as a result of ACE inhibitor disruption of the normal regulation of renal perfusion. Angiotensin receptor blockers block angiotensin II binding to its AT_1 receptors. A lupus-like syndrome is associated with hydralazine use.

5. **The answer is B.** Secondary hypertension refers to elevated blood pressure attributed to a defined cause, including **oral contraceptive use**, hyperaldosteronism, primary renal disease, and renal vascular disease. In contrast, essential hypertension affects 90% to 95% of hypertensive patients. The etiology of essential hypertension is multifactorial, including both genetic and environmental factors, such as excess dietary salt and ethanol intake, and obesity.

CASE: PART 2

1. **The answer is E. A 52-year-old man who has exertional angina** would benefit from an HMG CoA reductase inhibitor. Lipid-lowering therapy reduces the incidence of cardiovascular events in patients with coronary artery disease. HMG CoA reductase inhibitors are contraindicated in women who are pregnant or may become pregnant, or who are nursing. They are also contraindicated in patients with cirrhosis because of the concern for potential hepato-toxicity.

2. **The answer is D. Aspirin, heparin, clopidogrel, and GPIIb/IIIa inhibitors** are indicated in preparation for percutaneous coronary intervention, in order to reduce platelet aggregation in the setting of epicardial artery occlusion. Aspirin and heparin in combination are more effective than either agent used alone. Clopidogrel, a platelet ADP-receptor antagonist, reduces recurrent coronary events in patients undergoing percutaneous coronary intervention. When coadministered with thrombolytics, clopidogrel increases the likelihood that the occluded vessel will remain open. GPIIb/IIIa inhibitors are not coadministered with thrombolytics because of the increased risk of bleeding. However, heparin should be administered when thrombolytic therapy is initiated. All of these agents in combination increase the risk of bleeding.

3. **The answer is B. β-receptor antagonists** are indicated for the treatment of patients with acute myocardial ischemia. They slow the rate of sinoatrial (SA) nodal firing and atrioventricular (AV) nodal conduction. By slowing the heart rate, β-receptor antagonists decrease myocardial oxygen demand in the setting of an imbalance between oxygen delivery and demand. β-receptor antagonists should not be administered in the setting of acute decompensated heart failure. Calcium channel blockers also slow AV nodal conduction and reduce myocardial contractility and systemic vascular resistance, all contributing to reduced myocardial oxygen demand. However, unlike β-receptor antagonists, calcium channel blockers have not been proven to provide a mortality benefit in the setting of coronary artery disease. Aspirin is an antiplatelet agent. Tenecteplase is a genetically engineered variant of tissue-type plasminogen activator. HMG CoA reductase inhibitors are lipid-lowering agents.

4. **The answer is B. Tolerance to the vasodilatory effect of nitrates complicates their long-term use.** Nitrate-free intervals may prevent the development of tolerance. Organic nitrates reduce preload by dilating systemic veins. They may also enhance coronary arterial flow by reducing coronary vasomotor tone. Nitrates improve exercise tolerance in patients with stable exertional angina. Headache is the most common adverse effect of nitrate therapy. Impotence is a potential adverse effect of β-receptor antagonist therapy.

5. **The answer is C. ACE inhibitors** and spironolactone (or eplerenone) are indicated for patients who have had a myocardial infarction, and who have left ventricular dysfunction. The general recommendations for the pharmacologic management of patients who have had a myocardial infarction includes aspirin, β-receptor antagonists, lipid-lowering agents, ACE inhibitors, spironolactone (or eplerenone), and clopidogrel (for patients who have undergone percutaneous coronary intervention).

CASE: PART 3

1. **The answer is C.** The initial treatment of patients with right ventricular heart failure consists of diuretic therapy (**furosemide**) to decrease intravascular volume and reduce preload. Nitrates would similarly venodilate and reduce preload. The most common cause of right ventricular heart failure is left ventricular heart failure, as noted in this case. Mr. N.'s left ventricle is dilated and thin with a reduced ejection fraction. In addition, his moderate mitral valve regurgitation contributes to excessive volume and pressure in the pulmonary vasculature, which can increase the afterload against which the right ventricle must pump. The compensatory response of the right ventricle is hypertrophy and dilation in an attempt to increase its stroke volume. Hydralazine is a systemic arterial vasodilator that would decrease left ventricular afterload. Dobutamine is a parenteral adrenergic agonist used in the treatment of patients with acute decompensated heart failure.

2. **The answer is B. Metoprolol and digoxin may cause symptomatic bradycardia** and conduction block through their combined negative chronotropic effects on the AV node. Digoxin is primarily renally excreted. Digoxin toxicity can occur in the setting of renal insufficiency.

3. **The answer is A. Milrinone** and inamrinone are phosphodiesterase inhibitors. They exert their effects by blocking the breakdown of cAMP and increasing intracellular calcium. This enhances myocyte contractility and **vasodilates both systemic arteries and veins;** therefore, these agents are commonly referred to as inodilators. **Their long-term use is associated with an increased incidence of mortality.** Nitrates are primarily venodilators, reducing preload. Long-term therapy as antihypertensives is complicated by the development of tolerance to their vasodilatory effects. Calcium channel blockers inhibit calcium-mediated arterial vascular smooth muscle contraction. ACE inhibitors prevent the conversion of angiotensin I to the vasoconstrictor, angiotensin II, the end product of renin release. β_2-receptor agonists enhance adrenergic tone at arterial vascular smooth muscle cells and promote muscle relaxation and vasodilation.

4. **The answer is E. Dobutamine** is a synthetic congener of epinephrine that acts primarily at cardiac β_1 adrenergic receptors to increase heart rate and contractility. It is administered intravenously. Digoxin and digitoxin are inotropes that can also be administered intravenously. Digoxin-specific antibodies are an antidote to cardiac glycoside toxicity. Inamrinone and milrinone can be administered intravenously. Minoxidil and hydralazine are vasodilating afterload reducers. Metoprolol is a β-receptor antagonist and negative inotrope. Although it is available in an intravenous formulation, it is not used to treat acute decompensated heart failure.

5. **The answer is D. Enjoying a big holiday meal** might contribute to an acute exacerbation of heart failure, or "holiday heart." Dietary indiscretion with excess sodium and fluid intake, medication noncompliance, myocardial ischemia, intercurrent illness, acute renal failure, or hepatic failure can all contribute to an acute exacerbation of heart failure.

IV

Principles of Endocrine Pharmacology

25

Pharmacology of the Hypothalamus and Pituitary Gland

TABLE 25-1   Anterior Pituitary Gland Cell Types, Hypothalamic Control Factors, and Hormonal Targets*

Anterior Pituitary Gland Cell Type	Stimulatory Hypothalamic Factors	Inhibitory Hypothalamic Factors	Pituitary Hormones Released	Major Target Organ	Target Gland Hormones
Somatotroph	GHRH, ghrelin	Somatostatin	GH	Liver	IGFs
Lactotroph	TRH	Dopamine, somatostatin	Prolactin	Mammary gland	None
Gonadotroph	GnRH	None known	LH and FSH	Gonads	Estrogen, progesterone, and testosterone
Thyrotroph	TRH	Somatostatin	TSH	Thyroid gland	Thyroxine and triiodothyronine
Corticotroph	CRH	None known	ACTH	Adrenal cortex	Cortisol, adrenal androgens

*Each anterior pituitary gland cell type responds to multiple hypothalamic stimulatory and inhibitory factors. Integration of these signals determines the relative extent of hormone release by the anterior pituitary gland. Each hormone has one or more specific target organs, which are, in turn, stimulated to release their own hormones. These target hormones cause feedback inhibition at the hypothalamus and anterior pituitary gland.

ACTH = adrenocorticotropic hormone; CRH = corticotropin-releasing hormone; GH = growth hormone; GHRH = growth hormone–releasing hormone; IGF = insulin-like growth factor; LH = luteinizing hormone; TSH = thyroid-stimulating hormone.

OBJECTIVES

- Understand hypothalamic and pituitary physiology, control, and regulation.

- Understand the pathophysiology and pharmacology associated with individual hypothalamic–pituitary–endocrine axes.

CASE 1

G.R. is a 54-year-old hard-driving sales executive. He travels constantly and prides himself on his high energy level and enthusiasm for surpassing his sales projections each quarter. Over the past 2 years, however, he has begun to feel increas-

ingly fatigued and has difficulty rushing the length of airport terminals. He has always had a muscular handshake, but lately he has also noticed that his company ring and wedding band are excessively tight. G.R. is also frustrated that he recently had to replace his entire dress shoe collection because his shoe size increased from 91\2 to 11. One afternoon while catching a flight back home, the man sitting next to G.R. says, ''I'm sorry to bring this up, but I can't help but noticing. I'm a medical doctor, and it looks to me like you might have acromegaly.''

QUESTIONS

1. The five hypothalamic–anterior pituitary–endocrine axes regulate numerous physiologic functions through the stimulation and inhibition of hormone release and subsequent effects on target organs. Which of the following normal physiologic axes is correctly described?

   A. Hypothalamic ghrelin stimulates anterior pituitary somatotrophs to secrete insulin-like growth factor (IGF).

   B. Hypothalamic gonadotropin-releasing hormone (GnRH) stimulates anterior pituitary lactotrophs to secrete prolactin.

   C. Hypothalamic somatostatin inhibits anterior pituitary thyrotrophs to reduce secretion of thyroid-stimulating hormone (TSH).

   D. Hypothalamic dopamine inhibits anterior pituitary somatotrophs to reduce secretion of growth hormone (GH).

   E. Hypothalamic corticotropin-releasing hormone (CRH) stimulates anterior pituitary gonadotrophs to secrete oxytocin.

G.R. scoffs at the idea that he may have any medical condition but mentions the encounter to his wife. At her prompting, G.R. goes to his doctor for further evaluation. A serum insulin-like growth factor (IGF-1) level is significantly elevated after correction for G.R.'s age, and his serum growth hormone (GH) level is 10 ng/ml (normal, < 1 ng/ml) after an oral glucose load of 75 mg. A magnetic resonance image (MRI) of his head reveals a pituitary adenoma with maximal diameter of 1.5 cm consistent with a diagnosis of acromegaly caused by a GH-secreting adenoma. After referral to an endocrinologist and neurosurgeon, G.R. elects to undergo trans-sphenoidal pituitary surgery. G.R. tolerates the surgery well, but his postoperative GH level remains elevated.

2. G.R.'s diagnostic work up included the measurement of serum levels of ILGF-1. Why is this measurement an appropriate screening test for acromegaly?

   A. Serum ILGF-1 is produced by the anterior pituitary somatotrophs under conditions of hypothalamic over-stimulation.

   B. Serum ILGF-1 is produced by the liver under conditions of anterior pituitary somatotroph over-secretion of GH.

   C. Serum ILGF-1 is produced by the liver under conditions of gigantism when the anterior pituitary is promoting hepatomegaly.

   D. Serum ILGF-1 is produced by the liver under conditions of anterior pituitary over-stimulation by ghrelin.

   E. Serum ILGF-1 is produced by the anterior pituitary under conditions of anterior pituitary over-stimulation by GH.

Based on the continued elevation in serum GH levels, G.R.'s endocrinologist recommends medical treatment with octreotide. G.R. tolerates the injections well, but he is annoyed by the need for injections every 8 hours, and airport security guards always make him put the needles in baggage. After 2 months of frequent injections, G.R. switches to a long-acting depot form of octreotide that is injected once a month. G.R. is much happier with the formulation, although he continues to experience mild nausea and bloating as an adverse effect of this medication.

3. After resection of his pituitary tumor, G.R. was initially treated with injections of octreotide, a synthetic long-acting peptide analogue of somatostatin. What is the mechanism of action of somatostatin in reducing elevated GH levels?

   A. Somatostatin decreases intracellular cyclic adenosine monophosphate (cAMP) in somatotroph cells and reduces their secretion of GH.

   B. Somatostatin inhibits growth hormone–releasing hormone (GHRH) binding to receptors on somatotroph cells and reduces their stimulation by GHRH.

   C. Somatostatin increases intracellular calcium concentrations in somatotroph cells and reduces their secretion of GH.

   D. Somatostatin increases intracellular calcium concentrations in the hypothalamus and reduces its secretion of GHRH.

   E. Somatostatin decreases intracellular cAMP in hepatocytes and reduces their release of ILGF-1.

After 6 months of depot octreotide injections, G.R.'s GH and ILGF-1 factor levels remain elevated. G.R. is frustrated at the lack of improvement of his biochemical assays but does feel that he has more energy than before treatment. G.R.'s endocrinologist recommends treatment with pegvisomant as an alternative medical approach to treating the effects of his elevated GH levels. G.R. begins monthly injections with pegvisomant. Six months later, G.R.'s ILGF-1 level is undetectable.

4. Why did G.R. have to receive injections of octreotide and pegvisomant, rather than taking the drugs orally?

   A. Peptide hormones and hormone antagonists are hepatically metabolized by first-pass metabolism.

   B. Peptide hormones and hormone antagonists are not activated when exposed to an acidic gastric pH.

   C. Peptide hormones and hormone antagonists promote antibody formation against normal hormones when they are administered orally.

   D. Peptide hormones and hormone antagonists can cause esophageal varices and bleeding.

   E. Peptide hormones and hormone antagonists are not absorbed from the intestine.

G.R. is again flying around the nation in pursuit of increased sales and stops in town just long enough to complete his yearly head MRI and liver function tests.

5. Why does G.R. have to be monitored with serial brain MRI while taking pegvisomant?
   A. Pegvisomant therapy is associated with reduced negative feedback on the posterior pituitary, and its subsequent enlargement.
   B. Pegvisomant therapy is associated with increased negative feedback on the hepatocytes, and subsequent hepatotoxicity.
   C. Pegvisomant therapy is associated with reduced negative feedback on hepatocytes, and subsequent hepatomegaly.
   D. Pegvisomant therapy is associated with the development of diabetes mellitus.
   E. Pegvisomant therapy is associated with reduced negative feedback on the anterior pituitary, and its subsequent enlargement.

■ CASE 2

Elaine is a 31-year-old woman who presents to her doctor with a complaint of unremitting headaches over the course of several months. She also notes the recent onset of irregular menses and some visual disturbances. Given her symptoms, her internist orders a serum prolactin level, which returns elevated. After a review of Ms. Y.'s medication list, her doctor adds thyroid function tests to her diagnostic laboratory screen. These studies all return with normal results. Ms. Y. undergoes brain MRI scanning, which reveals a pituitary tumor, and she is diagnosed with a pituitary prolactinoma.

QUESTIONS

1. What is the relationship of thyroid function and a patient's medication use to an elevated serum prolactin level?
   A. TSH and dopamine receptor agonists stimulate prolactin release.
   B. TSH and dopamine receptor antagonists stimulate prolactin release.
   C. Thyrotropin-releasing hormone (TRH) stimulates prolactin release, and phenothiazine antipsychotics provide negative feedback to its release.
   D. TRH and phenothiazine antipsychotics stimulate prolactin release.
   E. TRH provides negative feedback to prolactin release, and phenothiazine antipsychotics stimulate prolactin release.

Ms. Y. is referred to an endocrinologist to discuss potential therapies of her pituitary tumor. She is frightened of ''having brain surgery'' and decides to opt for medical therapy with bromocriptine. To limit potential adverse effects of this therapy, her endocrinologist administers bromocriptine at a low dose, which Ms. Y. takes orally at bedtime, then slowly increases her dose every 3 days, until she is taking bromocriptine 2.5 mg twice daily. Her serum prolactin levels are followed closely and show a slight reduction. However, after several months of therapy, Ms. Y. complains that the adverse effects of bromocriptine are preventing her from performing her usual job as a children's librarian.

2. How does bromocriptine contribute to a reduction in serum prolactin concentration?
   A. Bromocriptine is a TRH antagonist that suppresses lactotroph release of prolactin and TSH.
   B. Bromocriptine is a dopamine antagonist that competitively antagonizes the binding of phenothiazine antipsychotics.
   C. Bromocriptine is a dopamine agonist that inhibits the binding of prolactin on mammary gland cells.
   D. Bromocriptine is a dopamine agonist that suppresses TRH release from the hypothalamus.
   E. Bromocriptine is a dopamine agonist that suppresses lactotroph cell growth and inhibits release of prolactin.

Ms. Y. decides to undergo trans-sphenoidal resection of her pituitary prolactinoma. The procedure is uneventful and successful. After surgery, she is monitored closely. She is weighed daily, and the nurses carefully measure her oral and intravenous intake of fluids, as well as her urine output. Her serum electrolytes (sodium, potassium, and calcium), serum osmolarity, and urine-specific gravity are monitored twice daily. Two days after surgery, Ms. Y. notes that she is in the bathroom urinating ''constantly.'' She feels thirsty. Over the ensuing 12 hours, her urine output exceeds 300 cc/hr, and her measured serum sodium is elevated. The consulting neuroendocrinologist considers administering a medication to reverse this abnormal fluid balance. After therapy, Ms. Y. is feeling improved and is able to be discharged home 6 days after surgery.

3. Of the following combinations (drug : mechanism of action), which is most likely to be effective in treating Ms. Y.'s postoperative symptoms?
   A. demeclocycline : stimulates antidiuretic hormone (ADH) secretion from the posterior pituitary
   B. desmopressin : stimulates V_2 receptors in the nephron to increase water resorption
   C. conivaptan : antagonizes ADH effects at V_1 receptors in the nephron
   D. desmopressin : antagonizes ADH effects at V_2 receptors in the nephron
   E. demeclocycline : stimulates osmoreceptors in the hypothalamus to secrete oxytocin

4. Cosyntropin is a synthetic form of ACTH used to diagnose suspected cases of adrenal insufficiency. Administration of cosyntropin to patients with adrenal insufficiency will cause:
   A. no increase in plasma cortisol concentration
   B. no increase in ACTH release
   C. an increase in mineralocorticoid release
   D. an increase in plasma cortisol concentration
   E. an increase in ACTH release

5. Leuprolide is a peptide GnRH analogue that is used therapeutically in:
   A. induction of labor
   B. uterine atony
   C. androgen-dependent prostate cancer
   D. ovarian hyperstimulation syndrome
   E. oxytocin deficiency in nursing mothers

26

Pharmacology of the Thyroid Gland

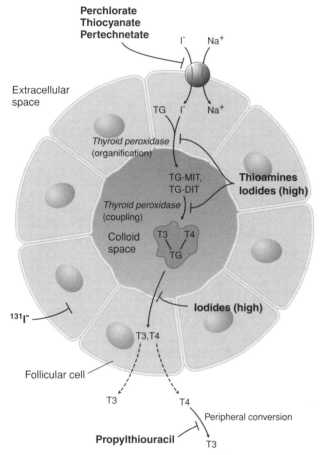

Figure 26-1. Pharmacologic Interventions Affecting Thyroid Hormone Synthesis. Anions with a molecular radius approximately equal to that of the iodide anion (I^-), such as perchlorate, thiocyanate, and pertechnetate, compete with iodide for uptake by the Na^+/I^- symporter. Radioactive $^{131}I^-$, when concentrated within thyroid cells, causes selective destruction of the thyroid gland. High levels of iodide transiently depress thyroid function by inhibiting organification, coupling, and proteolysis of thyroglobulin. Thioamines, such as propylthiouracil and methimazole, inhibit organification and coupling; propylthiouracil also inhibits peripheral conversion of T4 to T3. TG-DIT = thyroglobulin-diiodotyrosine; TG-MIT = thyroglobulin-monoiodotyrosine.

OBJECTIVES

■ Understand the physiologic regulation of thyroid hormone.

■ Understand the pharmacology, therapeutic uses, and adverse effects of agents used in the setting of altered thyroid hormone regulation.

■ CASE 1

Over the course of a few months, 45-year-old Diana L. notices a number of disconcerting changes in the way she feels and her general appearance. Ms. L. feels nervous all the time; small events make her jumpy. She also keeps the temperature unusually cold in her house, to the point where her husband and children begin to complain. Because of these symptoms and the occasional feeling that her heart "skips a beat," Ms. L. goes to see her doctor. After some questioning, he palpates her neck and notes that her thyroid gland is diffusely enlarged. He also notes that her eyes are more prominent than normal. Tests for thyroid hormone levels reveal high serum-free triiodothyronine (T3) and low thyrotropin (thyroid-stimulating hormone [TSH]). In addition, a test for TSH receptor antibody is positive.

QUESTIONS

1. Why was Ms. L.'s serum TSH level low, but her T3 concentration high?

A. High concentrations of T3 are not being converted to T4.

B. High concentrations of T3 are causing negative feedback on TSH production.

C. Low concentrations of TSH are causing preferential production of T3.

D. High concentrations of TSH are causing excessive T3 production.

E. Low concentrations of TSH are causing positive feedback on TRH release.

Ms. L. is diagnosed with Grave's disease, a form of hyper-thyroidism, and treated with methimazole. Although initially comforted by the fact that her doctor can explain her symptoms, she soon becomes discouraged because she does not notice any improvement for a couple of weeks. After 1 month, however, her symptoms begin to subside. Repeat tests confirm that her thyroid hormone levels are normalized. One year after starting treatment with methimazole, however, she begins to re-experience palpitations and feels anxious. Her doctor confirms that her thyroid hormone levels are again elevated despite methimazole therapy.

2. What is the mechanism of action of methimazole?
    A. Methimazole inhibits conversion of T4 to T3 in the liver.
    B. Methimazole inhibits thyroid peroxidase function and limits T4 and T3 production.
    C. Methimazole inhibits TSH stimulation of follicular cells.
    D. Methimazole inhibits iodine uptake into the follicular cells and limits T4 and T3 production.
    E. Methimazole inhibits release of pre-formed rT3 from the follicular cells.

After discussion with her doctor, Ms. L. elects to undergo treatment with radioactive iodide. She tolerates the treatment well, and testing over the next 3 years shows that she has normal thyroid hormone levels.

3. What features of the thyroid gland make radioactive iodide a generally safe and specific therapy for hyperthyroidism?
    A. The thyroid gland consists of cells with a low rate of turnover, which are not susceptible to radioactive toxicity.
    B. The thyroid gland competitively takes up iodide in the presence of ipodate.
    C. The thyroid gland selectively takes up and concentrates iodide.
    D. The thyroid gland shields other head and neck structures from potential radioactive toxicity.
    E. The thyroid gland takes up radioactive iodide, which destroys excess thyroglobulin and colloid.

Four years after radioactive iodide treatment, Ms. L. begins to develop symptoms that are the opposite of her original problems: she feels tired all the time, and she gains 30 pounds over the course of 6 months. Her doctor confirms that Ms. L. has developed hypothyroidism. He prescribes thyroxine (T4), which she now takes once a day, and she feels well again.

4. Why did Ms. L. develop hypothyroidism after treatment with radioactive iodide?
    A. Radioactive iodide depleted her normal stores of thyroglobulin and colloid.

    B. Radioactive iodide prevented future gastrointestinal absorption of dietary iodide.
    C. Hypothyroidism is the final disease manifestation of Grave's disease.
    D. Radioactive iodide killed all or most of her thyroid follicular cells.
    E. Radioactive iodide inhibited normal thyroid gland function through the Wolff–Chaikoff effect.

5. Levothyroxine is a pharmacologic replacement for missing endogenous thyroid hormone. Which of the following statements regarding levothyroxine is correct?
    A. Levothyroxine metabolism is inhibited by drugs which induce hepatic P450 enzyme function.
    B. Levothyroxine is a mixed isomeric formulation of T4 and T3, allowing for a more physiologic correction of hypothyroidism.
    C. Levothyroxine therapy causes elevated TSH levels.
    D. Levothyroxine is an L-isomer of T3 with a half-life of one day, allowing for periodic daily dose adjustments based on changing metabolic needs.
    E. Levothyroxine is an L-isomer of T4 with a half-life of 6 days, creating a circulating pool of thyroid "pro-drug" to buffer and normalize metabolic rates.

■ CASE 2

Lacey P. is a 72-year-old woman who is brought to the emergency department by ambulance when her neighbors become concerned that they have not seen her come out of her apartment in the mornings to collect her daily newspaper. Paramedics report that they found Mrs. P. confused, lying in her bed. There was evidence in the bedroom and bathroom that she had vomited dark brown material, and been incontinent of stool. They noted that the temperature in the apartment was quite cold for this January day.

Mrs. P. is confused and lethargic but is able to say that she has a medical history of "heart disease, high blood pressure, and low thyroid." Two weeks ago, she was diagnosed with a bladder infection and began taking antibiotics. However, the antibiotics have "aggravated her irritable bowel," and she has been vomiting and having diarrhea for the past 10 days. She has not been able to eat or drink or take her medications for at least 10 days.

On examination, Mrs. P. is a dehydrated-appearing elderly woman. Her vital signs are remarkable for a temperature of 95°F (35°C), a heart rate of 58 bpm, a respiratory rate of eight breaths/min., and a blood pressure of 86/52 mm Hg. Her lips and mucous membranes are very dry, her lung examination reveals coarse rhonchi bilaterally, and her abdomen is distended with diminished bowel sounds. Her extremities are edematous, and her skin is puffy and pale.

Intravenous access is obtained and laboratory studies, including blood and urine cultures, are sent. An electrocardiogram (ECG) shows sinus bradycardia with a prolonged QT interval and non-specific ST changes. A portable chest X-ray shows cardiomegaly and a right lower lobe consolidation consistent with aspiration pneumonia.

QUESTIONS

1. Based on Mrs. P.'s presentation, which of the following laboratory data are most consistent with her current illness?

    A. high TSH, high T3, high T4

    B. low TSH, high T3, high T4

    C. low TSH, high Tslg, low T3, low T4

    D. high TSH, high Tslg, high T3, high T4

    E. high TSH, low T3, low T4

2. Mrs. P. is treated with intravenous fluid resuscitation, broad-spectrum intravenous antibiotics, and passive rewarming before admission to the intensive care unit. Which of the following therapies is indicated?

    A. intravenous thyroxine

    B. β-receptor antagonists

    C. intravenous phenytoin

    D. oral cholestyramine

    E. intravenous infusion of thyroid-stimulating immunoglobulin

3. Patients with hyperthyroidism may be medically managed with thioamines. A potential complication of this therapy includes:

    A. induction of hepatic P450 enzymes

    B. agranulocytosis

    C. weight gain

    D. organification

    E. Hashimoto's thyroiditis

4. β-receptor antagonists are used in the treatment of thyroid storm. What is the rationale for the use of these medications in this disease?

    A. β-receptor antagonists inhibit release of TSH.

    B. β-receptor antagonists inhibit release of T4.

    C. β-receptor antagonists block sympathomimetic-like symptoms.

    D. β-receptor antagonists block oral levothyroxine absorption.

    E. β-receptor antagonists block iodide uptake into the follicular cells.

5. A number of pharmacologic agents can affect thyroid hormone homeostasis. Which of the following combinations (drug : interaction) is correct?

    A. amiodarone : diminished thyroid hormone production

    B. rifampin : enhanced hepatic metabolism of thyroid hormone

    C. methimazole : enhanced conversion of T3 to T4

    D. corticosteroids : decreased release of TSH

    E. sodium polystyrene sulfate : enhanced secretion of thyroid hormone into the gastrointestinal lumen

27

Pharmacology of the Adrenal Cortex

Figure 27-1. Hormone Synthesis in the Adrenal Cortex. The hormones of the adrenal cortex are steroids derived from cholesterol. The rate-limiting step in adrenal hormone biosynthesis is the modification of cholesterol to pregnenolone by side-chain cleavage enzyme. From this step, pregnenolone metabolism can be directed toward the formation of aldosterone, cortisol, or androstenedione. The flux of metabolites through each of these pathways depends on the tissue-specific expression of enzymes in the different cell types of the cortex and on the relative activity of the different synthetic enzymes. Note that several enzymes are involved in more than one pathway and that defects in these enzymes can affect the synthesis of more than one hormone. For example, a defect in steroid 21-hydroxylase prevents the synthesis of both aldosterone and cortisol. This overlap of synthetic activities also contributes to the nonselective action of glucocorticoid synthesis inhibitors such as trilostane. Aminoglutethimide and high levels of ketoconazole inhibit side-chain cleavage enzyme. Ketoconazole also inhibits 17, 20-lyase; trilostane inhibits 3β-hydroxysteroid dehydrogenase; and metyrapone inhibits steroid 11β-hydroxylase. Enzymes are shown as numbers: 11 = steroid 11β-hydroxylase; 17 = steroid 17α-hydroxylase; 21 = steroid 21-hydroxylase. ACTH = adrenocorticotropic hormone. Adapted from Cotran RS, Kumar V, Collins T, eds. Robbins Pathologic Basis of Disease, 6th Ed, Figure 26-27. Philadelphia: WB Saunders Company, 1999. With permission from Elsevier.

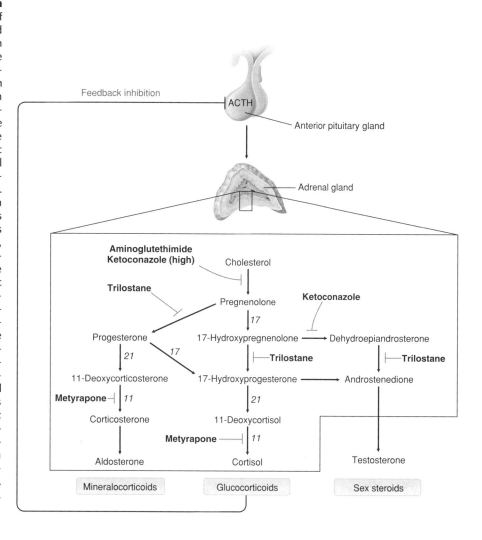

OBJECTIVES

- Understand the normal physiologic control and functions of adrenal hormones.
- Understand the pharmacologic indications and adverse effects of agents that affect glucocorticoid and mineralocorticoid pathways.

■ CASE 1

Johnny is 8 years old when he finds that he can barely catch his breath at times, especially while exercising. His asthma comes and goes, but no therapy seems to stop the asthma attacks completely. Although his doctor is concerned that it could stunt Johnny's growth, she eventually prescribes oral prednisone (a glucocorticoid analogue) and tells Johnny's parents to make sure he takes the medication every day.

After a few weeks, Johnny's asthma attacks subside, and he is able to have a fairly normal childhood. During this time, the doctor pays close attention to Johnny's linear growth.

QUESTIONS

1. Why are cortisol analogues such as prednisone used for treating asthma?
   A. Cortisol analogues reduce lung compliance.
   B. Cortisol analogues enhance oxygen utilization.
   C. Cortisol analogues enhance rib growth.
   D. Cortisol analogues promote lung maturation.
   E. Cortisol analogues reduce airway inflammation.

2. Why did the doctor monitor Johnny's linear growth?
   A. Chronic glucocorticoid use diverts calcium to soft tissue rather than to bone.
   B. Chronic glucocorticoid use prevents glucose uptake by bone.
   C. Chronic glucocorticoid use prevents bone mineralization, resulting in soft bones.
   D. Chronic glucocorticoid use slows linear bone growth, resulting in short stature.
   E. Chronic glucocorticoid use promotes bone resorption and pathologic fractures.

Two years later, Johnny's doctor decides that a new inhaled glucocorticoid could be a safer medication for him. Johnny switches to the inhaled glucocorticoid and discontinues oral prednisone. Three days later, he develops a respiratory infection and is brought to the emergency department with low blood pressure and a temperature of 103°F. Based on his history of prednisone use, Johnny is immediately given hydrocortisone (cortisol) intravenously, as well as a saline infusion.

3. Why did abrupt cessation of oral prednisone precipitate Johnny's clinical presentation in the emergency department?
   A. Johnny had acute adrenal insufficiency.
   B. Johnny had acute prednisone withdrawal.
   C. Johnny had an acute exacerbation of asthma.
   D. Johnny had an acute allergic reaction to an inhaled glucocorticoid.
   E. Johnny had acute fever and dehydration.

Johnny recovers, and for the next 6 months slowly tapers his oral prednisone dose with continued use of the inhaled glucocorticoid. Eventually, he is able to take the inhaled glucocorticoid alone as an effective therapy for his asthma.

4. Why are inhaled glucocorticoids safer than oral glucocorticoids for long-term treatment of asthma?
   A. Inhaled glucocorticoids limit the development of oro-

pharyngeal candidiasis and the resultant bronchial irritation it causes.
   B. Inhaled glucocorticoids deliver the drug locally to limit long-term exacerbations of asthma.
   C. Inhaled glucocorticoids deliver the drug locally to limit long-term systemic glucocorticoid exposure.
   D. Inhaled glucocorticoids deliver a greater percentage of each drug dose to the lung.
   E. Inhaled glucocorticoids are activated by first-pass metabolism in the liver to exert a more potent drug effect.

5. Which of the following agents has both glucocorticoid and mineralocorticoid activity?
   A. prednisone
   B. fludrocortisone
   C. dexamethasone
   D. mifepristone
   E. aldosterone

 CASE 2

In November, 1955, the *Journal of the American Medical Association* (*JAMA*) published a letter to the editor of a case of a 37-year-old man with Addison's disease who had been managed for several years with exogenous corticosteroid replacement. The patient also had a history of significant back pain and was advised to undergo lumbosacral fusion after orthopedic consultation. Surgical intervention was thought to be exceedingly dangerous in this case because of the patient's adrenal cortical insufficiency and the trauma involved in the operation.

QUESTIONS

1. What normal physiologic functions are under the control of cortisol?
   A. Cortisol mobilizes amino acid in response to a prolonged fast.
   B. Cortisol promotes glucose uptake by muscle cells in response to trauma.
   C. Cortisol promotes glycogen synthesis by the liver in response to severe infection.
   D. Cortisol promotes lipolysis in response to a large meal.
   E. Cortisol enhances the inflammatory response to inhaled irritants.

The *JAMA* report continued that because the patient would be nearly incapacitated by his back pain without surgical intervention, it was decided to undergo two operations on his back. The patient suffered some complications postoperatively, but no Addisonian crisis occurred.

2. What is a clinical effect of hypoaldosteronism in Addison's disease?
   A. hair loss
   B. lower extremity edema
   C. hypertension
   D. hypotension
   E. muscle spasm

The patient in the above report is widely suspected to have been President John F. Kennedy. Many historical writings have commented on Kennedy's ''year-round'' tan.

3. What is the etiology of increased skin pigmentation in patients with primary hypoadrenalism?
   A. Anterior pituitary adenomas release excessive melanocyte-stimulating hormone (MSH) to stimulate MSH receptors in the skin.
   B. High concentrations of both adrenocorticotropic hormone (ACTH) and MSH stimulate MSH receptors in the skin.
   C. High concentrations of MSH are secreted by the adrenal cortex in response to ACTH stimulation.
   D. Low concentrations of aldosterone promote renal sparing of MSH proteins.
   E. Frequent sun exposure is necessary to promote vitamin D synthesis in the setting of glucocorticoid excess.

4. Which of the following statements regarding aldosterone, spironolactone, and potassium is correct?
   A. Potassium loading decreases aldosterone synthesis, reversing the therapeutic effects of spironolactone.
   B. Spironolactone potentiates the effects of excess aldosterone in causing hyperkalemic acidosis.
   C. Spironolactone antagonizes the physiologic activity of aldosterone, which is to cause sodium retention and potassium excretion.
   D. Aldosterone promotes renal sodium and potassium wasting, which is reversed by the therapeutic action of spironolactone.
   E. Hyperaldosteronism leads to hyperkalemia, which is reversed by the administration of spironolactone.

5. The treatment of patients with secondary adrenal insufficiency includes replacement with:
   A. ketoconazole
   B. spironolactone
   C. fludrocortisone
   D. hydrocortisone
   E. fluticasone

28

Pharmacology of Reproduction

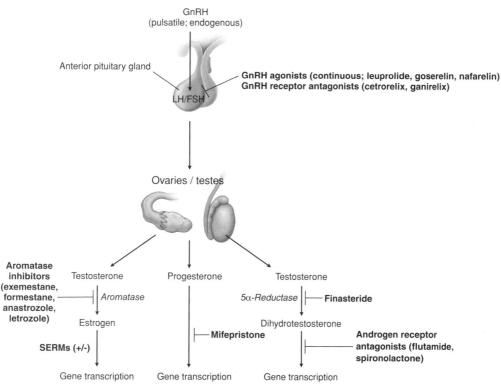

Figure 28-1. Pharmacologic Modulation of Gonadal Hormone Action. Pharmacologic modulation of gonadal hormone action can be divided into inhibitors of hormone synthesis and hormone receptor antagonists. Continuous administration of gonadotropin-releasing hormone (GnRH) suppresses luteinizing hormone (LH) and follicle-stimulating hormone (FSH) release from the anterior pituitary gland, preventing gonadal hormone synthesis. GnRH receptor antagonists (cetrorelix, ganirelix) are also used for this purpose. Finasteride inhibits the enzyme 5α-reductase, preventing conversion of testosterone to the more active dihydrotestosterone. Aromatase inhibitors (exemestane, formestane, anastrozole, letrozole) inhibit production of estrogens from androgens. A number of hormone receptor antagonists prevent the action of endogenous estrogens (some selective estrogen receptor modulators [SERMs]), androgens (flutamide, spironolactone), and progesterone (mifepristone).

OBJECTIVES

▪ Understand the physiology and pathophysiology of reproductive hormone control.

▪ Understand the pharmacology of, indications for, and adverse effects of agents that modulate reproductive hormone synthesis and function.

▪ CASE 1

Amy J. first notices that her hair is thinning somewhat during her teenage years. Even though she loses some hair on her scalp, Ms. J. notices excessive hair growth on her face; she sometimes has to shave to remove inappropriate hair growth. At age 24, she goes to her doctor complaining of both her hair problem and the fact that her periods are irregular. On further questioning, the doctor discovers that the longest interval between her menstrual cycles has been 6 months and the shortest 22 days. When Ms. J. does have periods, they are heavy and last for more than her previous average of 5 days. The increased hair growth on her face, extremities, abdomen, and breasts had begun around age 15. Ms. J. also reports a problem with being overweight since high school, although in middle school she had been extremely active in soccer, field hockey, and swimming. The doctor orders several tests and finds that Ms. J. has mildly elevated free and total testosterone levels and an increased ratio of plasma luteinizing hormone (LH) to follicle-stimulating hormone (FSH). Based on these findings, the doctor tells Ms. J. that she probably has a disorder called polycystic ovarian syndrome (PCOS).

QUESTIONS

1. What is the pathophysiologic link between excessive hair growth and infertility in polycystic ovarian syndrome?
   A. Increased androgen levels stimulate excessive hair growth, while also limiting luteinizing hormone (LH) and FSH production,
   B. Increased LH and androgen levels inhibit ovulation, while increased androgen levels stimulate excessive hair growth.
   C. Increased LH stimulates Leydig cells to increase the production of androgens, which stimulate excessive hair growth.
   D. Increased LH to FSH ratios enhance the aromatization of androgens to estrogens, and stimulate excessive hair growth and inhibit ovulation.
   E. Increased androgen levels stimulate excessive hair growth and are converted to LH, which inhibits ovulation.

Ms. J.'s doctor recommends combination estrogen-progestin oral contraceptives to regularize her menstrual cycles. He also prescribes spironolactone to reduce her problems with hair growth and balding.

2. Which of the following statements regarding oral contraceptives is correct?
   A. Estrogen-only contraceptives are favored because they limit the androgenic adverse effects of progestins.
   B. The use of oral contraceptives for more than 10 years significantly increases a woman's risk of developing breast cancer.
   C. Mifepristone is a third-generation progestin-only agent that minimizes the risk of developing estrogen-associated endometrial cancer.
   D. Biphasic and triphasic contraceptive formulations maintain a constant low dose of estrogen and progestin, but vary the concentration of androstenedione.
   E. The combination of estrogen and a progestin suppresses gonadotropin-releasing hormone (GnRH), LH, and FSH secretion, suppressing follicle growth and ovulation.

3. How will the effects of oral contraceptives help regularize Ms. J.'s menstrual cycles?
   A. Estrogen-containing oral contraceptives will replace the lack of estrogen being secreted by ovarian follicles.
   B. Estrogen-progestin oral contraceptives will suppress ovarian production of testosterone.
   C. Progestin-only oral contraceptives will prevent ovulation and redistribute excessive hair growth to the scalp.
   D. Estrogen-progestin oral contraceptives will permanently antagonize the end-organ effects of androgens.
   E. Estrogen-containing oral contraceptives will block the effects of LH on the granulosa cells.

4. Why was spironolactone prescribed to reduce Ms. J.'s hair problem?
   A. Spironolactone promotes hair growth.
   B. Spironolactone is an aldosterone antagonist.
   C. Spironolactone is an androgen antagonist.
   D. Spironolactone enhance the degradation of androgens.
   E. Spironolactone enhances the renal elimination of excessive androgens.

5. The LH and FSH surges cause
   A. ovulation
   B. corpus luteum involution
   C. endometrial secretion
   D. follicular release of activin
   E. endometrial secretion of human chorionic gonadotropin (hCG)

■ CASE 2

A 26-year-old male amateur bodybuilder (222 pounds; 5 foot, 11 inches) with no medical history suddenly collapses in the gym. He is incontinent of urine, develops agonal respirations, and then cardio-pulmonary arrest. Despite advanced cardiac life support measures, the patient expires at the hospital. An autopsy report notes gynecomastia, testicular atrophy, and an acneiform rash over the patient's face and torso. The autopsy pathology findings include mildly atherosclerotic coronary arteries, a heart weight of 515 g (normal, 250 g), and concentric left ventricular hypertrophy. The patient had just completed a 3-month cycle of anabolic androgenic steroids, including methenolone (a dihydrotestosterone derivative) and veterinarian-grade testosterone enanthate.

QUESTIONS

1. What is the physiologic relationship between this patient's use of exogenous testosterone and the development of gynecomastia and testicular atrophy?

A. Exogenous testosterone suppresses the effects of gonadotropins on the testicular cells, causing testicular atrophy, and is converted to estrogen, causing gynecomastia.

B. Exogenous testosterone causes prostatic hypertrophy, which increases pressure on testicular cells, causing testicular atrophy, and is converted to estrogen, causing gynecomastia.

C. Exogenous testosterone overstimulates testicular cells, causing premature aging and atrophy, and overstimulates breast tissue cells, causing gynecomastia.

D. Exogenous testosterone causes hyperlipidemia, which contributes to inadequate testicular blood flow and atrophy, while promoting lipid deposits in breast tissue.

E. Exogenous testosterone suppresses the effects of gonadotropins on the testicular cells and breast tissue cells, causing testicular atrophy and reactive breast engorgement.

2. Aging men with both symptoms of hypogonadism *and* low plasma testosterone levels may be administered androgen replacement therapy. Which of the following statements regarding androgen replacement therapy is correct?

A. Oral testosterone must be administered on an empty stomach to facilitate its absorption.

B. Testosterone replacement therapy can contribute to the development of testicular cancer.

C. Transdermal testosterone patches must be applied every 2 to 4 weeks to achieve physiologic replacement levels of testosterone.

D. Intramuscular testosterone administration is contraindicated because of rapid hepatic metabolism of the drug.

E. Daily application of a testosterone topical gel formulation reaches physiologic replacement levels of testosterone after 1 month of application.

3. Finasteride is approved for the treatment of patients with benign prostatic hyperplasia. By what mechanism does finasteride reduce the rate of prostatic enlargement?

A. Finasteride blocks type II 5α-reductase conversion of testosterone to dihydrotestosterone in prostatic cells, slowing their growth.

B. Finasteride blocks the release of gonadotropins, preventing their stimulation of prostatic cells and slowing their growth.

C. Finasteride is a direct competitive antagonist at the androgen receptor in prostatic cells, slowing their growth.

D. Finasteride blocks the aromatase conversion of estrogens to androgens, limiting the effect of dihydrotestosterone on prostatic cells, slowing their growth.

E. Finasteride stimulates estrogen receptors to overcome the growth effects of androgens on prostatic cells, slowing their growth.

4. Selective estrogen receptor modulators (SERMs) inhibit estrogenic effects in some tissues while promoting estrogenic effects in others. Which of the following combinations (SERM : pharmacologic effect) is correct?

A. tamoxifen : estrogen antagonist in breast and endometrial tissues

B. tamoxifen: estrogen antagonist in breast but agonist in endometrial tissue

C. raloxifene : estrogen antagonist in breast and bone tissues

D. raloxifene : estrogen agonist in breast but antagonist in endometrial tissue

E. clomiphene : estrogen antagonist in hypothalamus and bone tissue

5. Estrogen replacement therapy is associated with the development of:

A. endometriosis

B. uterine atrophy

C. ovarian cancer

D. thromboembolic disease

E. coronary artery disease

29

Pharmacology of the Endocrine Pancreas

OBJECTIVES

■ Understand the physiologic controls and pathophysiologic states that affect energy homeostasis.

■ Understand the pharmacology of, indications for, and adverse effects of various agents used to treat hyperglycemia in Type I and Type II diabetes mellitus.

■ CASE 1

At her annual checkup, 55-year-old Mrs. S. complains of fatigue and frequent urination (polyuria), even at night. She also reports drinking large volumes of fluids (polydipsia) to quench her thirst. Although these symptoms have been "going on for a while" and are getting worse, Mrs. S. has difficulty pinpointing their exact onset. She denies other urinary symptoms such as pain on urination, blood in her urine, dribbling, and incontinence. Her medical history is remarkable for hyperlipidemia of 10 years' duration. Both of her parents died of coronary heart disease in their early 60s.

On physical examination, Mrs. S. is moderately obese but otherwise appears well. Glucose is detected in her urine, but proteins and ketones are not. Her blood tests are significant for elevated glucose (240 mg/dL); elevated total cholesterol (340 mg/dL); and HbA1c, a measure of glucose covalently bound to hemoglobin, of 9.2%. The physician explains to Mrs. S. that she has Type II diabetes mellitus. In this disease, the body fails to respond normally to insulin (insulin resistance) and cannot produce a sufficient amount of insulin to overcome this resistance.

QUESTIONS

1. What are the cellular and molecular actions of insulin?
   A. Insulin binds to its receptor on hepatocytes and stimulates the activity of glycogen synthase.
   B. Insulin binds to the GLUT4 receptor on adipose cells and promotes the activity of hormone sensitive lipase.
   C. Insulin binds to its receptor on muscle cells and promotes amino acid synthesis.
   D. Insulin binds to hemoglobin and reverses its glycosylation by excess circulating glucose.
   E. Insulin promotes the renal excretion of excess glucose.

2. Which of the following statements regarding the etiologies of Type I and Type II diabetes mellitus is correct?
   A. Type II diabetes mellitus is caused by a genetic predisposition to obesity and pancreatic α-cell failure.
   B. Type II diabetes mellitus is caused by the development of pancreatic β-cell resistance to post-prandial plasma glucose concentrations.
   C. Type II diabetes mellitus is caused by a viral infection, which promotes the production of autoantibodies, and the destruction of pancreatic β-cells.
   D. Type I diabetes mellitus is caused by a viral infection, which specifically targets and destroys gastrointestinal cells, including the pancreatic β-cells.
   E. Type I diabetes mellitus is caused by the autoimmune destruction of pancreatic β-cells in patients with a genetic predisposition to the formation of autoantibodies.

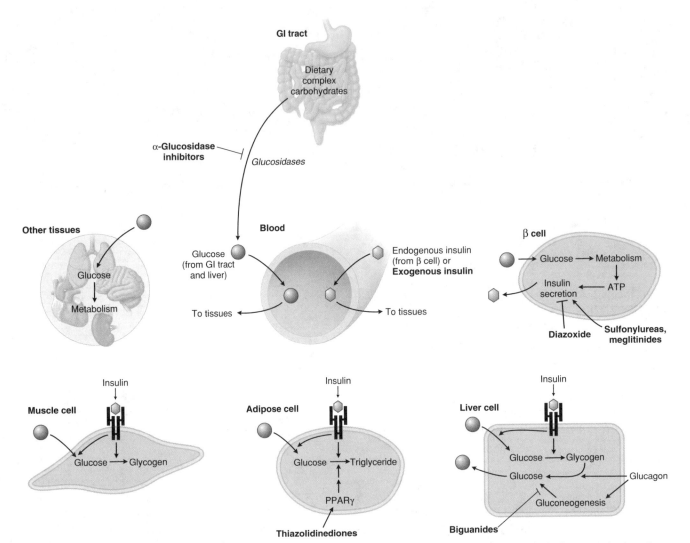

Figure 29-1. Physiologic and Pharmacologic Regulation of Glucose Homeostasis. Dietary complex carbohydrates are broken down to simple sugars in the gastrointestinal (GI) tract by the action of glucosidases; simple sugars are then absorbed by GI epithelial cells and transported into the blood. Glucose in the blood is taken up by all metabolically active tissues in the body. In pancreatic β cells, glucose metabolism increases levels of cytosolic adenosine triphosphate (ATP), which stimulates insulin secretion. Insulin then acts on plasma membrane insulin receptors in target tissues (muscle, adipose, liver) to increase glucose uptake and storage as glycogen or triglyceride. Glucose is also taken up by other cells and tissues to fuel metabolism. In muscle cells, insulin promotes glucose storage as glycogen. In adipose cells, insulin promotes glucose conversion to triglycerides. Peroxisome proliferator-activated receptor γ (PPARγ) also promotes the conversion of glucose to triglycerides in adipose cells. In liver cells, insulin promotes glucose storage as glycogen. Glucagon promotes both gluconeogenesis and the conversion of glycogen back to glucose; glucose generated by gluconeogenesis or from glycogen is transported out of the liver cell into the blood. Note that glucose from dietary complex carbohydrates and insulin secreted by pancreatic β cells both enter the liver in high concentrations through the portal circulation (not shown). Pharmacologic interventions that decrease blood glucose levels include inhibiting intestinal β-glucosidases; administering exogenous insulin; using sulfonylureas or meglitinides to augment secretion of insulin by β cells; and using biguanides or thiazolidinediones to enhance the action of insulin in liver or adipose cells, respectively. Glucagon like peptide-1 (GLP-1) mimetics decrease blood glucose levels by several complementary mechanisms (not shown). Diazoxide inhibits insulin secretion from pancreatic β cells.

3. Mrs. S. has both blood glucose and HbA1c levels measured during her annual appointment. What do these test results indicate about blood glucose concentrations?

   A. An elevated blood glucose level indicates a recent carbohydrate-rich meal while an elevated HbA1c indicates that glucose control has been adequate over the preceding months.

   B. A low blood glucose level indicates good recent glucose control, while a low HbA1c indicates that the patient suffers from acute hemolytic anemia.

   C. A low blood glucose level indicates good recent glucose control, while an elevated HbA1c indicates that glucose has been elevated over the preceding months.

   D. An elevated blood glucose level indicates poor recent glucose control, while a low HbA1c indicates that the patient is at risk of diabetic complications.

   E. Elevated blood glucose and HbA1c levels indicate that the patient recently discontinued his or her insulin use.

The physician discusses with Mrs. S. the importance of decreasing her caloric intake and increasing her exercise to improve her metabolic state. The physician also prescribes metformin (a biguanide) to treat her diabetes.

4. In addition to alleviating her polyuria and polydipsia, why is it important to control Mrs. S.'s diabetes (What acute and chronic complications could arise)?

A. Mrs. S. is at risk for developing starvation ketosis.

B. Mrs. S. is at risk for developing glycosylation of atrophied skeletal muscles.

C. Mrs. S. is at risk for developing atherosclerotic heart disease.

D. Mrs. S. is at risk for osmotic diarrhea.

E. Mrs. S. is at risk for developing acute HbA1c hemolysis.

5. Mrs. S. was prescribed metformin, a biguanide, as an initial treatment for her diabetes. How do the mechanisms of action of different pharmacologic therapies for diabetes influence the decision about which therapy to institute?

A. Biguanides block adenosine monophosphate (AMP)–dependent protein kinase and inhibit hepatic gluconeogenesis, but should not be used in patients with high-protein diets.

B. Biguanides block AMP-dependent protein kinase and inhibit hepatic gluconeogenesis, but do not contribute to weight gain in obese patients.

C. α-Glucosidase inhibitors enhance the intestinal breakdown of ingested carbohydrates, but should not be used in patients with short-gut syndrome.

D. Sulfonylureas stimulate pancreatic β-cell insulin release, but also promote muscle wasting and should not be used in patients with myopathies.

E. Sulfonylureas improve insulin sensitivity in adipose tissue by modulating the transcription of genes, but promote weight gain in obese patients.

■ CASE 2

In 1933, Bill is 4 years old when he abruptly becomes ill with loss of appetite, nausea, and generalized weakness. His parents note that he is sleeping a lot. They bring him to their family doctor, where a urine test shows a large amount of glucose. His blood glucose is elevated, greater than 400 mg/dL. He is diagnosed with diabetes mellitus. Fortunately for Bill and his family, they live just outside of Boston, Massachusetts, and his parents take him to Dr. Elliott P. Joslin, M.D. for an evaluation. Dr. Joslin, a diabetes specialist in practice since 1898, has been treating diabetic children with the newly identified and isolated protein, insulin. Bill is treated with injections of insulin derived from calf pancreas. His mother is very strict about what he is allowed to eat, weighing and limiting the portion of carbohydrates in his diet.

QUESTIONS

1. Insulin was first isolated from an extract of dog pancreas in the summer of 1921. For the majority of the 20th century, diabetic patients were treated with insulin derived from beef or porcine sources. What is a potential disadvantage of this therapy?

A. Non–human-derived insulin must be administered parenterally.

B. Non–human-derived insulin is less effective than human insulin.

C. Non–human-derived insulin can cause potential immunologic reactions.

D. Non–human-derived insulin is easier to obtain commercially.

E. Non-human-derived insulin promotes weight gain.

2. Today several types of exogenous insulin preparations are available to treat hyperglycemia. They are classified by their onset and duration of action. Which of the following combinations (insulin type : duration of action) is correct?

A. Lispro : intermediate acting (16–24 hours)

B. Glargine : long acting (18–24 hours)

C. Lente : short acting (6–8 hours)

D. Regular : ultrarapid acting (3–4 hours)

E. Semilente : long acting (24–36 hours)

In 1969, Bill, now 40 years old, begins to develop complications of his diabetes, including retinopathy, which is treated with a newly researched therapy, laser photocoagulation, at the Joslin Center. That summer, his younger brother, Al, age 36, becomes ill with a severe throat infection, subsequently develops hyperglycemia, and is diagnosed with diabetes mellitus. The family is surprised. Al had taken note of Bill's requirements for insulin and careful diet, and had kept himself thin and fit.

3. Which of the following statements regarding the new diagnosis of diabetes mellitus is correct?

A. Maturity-onset diabetes in the young (MODY) is associated with an inherited mutation in β-cell transcription factors, causing a predisposition to early β-cell failure.

B. Type I diabetes becomes clinically symptomatic when all of the pancreatic β-cells have been destroyed.

C. Newly diagnosed Type I diabetic patients have elevated serum glucose, but low ketone bodies and bicarbonate levels.

D. Newly diagnosed Type II diabetic patients have elevated serum glucose and ketone bodies, but low bicarbonate levels.

E. Type II diabetes abruptly becomes clinically symptomatic when the body mass index (a measure of body fat based on height and weight) approaches 30.

4. Which of the following agents increases insulin secretion?
   A. Miglitol
   B. neutral protamine Hagedorn (NPH) insulin
   C. Meglitinides
   D. Rosiglitazone
   E. Pioglitazone

5. Glucagon is one of the "counterregulatory" hormones that can be used for the treatment of hypoglycemia. What is its mechanism of action?
   A. Glucagon stimulates leptin release.
   B. Glucagon stimulates somatostatin release.
   C. Glucagon enhances renal reabsorption of tubular glucose.
   D. Glucagon stimulates epinephrine secretion.
   E. Glucagon promotes glycogenolysis and gluconeogenesis.

30

Pharmacology of Bone Mineral Homeostasis

TABLE 30-1 Mechanisms, Clinical Features, and Treatments for Common Diseases of Bone Mineral Homeostasis

Disease	Mechanism	Clinical Features	Treatment

Osteoporosis
  Senile
  Postmenopausal
	Bone resorption > bone formation
	
	↓ Estrogen
		Fragile bone
		Vulnerable to fracture
			Calcium
			Vitamin D
			Bisphosphonates
			Raloxifene (SERM)
			  (selective estrogen
			  receptor modulator)
			Calcitonin
			PTH

Chronic kidney disease	↓ Excretion of phosphate ↓ Production of 1,25(OH)$_2$D (1,25-dihydroxy vitamin D) (calcitriol)	Osteomalacia Osteitis fibrosa cystica	Phosphate restriction Active vitamin D Calcimimetics

Rickets
  Nutritional
 	
  Vitamin D resistant
 	
  Type I vitamin D
    dependent
  Type II vitamin D
    dependent
	
	Inadequate sunlight or dietary ↓ vitamin D
	
	Defect in renal reabsorption of phosphate and
	  production of vitamin D
	↓ Production of 1,25(OH)$_2$D
	
	Defective receptors for 1,25(OH)$_2$D
		Skeletal deformities in children
		Osteomalacia in adults
			
			Vitamin D
			
			Oral phosphate
			Calcitriol
			Oral phosphate
			Calcitriol
			Calcitriol (high dose)

Primary hyperparathyroidism	↑ PTH (parathyroid hormone) → ↑ bone
	  resorption → hypercalcemia
		Osteoporosis
		Nephrolithiasis
		Osteitis fibrosa cystica
		Depression
			Surgical removal
			Calcimimetic agents
			  (investigational)

Familial hypocalciuric hypercalcemia (FHH)	Mutation in Ca^{2+}-sensing receptor	Hypocalciuria Hypercalcemia Hypermagnesemia	None

Hypoparathyroidism	Decreased activity or absence of the
	  parathyroid gland; → hypocalcemia and
	  hyperphosphatemia
		Neuromuscular excitability
		Tetany
		Depression
			Calcium
			Vitamin D

Pseudohypoparathyroidism	Impaired response to PTH → hypocalcemia	Short stature Short metacarpals	Calcium Vitamin D
Paget's disease	↑ Local bone turnover	Bone pain Hearing loss High-output cardiac failure	Bisphosphonates Calcitonin

OBJECTIVES

■ Understand the physiologic control of bone mineral homeostasis.

■ Understand the pharmacology, therapeutic uses, and adverse effects of agents used in pathologic conditions of bone mineral homeostasis.

■ CASE 1

M.S. is a 60-year-old caucasian woman who comes to her physician with the recent onset of low back pain that began when she unexpectedly stepped into a pothole. She is otherwise in good health.

Her menstrual periods ceased when she was 54 years old. She had little in the way of postmenopausal symptoms and never took hormone replacement therapy. Menarche was at age 11 years. She has one child who was born when M.S. was 38 years old. Her mother died at age 55 years with breast cancer, and her sister, age 58 years, was recently diagnosed with breast cancer. The patient is moderately active and plays tennis for 1 hour about once a week. Her father and maternal aunt died in their 60s with coronary artery disease.

On physical examination, she has point tenderness over lumbar vertebra L1. Her weight is 135 pounds, and she is 64 inches tall, but she believes she has lost some height over the past year. Laboratory studies are all within normal limits. A lateral X-ray of the spine shows a compression fracture of L1 and generalized osteopenia. Measurement of bone mineral density (BMD) at the spine and hip reveals values that are 2.6 standard deviations below the healthy peak female value.

QUESTIONS

1. Numerous risk factors are associated with the development of osteoporosis according to the case, which of the following risk factors puts M.S. at particularly high risk at osteoporosis?
   A. M.S. is Caucasian.
   B. M.S. is thin.
   C. M.S. smokes.
   D. M.S. has a family history of breast cancer.
   E. M.S. has hypothyroidism.

Her physician diagnoses postmenopausal osteoporosis and a recent compression fracture of L1.

2. Postmenopausal women have a rapid loss of bone mineral density and bone mass. What is the mechanism of action of estrogen in preventing bone loss in pre-menopausal women?

   A. Estrogen promotes osteoblast maturation, while promoting osteoclast apoptosis.
   B. Estrogen prolongs osteoblast function, while inhibiting osteoclast function.
   C. Estrogen suppresses osteoclast production, of cytokines, which amplify osteoclast activity.
   D. Estrogen promotes osteoblast production of cytokines, which inhibit osteoclast activity.
   E. Estrogen hyperstimulates osteoblast activity, while promoting osteoclast apoptosis.

M.S. asks her physician to discuss with her the available therapeutic options, and is particularly interested in the potential risks and benefits of each option.

3. As with most pharmacologic therapies, treatment options for M.S.'s osteoporosis include both benefits and potential risks. Which of the following statements regarding potential therapies is correct?
   A. Alendronate will reduce bone loss but will place M.S. at risk for gastric ulcer formation and hemorrhage.
   B. Raloxifene will reduce bone loss but will place M.S. at risk for hypercholesterolemia and coronary artery disease.
   C. Hormone replacement therapy will reduce bone loss but will place M.S. at increased risk for venous thromboembolic disease.
   D. Hormone replacement therapy will enhance new bone growth but will place M.S. at increased risk of breast cancer.
   E. Parathyroid hormone (PTH) will enhance new bone growth but will place M.S. at risk for long-term aluminum neurotoxicity.

M.S. decides to take oral alendronate, a bisphosphonate, for treatment of her osteoporosis. She is cautioned by her physician to take her medication early in the morning on an empty stomach with a large glass of water, and to sit upright for 30 minutes after taking her medication to reduce the chance of esophageal irritation.

4. Which of the following statements regarding bisphosphonates is correct?
   A. Bisphosphonates are bone anabolic agents.
   B. Bisphosphonates concentrate in bone matrix, where they cannot be resorbed by osteoclasts.
   C. Bisphosphonates disrupt the mevalonate pathway and promote osteoblast apoptosis.
   D. Bisphosphonates disrupt the mevalonate pathway and limit osteoclast acid secretion.
   E. Bisphosphonates increase spine and hip bone mineral density but do not decrease the risk of fractures.

5. Hyperparathyroidism in chronic renal insufficiency is associated with:

A. enhanced PTH metabolism and turnover

B. hypophosphatemia

C. hypercalcemia

D. decreased production of 1,25(OH)$_2$D (calcitriol)

E. decreased production of 25(OH)D (calcifediol)

 CASE 2

Joshua Z. is a 52-year-old man whose wife brings him to his primary care physician, Dr. Greene, for an evaluation. Although Mr. Z. says he is ''just tired'' from overwork, his wife relates that he has persistently complained of back, hip, and left ankle pain for the past month. During the past week, she has found him asleep in his reading chair shortly after dinner. (He is usually a night owl and stays up late to watch old movies on cable.) This past weekend, he went back to bed after breakfast and slept for 6 hours. She notes he seems very weak, is limping on his left side, has been complaining of nausea, and has not been eating well for the past few days. Mr. Z. agrees that he feels generally nauseated much of the time recently and attributes it to constipation. (He has not had a bowel movement in four or 5 days.)

Dr. Greene finds Mr. Z. to be unusually less alert than normal and slow in his responses. His mucous membranes are somewhat dry and pale. His thyroid is not enlarged. His cardiac and pulmonary examinations are normal, but his abdomen is slightly distended with diminished bowel sounds. His muscle strength is globally decreased. Of great concern to her is the presence of fairly diffuse bony tenderness, most marked over his lumbar spine, left pelvis, and left ankle.

Dr. Greene orders several laboratory tests and sends Mr. and Mrs. Z. downstairs to the clinic radiology suite for several X-rays. Forty minutes later, she receives a call from the radiologist informing her that Mr. Z. has tripped while maneuvering around the X-ray table and has fallen and broken his left distal tibia. He is being loaded onto an ambulance to take him to the emergency department. The radiologist also reports that Mr. Z.'s radiographs are very worrisome; the left ankle radiograph taken just before his fall showed a large lytic lesion in his distal tibia. He suspects that the fracture is pathologic in nature, related to a bony malignancy. Review of the other X-rays confirms multiple lytic lesions in the left iliac crest and the lumbar vertebrae.

QUESTIONS

1. PTH is the most important endocrine regulator of calcium homeostasis. Which of the following is a function of PTH?

A. PTH increases renal calcium and phosphate reabsorption.

B. PTH inhibits the function of osteoclast differentiation factor (RANKL), inhibiting osteoclast activity.

C. PTH increases renal calcium reabsorption and decreases renal phosphate reabsorption.

D. PTH stimulates cell surface PTH receptors on osteoblasts, inhibiting their function.

E. PTH increases gastrointestinal absorption of calcitriol.

In the emergency department, Mr. Z.'s ankle is immobilized to maintain vascular integrity to the distal extremity and to limit pain from movement of the fracture site. Intravenous access is established, and laboratory studies are ordered. He receives intravenous morphine sulfate for his pain. Laboratory studies reveal anemia and an elevated serum calcium concentration of 12.3 mg/dL. Intravenous fluids are administered. A head computed tomography scan shows no intracerebral injury after his fall, but several lytic lesions are noted in the skull seen on the bony windows of his images. Mr.Z. is consulted to the orthopedic surgery service and admitted to the medical service for a workup of malignancy.

2. What is hypercalcemia of malignancy?

A. Hypercalcemia of malignancy is caused by enhanced gastrointestinal absorption of calcium by intestinal adenomas.

B. Hypercalcemia of malignancy is caused by the production of excessive calcitriol by renal cell carcinomas.

C. Hypercalcemia of malignancy is caused by the activity of osteoclastic sarcomas.

D. Hypercalcemia of malignancy is caused by parathyroid tumors.

E. Hypercalcemia of malignancy is caused by tumor production of PTH-related peptide (PTHrP).

Mr. Z.'s workup reveals a monoclonal globulin spike on serum protein electrophoresis, and Bence Jones protein (lambda light chains) in his urine. A bone marrow biopsy shows approximately 30% plasma cells. He is diagnosed with multiple myeloma. Dr. Greene consults an oncologist to assist in his therapy, which will consist of chemotherapy and radiation therapy to the skeletal areas of bony pain and lytic lesions. An orthopedist discusses the optimal management of his pathologic tibia fracture. In addition, his hypercalcemia is treated.

3. Which of the following agents is the most appropriate therapy for hypercalcemia of malignancy?

A. fluoride

B. teriparatide

C. oral alendronate

D. intravenous pamidronate

E. calcitonin

4. Calcitriol is the dihydroxylated form of vitamin D_3. What is a potential adverse effect of calcitriol therapy?
   A. Administration of calcitriol in the presence of hyperphosphatemia can cause an excessive increase in plasma calcium and phosphate.
   B. Administration of calcitriol in the presence of hyperphosphatemia can cause acute renal failure.
   C. Administration of calcitriol in the presence of hyperphosphatemia can precipitate calcium chloride stones in the renal collecting system.
   D. Administration of calcitriol in the presence of PTH will enhance its conversion to the relatively inactive form, paracalcitol.

E. Intravenous administration of calcitriol causes painful venous irritation.

5. Surgical thyroidectomy sometimes results in hypoparathyroidism. What is the result of low PTH?
   A. hypocalcemia
   B. hyperphosphatemia
   C. elevated PTHrP
   D. enhanced fluoride excretion by the kidney
   E. enhanced hepatic storage of calcitriol

ANSWERS TO SECTION IV

CHAPTER 25 ANSWERS

CASE 1

1. **The answer is C. Hypothalamic somatostatin inhibits anterior pituitary thyrotrophs, to reduce secretion of TSH.** Hypothalamic ghrelin and GHRH both stimulate somatotrophs to secrete GH. Insulin-like growth factors, (IGFs) are secreted by the liver in response to GH. Hypothalamic somatostatin inhibits somatotrophs, to reduce secretion of GH. Normally, dopamine stimulates GH release from the anterior hypothalamus, but in the case of acromegaly, there is a paradoxical decrease in GH secretion in response to dopamine. This is why dopamine analogues are sometimes used as adjuvant therapy in the treatment of patients with acromegaly. Hypothalamic GnRH stimulates gonadotrophs to secrete LH and FSH. Lactotrophs secrete prolactin. Hypothalamic CRH stimulates corticotrophs to secrete ACTH. Oxytocin is released by the posterior pituitary.

2. **The answer is B. Serum ILGF-1 is produced by the liver under conditions of anterior pituitary somatotroph oversecretion of GH.** Growth hormone excess usually results from a somatotroph adenoma and oversecretion of GH. Gigantism occurs under conditions of excess GH secreted before closure of the epiphyses, resulting in excessive longitudinal bone growth in children. Acromegaly is the result of excess serum GH after closure of the epiphyses, resulting in large facial structures, macroglossia, and hepatomegaly. Ghrelin and GHRH from the hypothalamus both stimulate GH release from the anterior pituitary.

3. **The answer is A. Somatostatin decreases intracellular cAMP in somatotroph cells and reduces their secretion of GH.** Decreased intracellular cAMP and subsequent decreased calcium concentrations inhibit the release of GH from somatotroph cells.

4. **The answer is E. Peptide hormones and hormone antagonists are not absorbed from the intestine.** As proteins, they are digested by local proteases into their constituent amino acids. Therefore, they must be administered by a non-oral route. The somatostatin analogue, octreotide, is also used in the treatment of patients with esophageal varices and some hormone-secreting tumors.

5. **The answer is E. Pegvisomant therapy is associated with reduced negative feedback on the anterior pituitary,** and subsequent pituitary enlargement. As a GH analogue, pegvisomant is a competitive antagonist of GH binding to its receptor. Pegvisomant binds to the transmembrane GH receptor but does not cause intracellular signaling. It reduces the release of ILGF-1 and decreases the IGF-mediated negative feedback on the anterior pituitary. Without this negative feedback, the anterior pituitary somatotrophs increase GH release, and in a small number of patients, the underlying pituitary adenoma may increase in size. Pegvisomant therapy has also been associated with elevations of hepatic aminotransferases. Pegvisomant is being investigated as a possible therapy to prevent the late complications of diabetes mellitus.

CASE 2

1. **The answer is D. TRH and phenothiazine antipsychotics stimulate prolactin release** and are associated with elevated serum prolactin concentrations. Lactotroph cells in the anterior pituitary are under tonic inhibition by dopamine from the hypothalamus. Therefore, dopamine receptor antagonists, such as phenothiazine antipsychotic agents (trifluoperazine), butyrophenones (haloperidol), metoclopramide, and reserpine, may all be associated with elevated prolactin levels.

2. **The answer is E. Bromocriptine is a dopamine agonist that suppresses lactotroph cell growth and inhibits release of prolactin.** Because the lactotrophs are under tonic inhibition by the presence of dopamine, this synthetic dopamine agonist is an established medical therapy for small prolactinomas. Its use shrinks microadenomas and reduces prolactin levels in 80% of patients. Bromocriptine can be administered orally. Many of its adverse effects are related to its dopamine agonist effect. This is why the initial dose should be low and slowly titrated upward, while patients' prolactin levels and symptoms are monitored. Other synthetic dopamine receptor agonists include pergolide and cabergoline. Prolactin release is not regulated by a negative feedback system because the mammary gland does not secrete hormones when prolactin binds to its receptors.

3. **The answer is B. desmopressin : stimulates V_2 receptors in the nephron to increase water resorption.** Ms. Y.'s postoperative symptoms of excessive urine volumes, hypernatremia, and thirst are caused by diabetes insipidus. Neurogenic diabetes insipidus is caused by a deficiency in ADH secretion by the posterior pituitary, often after manipulation of the stalk or posterior pituitary during transsphenoidal resection of anterior pituitary microadenomas. The incidence ranges from 16% to 30%. In most cases, it is transient. Desmopressin is an ADH analogue that stimulates V_2 receptors to enhance water resorption. In contrast to neurogenic diabetes insipidus, nephrogenic diabetes insipidus is caused by a mutation in the V_2 receptor such that it is no longer stimulated by ADH. Demeclocycline and lithium are pharmacologic treatments for the syndrome of inappropriate ADH (SIADH.) Conivaptan is an ADH antagonist approved for the treatment of euvolemic hyponatremia and heart failure.

4. **The answer is A.** Administration of cosyntropin to patients with adrenal insufficiency will cause **no increase in plasma cortisol concentration**.

5. **The answer is C. Androgen-dependent prostate cancer** can be treated with the GnRH analogue, leuprolide. Leuprolide, histrelin, and goserelin are administered as injections. Nafarelin is a nasal spray. Longer acting analogues are used to suppress production of sex hormones by desensitizing the pituitary glad to the stimulating effect of the releasing factor. Other diseases treated with GnRH agonists include endometriosis, uterine fibroids, and precocious puberty.

CHAPTER 26 ANSWERS

CASE 1

1. **The answer is B. High concentrations of T3 are causing negative feedback on TSH production.** The hypothalamic–pituitary–thyroid axis is controlled by negative feedback on releasing factors by organ-specific hormones. Ms. L. has Grave's disease, characterized by the presence of thyroid-stimulating immunoglobulin (TSH receptor antibody), which binds to TSH receptors and stimulates unregulated production of thyroid hormone. Release of T4 and T3 from the follicular cells is increased. T4 is deiodonated to T3 in the periphery. Elevated concentrations of T3 inhibit further TSH release from the anterior pituitary thyrotroph cells.

2. **The answer is B. Methimazole inhibits thyroid peroxidase function and limits T4 and T3 production.** Thyroid peroxidase oxidizes iodide to a reactive intermediate, which couples with tyrosine in the initial steps of thyroid hormone synthesis. Thyroid peroxidase also catalyzes monoiodotyrosine (MIT) and diiodotyrosine (DIT) coupling to create T3 and T4. Propylthiouracil, another thioamine, also inhibits thyroid peroxidase function. It also inhibits the peripheral conversion of T4 to T3 by deiodinase enzymes. Reverse triiodothyronine (rT3) is an inactive form of thyroid hormone.

3. **The answer is C. The thyroid gland selectively takes up and concentrates iodide** as part of its normal function. The radioactive iodide isotope ($^{131}I^-$) is also taken up and concentrated in thyroid follicular cells, where its emission of β particles causes selective local destruction of the thyroid gland. Ipodate is a radiocontrast agent that inhibits the conversion of T4 to T3. It is no longer commercially available.

4. **The answer is D. Radioactive iodide killed all or most of her thyroid follicular cells.** This therapy is an alternative to surgical thyroidectomy. However, it is sometimes difficult to determine what dose of radioactive iodide will be sufficient to result in a euthyroid state. Hypothyroidism is a potential consequence of radioactive iodide therapy. The Wolff-Chaikoff effect is a negative feedback effect of high intrathyroidal inorganic iodide that results in the inhibition of normal thyroid gland hormone synthesis. This effect is reversible and transient.

5. **The answer is E. Levothyroxine is an L-isomer of T4 with a half-life of 6 days, creating a circulating pool of thyroid "prodrug" to buffer and normalize metabolic rates.** This is in contrast to T3, which has a half-life of 1 day. As a replacement for endogenous thyroid hormone, levothyroxine causes a decline in TSH levels through negative feedback on the anterior pituitary. The efficacy of therapy is monitored by assaying plasma TSH levels. Levothyroxine metabolism is enhanced by drugs (e.g., rifampin, phenytoin, phenobarbital) that induce hepatic P450 enzyme function.

CASE 2

1. **The answer is E.** Mrs. P.'s presentation is suggestive of myxedema, a life-threatening form of profound hypothyroidism. In this setting, laboratory analysis would reveal **high TSH, low T3, and low T4**. Myxedema is a rare

complication of hypothyroidism. Symptoms include confusion and lethargy, hypothermia, bradycardia, gastrointestinal ileus, and edema. Myxedema occurs more often in elderly women over 60 years of age, more often in the winter months. Precipitants of myxedema include gastrointestinal bleeding, cold exposure, infections, cerebrovascular accident, trauma, and the use of certain medications, such as barbiturates, lithium, narcotics, phenothiazines, and phenytoin. Low circulating thyroid hormone stimulates the anterior pituitary to release TSH. However, in patients with preexisting hypothyroidism, the thyroid gland is unable to respond to the effect of TSH. TsIg is an antibody that binds to the TSH receptor and stimulates the synthesis and release of thyroid hormone in Grave's disease.

2. **The answer is A. Intravenous thyroxine** is indicated for the treatment of patients with myxedema. There is some controversy in the literature regarding the use of intravenous T3 versus T4 in this disease. However, T4 is generally accepted as a safe treatment for myxedema because of the risk of cardiac arrhythmia and ischemia associated with administration of T3, the active form of thyroid hormone. Intravenous corticosteroids are often administered in the setting of myxedema until coexisting adrenal insufficiency is ruled out through the measurement of a random serum cortisol level. β-receptor antagonists are used in the treatment of thyroid storm. Phenytoin can cause subtherapeutic levothyroxine levels because of its induction of hepatic P450 enzymes, and induced levothyroxine metabolism. Oral cholestyramine decreases the absorption of levothyroxine.

3. **The answer is B. Agranulocytosis**, allergic hepatitis, and vasculitis are rare, but potential complications of propylthiouracil and methimazole therapy. More common adverse effects of thioamines include a pruritic rash and arthralgias. Propylthiouracil can also cause hypoprothrombinemia and bleeding. Because these agents prevent thyroid hormone production and release, compensatory TSH stimulation of the thyroid gland can lead to goiter formation. Hashimoto's thyroiditis is an autoimmune-related form of hypothyroidism, one common symptom of which is weight gain. Organification is the process by which thyroglobulin becomes iodinated during the synthesis of thyroid hormone.

4. **The answer is C. β-receptor antagonists block sympathomimetic-like symptoms** associated with hyperthyroidism. Symptoms of tachycardia, tremor, and anxiety are similar to nonspecific β-adrenergic stimulation. β-receptor antagonists also reduce peripheral conversion of T4 to T3, but this effect is not considered to be clinically relevant in the treatment of thyroid storm.

5. **The answer is A. Amiodarone is associated with diminished thyroid hormone production** because of its release of iodide. Increased plasma iodide is concentrated in the thyroid gland, resulting in negative feedback on thyroid hormone synthesis through the Wolff-Chaikoff effect. Amiodarone also inhibits the conversion of T4 to T3, and increases the peripheral production of inactive rT3. Amiodarone is also associated with the development of hyperthyroidism by causing an increased iodide load and increased hormone production, by the induction of an autoimmune thyroiditis, and by acting as a homologue at thyroid hormone receptors. Rifampin induces hepatic P450 enzymes, which increases the metabolism of levothyroxine. Methimazole inhibits thyroid hormone production by inhibiting the action of thyroid peroxidase. Corticosteroids inhibit conversion of T4 to T3 by deiodinase. Sodium polystyrene sulfate is a resin that may decrease the gastrointestinal absorption of levothyroxine.

CHAPTER 27 ANSWERS

CASE 1

1. **The answer is E. Cortisol analogues reduce airway inflammation** by inhibiting both cytokine release and prostaglandin production. The cortisol analogue dexamethasone is administered to promote fetal lung maturation.

2. **The answer is D. Chronic glucocorticoid use slows linear bone growth, resulting in short stature** in children who take glucocorticoids through adolescence. Glucocorticoids inhibit vitamin D–mediated calcium absorption. This results in a compensatory increase in PTH release, which promotes bone resorption. Glucocorticoids also suppress osteoblast function. Osteoporosis can develop as a result of these effects.

3. **The answer is A. Johnny had acute adrenal insufficiency** as a result of prolonged administration and abrupt withdrawal of exogenous glucocorticoids. His daily use of prednisone caused the secretion of ACTH to become negligible (through negative feedback on the hypothalamic–pituitary axis). This resulted in adrenal cortical atrophy. He was unable to produce sufficient cortisol in response to the stress of infection, putting him at risk for the development of sepsis and death. Exogenous glucocorticoid therapy should be tapered slowly because it can take months to regain normal hypothalamic–pituitary–adrenal function.

4. **The answer is C. Inhaled glucocorticoids deliver the drug locally to limit long-term systemic glucocorticoid exposure,** while maximizing the amount of glucocorticoid activity at the mucosal surface of the pulmonary bronchioles. The goal is to control pulmonary inflammation while limiting the potential adverse effects of chronic systemic glucocorticoid use. Although inhaled preparations deliver only about 20% of the glucocorticoid dose to the lung, the remainder, which is swallowed, is inactivated by first-pass hepatic metabolism, further limiting systemic exposure to the active drug. Oropharyngeal candidiasis is a potential complication of inhaled glucocorticoid use because of the immunosuppressive effect of glucocorticoids on normal flora within the oral cavity.

5. **The answer is B. Fludrocortisone** has both glucocorticoid and mineralocorticoid activity. Prednisone and dexamethasone are glucocorticoids. Mifepristone is a progesterone receptor antagonist that also blocks the glucocorticoid receptor at high doses.

CASE 2

1. **The answer is A.** Cortisol has both metabolic and antiinflammatory effects. **Cortisol mobilizes amino acid in response to a prolonged fast,** in order to maintain glucose concentrations (via hepatic gluconeogenesis). It also increases blood glucose by antagonizing insulin action, and increases serum free fatty acid concentrations by promoting lipolysis. The increase in these nutrients maintains energy homeostasis during stress ensuring adequate nutrient delivery to critical organs, such as the brain and heart. Patients with Addison's disease who are exposed to stresses such as trauma, surgery, severe infection, or prolonged fasting may not have the capacity to respond physiologically because of inadequate endogenous cortisol production. Exogenous replacement glucocorticoids are necessary under these conditions.

2. **The answer is D. Hypotension** could result from hypoaldosteronism. Aldosterone normally enhances renal sodium reabsorption and potassium secretion in the distal nephron. Inadequate aldosterone concentrations can cause sodium wasting, volume loss, and hyperkalemic acidosis. In contrast, excess aldosterone can cause sodium retention, volume expansion, edema, and hypertension. Concomitant hypokalemia can cause muscle spasm.

3. **The answer is B. High concentrations of both ACTH and MSH stimulate MSH receptors in the skin**, promoting melanogenesis and increased skin pigmentation. Patients with primary hypoadrenalism do not produce cortisol, which would normally have a negative feedback effect on CRH production by the hypothalamus, and ACTH production by the anterior pituitary. The resulting CRH stimulation of pituitary corticotrophs causes them to synthesize proopiomelanocortin (POMC), the precursor of both ACTH and γ-melanocyte–stimulating hormone MSH.

4. **The answer is C. Spironolactone antagonizes the physiologic activity of aldosterone, which is to cause sodium retention and potassium excretion.** Spironolactone is a competitive antagonist at the mineralocorticoid receptor, and is used as a potassium-sparing diuretic. Potassium loading increases aldosterone synthesis. Hyperaldosteronism leads to potassium wasting, volume expansion, and hypertension.

5. **The answer is D.** The treatment of patients with secondary adrenal insufficiency includes replacement with **hydrocortisone** (or other glucocorticoids). These patients have decreased ACTH levels, which decreases the synthesis of cortisol and sex hormones, but does not alter levels of aldosterone. Aldosterone production is primarily regulated by the renin–angiotensin system and serum potassium concentrations. Therefore, mineralocorticoid replacement with fludrocortisone is not necessary. Fluticasone is an inhaled glucocorticoid used in the treatment of patients with asthma. Spironolactone is a mineralocorticoid antagonist. Ketoconazole inhibits steroidogenesis, and would be contraindicated in this setting.

CHAPTER 28 ANSWERS

CASE 1

1. **The answer is B. Increased LH and androgen levels inhibit ovulation, and increased androgen levels stimulate excessive hair growth.** The increased pituitary secretion of LH stimulate ovarian thecal cells to synthesize increased amounts of masculinizing androgens such as testosterone. Increased LH and androgen levels prevent normal follicle growth and the secretion of estrogen. The lack of a large dominant follicle and insufficient estrogen production prevents the LH surge and ovulation. The hormonal derangements of PCOS may be caused by a primary increase in LH pulses, an effect of increased insulin secretion on sex hormones in obesity-related insulin resistance, and/or a primary dysregulation of sex hormone synthesis in the thecal cell. The enzyme aromatase converts androgens to estrogens in the ovary, adipose tissue, hypothalamic neurons, and muscle. Aromatase activity is influenced by FSH, seasonal variation, and several drugs. In males, LH stimulates testicular Leydig cells to increase the production of androgens. Testosterone provides negative feedback on hypothalamic GnRH secretion and anterior pituitary LH and FSH release.

2. **The answer is E. The combination of estrogen and a progestin suppresses GnRH, LH, and FSH secretion, suppressing follicle growth and ovulation.** Secondary mechanisms of inhibiting pregnancy include the inhibition of fallopian tube peristalsis, reduced endometrial receptivity to blastocyst implantation, and thickening of cervical mucus secretions that result in reduced sperm transport to the fallopian tubes. Estrogen-only contraceptives are associated with an increased risk of developing endometrial cancer. For women with a uterus, estrogen is always used in combination with a progestin. Studies have not shown a change in the incidence of breast cancer associated with oral contraceptive use. The use of oral contraceptives is associated with an increase in gallbladder disease and thromboembolic events. The oral contraceptive associated increase in thromboembolic events is especially marked in smokers older than age 35 years. Biphasic contraceptive formulations maintain a constant dose of estrogen and vary the amount of progestin over the cycle, while triphasic formulations vary the dose of both estrogen and progestin. Mifepristone is a progesterone receptor antagonist used to induce first-trimester abortion.

3. **The answer is B. Estrogen–progestin oral contraceptives will suppress ovarian production of testosterone.** All estrogen-progestin and progestin-only oral contraceptives prevent ovulation. They do not reverse excessive hair growth or antagonize the end-organ effects of androgens. LH stimulates the ovarian thecal cells to produce androstenedione.

4. **The answer is C. Spironolactone is an androgen antagonist.** It acts by competitively inhibiting the binding of endogenous androgens to the androgen receptor. This would limit the masculinizing effects of testosterone, including excessive hair growth. Spironolactone is also an aldosterone antagonist, accounting for its actions as a potassium-sparing diuretic agent. This action, however, would not have any effect on Ms. J.'s hair growth.

5. **The answer is A.** The LH and FSH surge cause **ovulation**. In the absence of pregnancy and secretion of hCG, the corpus luteum is pre-programmed to undergo involution through apoptotic processes. Endometrial secretory changes are caused by the sequential stimulation of estrogen, followed by estrogen plus progesterone. The endometrium does not secrete hCG.

CASE 2

1. **The answer is A. Exogenous testosterone suppress the effects of gonadotropins on the testicular cells, causing testicular atrophy, and is converted to estrogen, causing gynecomastia.** It suppresses the release of GnRH from the hypothalamus and LH and FSH from the anterior pituitary. The lack of LH and FSH inhibits the normal function of testicular Leydig and Sertoli cells, causing azoospermia and testicular atrophy. Androgens are converted to estrogen by aromatase, increasing plasma estrogen and causing gynecomastia. Other adverse effects of high plasma androgens include erythrocytosis, acne, and hyperlipidemia. Androgenic steroid use is associated with toxicity to multiple organ systems, causing muscle hypertrophy, hypertension, dysrhythmias, and myocardial ischemia. Death is usually attributable to the pathologic effects on the cardiovascular system. Estimates of androgenic steroid users number 1 million, with an estimated $500 million spent on the sale of illegal androgenic steroids. Nearly 4000 websites advertise their use and the means to obtain them. Androgenic steroids were categorized as schedule III controlled substances in the United States in 1990.

2. **The answer is E.** Testosterone replacement therapy can be administered intramuscularly every 2 to 4 weeks, as a transdermal patch, as a transbuccal tablet, and as a topical gel. **Daily application of a testosterone topical gel formulation reaches physiologic replacement levels of testosterone after 1 month of application.** Oral testosterone is less effective because of high first-pass metabolism of testosterone by the liver. Testosterone should not be administered to men

with prostate cancer because it can stimulate tumor growth.

3. **The answer is A. Finasteride blocks type II 5α-reductase conversion of testosterone to dihydrotestosterone in prostatic cells, slowing their growth.** Dihydrotestosterone is the most active androgen, binding to the androgen receptor with ten time's higher affinity than testosterone. Finasteride inhibits the local effects of androgens on prostatic tissue and causes a reduction in prostate size. GnRH agonists, such as leuprolide and goserelin, block the pituitary secretion of LH, suppress testicular testosterone production, and are used to treat androgen-dependent prostate tumors. Flutamide is a direct competitive antagonist at the androgen receptor, and is approved for the treatment of patients with metastatic prostate cancer. Aromatase inhibitors include anastrozole, letrozole, exemestane, and formestane. These agents block the conversion of androgens to estrogens and inhibit the growth of estrogen-dependent tumors, such as breast cancer.

4. **The answer is B.** Some selective estrogen receptor modulators are mixed agonists and antagonists, on a tissue-specific basis. This allows for tissue-specific modulation of estrogen effects. For example, **tamoxifen is an estrogen antagonist in breast tissue but an agonist in endometrial tissue**. It inhibits the growth of estrogen-dependent breast cancers but has been associated with an increased incidence of endometrial cancer. Raloxifene is an estrogen antagonist in both breast and endometrial tissue but an agonist in bone. It has been used to prevent breast cancer in high-risk women, while limiting estrogen stimulation of endometrial tissue and promoting the protective effects of estrogen on bone. Clomiphene is an estrogen antagonist in the hypothalamus and anterior pituitary, and an agonist in the ovary. Clomiphene increases pituitary secretion of FSH and LH, and is used to induce ovulation.

5. **The answer is D.** Estrogen replacement therapy is associated with an increased risk of **thromboembolic disease**. Estrogen replacement must be combined with a progestin to prevent the induction of endometrial cancer in women with a uterus. The Women's Health Initiative study found that estrogen treatment alone did not increase the risk of coronary heart disease or breast cancer, but did increase the risk of stroke and thromboembolic disease, while decreasing the risk of osteoporotic fractures. In patients who received estrogen-progestin replacement therapy, there was an increase in cardiovascular events, breast cancer, and stroke.

CHAPTER 29 ANSWERS

CASE 1

1. **The answer is A.** Insulin is the major energy storage hormone, promoting the uptake of glucose, amino acids, and triglycerides in response to elevated plasma glucose concentrations. **Insulin binds to its receptor on hepatocytes and stimulates the activity of glycogen synthase** and the action of fatty acid synthase. These enzymes promote the storage of glucose and fatty acids. Similarly, in muscle and adipose cells, insulin stimulates the movement of the glucose transporter GLUT4 to the cell surface to enhance glucose and amino acid uptake. Glucose is stored as glycogen, and amino acids are used in protein synthesis. In adipose cells, insulin stimulates the activity of lipoprotein lipase and fatty acid and triglyceride uptake. Insulin is degraded by insulinase in the liver and kidney. Its half-life can be prolonged in patients with renal insufficiency.

2. **The answer is E. Type I diabetes mellitus is caused by the autoimmune destruction of pancreatic β cells in patients with a genetic predisposition to the formation of autoantibodies.** The genetic predisposition to Type I diabetes maps to alleles on chromosome 6, which code for major histocompatibility complex proteins involved with antigen presentation. Environmental factors also influence the development of Type I diabetes. A prodromal "flu-like" illness often occurs before the onset of clinical symptoms of hyperglycemia. This syndrome may represent a triggering viral illness or the clinical symptoms of the destructive autoimmune inflammatory reaction. Type II diabetes mellitus is associated with a genetic predisposition to obesity, insulin resistance, and pancreatic β-cell failure.

3. **The answer is C. A low blood glucose indicates good recent glucose control, while an elevated HbA1c indicates that glucose has been elevated over the preceding months.** The glycosylation of hemoglobin occurs at a rate that is proportional to the blood glucose concentration. Therefore, HbA1c concentrations are an indication of the average blood glucose over the lifespan of the erythrocyte, (120 days). In this case, Mrs. S.'s glucose testing indicates that her blood glucose has been elevated for several months. An HbA1c greater than 7.5% is associated with an increased rate of diabetic complications. When the erythrocyte lifespan is reduced (e.g., in patients with hemolysis), the HbA1c value may be misleading.

4. **The answer is C. Mrs. S. is at risk for developing atherosclerotic heart disease**, retinopathy, nephropathy, and neuropathy as a result of chronically elevated blood glucose levels. Acute complications of Type II diabetes mellitus include hyperglycemic hyperosmotic nonketotic coma. This is in contrast to diabetic ketoacidosis, which is more often an acute complication of Type I diabetes mellitus. Excess glucose in the renal tubules is unable to be reabsorbed and acts as an osmotic diuretic, contributing to polyuria.

5. **The answer is B. Biguanides block AMP-dependent protein kinase and inhibit hepatic gluconeogenesis, but do not contribute to weight gain in obese patients.** These agents also block the breakdown of fatty acids and inhibit glycogenolysis, and increase insulin signaling. Their overall effect is an increase in insulin sensitivity. Unlike the sulfonylureas, the thiazolidinediones, and exogenous insulin, biguanides do not promote weight gain. However, they can contribute to the development of lactic acidosis under conditions that predispose patients to metabolic acidosis. α-Glucosidase inhibitors competitively inhibit the activity of glucosidase in the brush border of the intestine, and increase the time required for the postprandial absorption of carbohydrates. They are contraindicated in patients with inflammatory bowel disease but are not associated with weight gain. Sulfonylureas stimulate pancreatic β-cell insulin release and can cause hypoglycemia. Thiazolidinediones enhance insulin sensitivity in adipose tissue by modulating PPARγ-control of gene transcription.

CASE 2

1. **The answer is C. Non–human-derived insulin can cause potential immunologic reactions.** Recombinant DNA techniques have enabled the production of biosynthetic human insulin, which is used by the majority of diabetic patients today. Insulin is a protein that is degraded in the gastrointestinal tract, and cannot be administered orally. It can be administered parenterally, via subcutaneous injection or intravenous infusion. Insulin can also be administered via the pulmonary tissues as an inhalational powder. Because insulin promotes the uptake of glucose into adipose tissue, all insulin preparations can promote weight gain, especially in insulin-resistant patients. Exogenous insulin administration is the only treatment for patients like Bill with Type I diabetes. Before the isolation of insulin as a specific treatment for Type I diabetes, patients were managed with "starvation diets" consisting of extremely low carbohydrate and high fat intake to limit their serum glucose. Most died within months to several years of their diagnosis.

2. **The answer is B. Glargine : long-acting (18–24 hours).** Insulin preparations are categorized based on their onset and duration of action. These factors also contribute to the individual regimens of insulin used to achieve glycemic control in relation to patient meals, exercise activity, and illness. Lispro insulin is a monomeric form of insulin designed for an ultrarapid onset and short duration of action (3–4 hours), and can be injected minutes before the patient eats a meal. Regular and semilente insulin are short-acting preparations with durations of action of 6 to 8 and 8 to 12 hours, respectively. They are also used to control glucose concentrations in relation to meals but must be administered approximately 1 hour before eating. Lente and NPH

insulin preparations are intermediate acting with durations of action of 16 to 24 hours. Ultralente and glargine insulins are long acting with durations of action of 24 to 36 and 18 to 24 hours, respectively. Intermediate- and long-acting insulins provide basal insulin and overnight glycemic control.

3. **The answer is A. Maturity-onset diabetes in the young (MODY) is associated with an inherited mutation in β-cell transcription factors, causing a predisposition to early β-cell failure.** This early-onset form of Type II diabetes occurs in "lean" patients who have a strong disposition to β-cell failure. Mild or early Type II diabetes can be unmasked in predisposed patients during periods of sudden insulin resistance. The majority of Type II diabetic patients are obese. Their pancreatic β-cells still produce insulin, but their peripheral tissues are insulin resistant. The onset of clinical symptoms is generally gradual, and the patient may be diagnosed when elevated serum glucose is measured on routine laboratory screening. Type I diabetes becomes clinically symptomatic when 85% of the pancreatic β-cells have been destroyed. The onset of clinical symptoms is usually abrupt. Newly diagnosed Type I diabetic patients often have elevated serum glucose and ketone bodies, but low bicarbonate, consistent with diabetic ketoacidosis.

4. **The answer is C. Meglitinides** stimulate insulin release by binding to sulfonylureas receptor 1 (SUR1) and inhibiting the β-cell K^+/ATP channel. Sulfonylureas act similarly. Both of these agents cause β-cell membrane depolarization, calcium influx, and exocytosis of insulin-containing vesicles. Exenatide is a GLP-1 agonist that also induces insulin secretion and inhibits glucagon secretion. Miglitol is a "starch-blocker" carbohydrate analogue. Neutral protamine Hagedorn insulin is NPH insulin. Rosiglitazone and pioglitazone are thiazolidinediones that enhance insulin sensitivity at target tissues. Biguanides also increase peripheral tissue sensitivity to insulin.

5. **The answer is E. Glucagon promotes glycogenolysis and gluconeogenesis.** It also promotes lipolysis. All of these actions have the catabolic effect of mobilizing energy sources in response to low plasma glucose. Glucagon is secreted by pancreatic α-cells in response to low glucose and sympathetic nervous system activity. (Norepinephrine and epinephrine are also counterregulatory hormones.) Glucagon is degraded in the liver and kidneys. Leptin is a hormone of adipocytes that regulates long-term energy balance and the neuroendocrine response to energy storage, based on total fat mass. Somatostatin inhibits the secretion of insulin, glucagon, thyroid-stimulating hormone, and growth hormone when plasma glucose is elevated.

CHAPTER 30 ANSWERS

CASE 1

1. **The answer is A.** M.S. has multiple risk factors associated with the development of osteoporosis. **M.S. is caucasian.** Caucasian and Asian women are at slightly greater risk of osteoporosis compared with women of other ethnicities. Advanced age, female gender, being postmenopausal, and a history of fracture as an adult are associated with increased risk of osteoporosis. Inadequate weight-bearing exercise is also associated with osteoporosis. Small-boned, thin women weighing less than approximately 125 pounds are at greater risk, as are tobacco and excessive ethanol users, and patients with hyperthyroidism. Several drugs, including thyroid hormone, aluminum-containing antacids, glucocorticoids, and anticonvulsants, are associated with osteoporosis.

2. **The answer is B. Estrogen prolongs osteoblast function, while inhibiting osteoclast function.** Estrogen suppresses the transcription of genes for cytokines, which are normally released by osteoblasts. These cytokines, such as interleukin-6 (IL-6), normally induce osteoclast proliferation, maturation, and activation. This process is prevented by estrogen. In addition, estrogen also increases the lifespan of osteoblasts and osteocytes, and promotes osteoclast apoptosis.

3. **The answer is C. Hormone replacement therapy will reduce bone loss but will place M.S. at increased risk for venous thromboembolic disease**, cardiovascular disease, and breast cancer, given her strong family history of the same. Therefore, hormone replacement therapy would not be a good choice for this patient. Raloxifene, a selective estrogen receptor modulator (SERM), will reduce bone loss, lower low-density lipoprotein cholesterol, and possibly decrease the risk of heart disease. However, as an estrogen analogue, raloxifene can still increase the risk of thromboembolism. Alendronate is a bisphosphonate that will reduce bone loss. The bisphosphonates are associated with esophagitis and esophageal erosion. Parathyroid hormone will enhance new bone growth. As a peptide, it is not bioavailable in an oral form and must be administered as a subcutaneous injection. Aluminum hydroxide is a phosphate binder used in the treatment of secondary hyperparathyroidism and chronic renal insufficiency. Its chronic use can lead to neurotoxicity, chronic anemia, and osteomalacia.

4. **The answer is D. Bisphosphonates disrupt the mevalonate pathway and limit osteoclast acid secretion** by inhibiting the osteoclast H^+-ATPase. They concentrate in, and are incorporated in bone matrix, where they are eventually internalized by osteoclasts during the process of remodeling. After they are taken up intracellularly, bisphosphonates disrupt normal protein function in cellular signaling and ultimately lead to osteoclast apoptosis. Bisphosphonates are anti-resorptive agents that are approved for the treatment and prevention of osteoporosis. Clinical trials show that their use is associated with increased spine and hip bone mineral density, and a decreased risk of vertebral and nonvertebral fractures.

5. **The answer is D.** Hyperparathyroidism in chronic renal insufficiency is associated with a **decreased production of 1,25(OH)$_2$D (calcitriol)**. Normally, cholecalciferol synthesized in the skin under exposure to ultraviolet radiation in sunlight is stored and converted to 25(OH)D (calcifediol) in the liver. Calcifediol is hydroxylated in the proximal renal tubules to calcitriol. This reaction does not occur in patients with chronic kidney disease. The result of inadequate vitamin D is a decreased absorption of dietary calcium from the small intestine, and hypocalcemia. Hypocalcemia stimulates PTH synthesis and secretion and suppresses PTH degradation. Hyperphosphatemia is a result of decreased renal excretion of phosphate, and exacerbates hypocalcemia by altering the equilibrium for hydroxyapatite formation and dissolution. Calcium phosphate can precipitate extravascularly and cause tissue damage.

CASE 2

1. **The answer is C. PTH increases renal calcium reabsorption and decreases renal phosphate reabsorption.** This is the most rapid physiologic effect of PTH in increasing plasma calcium levels. PTH also has a direct effect on bone cells by stimulating osteoblast expression of osteoclast differentiation factor (RANKL). RANKL subsequently promotes the maturation of osteoclast precursors, which then increase bone resorption and the liberation of calcium. PTH increases gastrointestinal absorption of calcium indirectly by stimulating the kidney to increase the production of activated vitamin D,

calcitriol. PTH has a differential effect, based on its intermittent versus continuous stimulation of its bone cell receptors: continuous PTH activity promotes osteoclastic activity and intermittent PTH activity promotes osteoblastic activity.

2. **The answer is E. Hypercalcemia of malignancy is caused by tumor production of parathyroid hormone-related peptide (PTHrP).** This peptide is structurally and functionally related to PTH, similarly increasing serum calcium concentration.

3. **The answer is D. Intravenous pamidronate** and zoledronate, both bisphosphonates, are approved for the treatment of hypercalcemia of malignancy. They inhibit the mevalonate pathway in osteoclasts and inhibit the accelerated bone resorption associated with PTHrP-mediated osteoclast hyperstimulation. Oral alendronate, risedronate, and ibandronate are approved for the treatment and prevention of osteoporosis. Calcitonin also decreases the resorptive activity of osteoclasts, but at a slower rate. Fluoride is a bone anabolic agent that is a mitogen for osteoblasts and increases trabecular bone mass. Teriparatide is PTH(1–34), an exogenously administered PTH analogue.

4. **The answer is A. Administration of calcitriol in the presence of hyperphosphatemia can cause an excessive increase in plasma calcium and phosphate.** Calcitriol is able to increase plasma calcium concentrations within 24 to 48 hours of administration. Calcium absorption from the intestine can be increased by as much as 600 mg/day in the presence of calcitriol. However, it should not be administered until hyperphosphatemia has been controlled because of the risk of excessively high calcium and phosphate levels as a result of its administration. Paracalcitol is a synthetic analogue of vitamin D that may lower PTH levels without significantly increasing plasma calcium levels. Intravenous administration of calcium chloride can cause painful venous irritation.

5. **The answer is A. Hypocalcemia** and hypophosphatemia are a result of hypoparathyroidism. PTHrP is associated with hypercalcemia of malignancy. Cholecalciferol and ergocalciferol are stored in the liver or converted to calcifediol. Calcifediol is converted to calcitriol, the active form of vitamin D, in the kidney.

V

Principles of
Chemotherapy

31

Principles of Antimicrobial and Antineoplastic Pharmacology

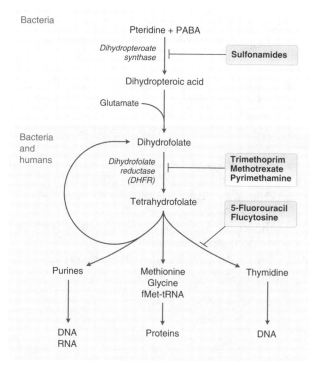

Figure 31-1. Folate Synthesis and Functions. Folate synthesis begins with the formation of dihydropteroic acid from pteridine and para-aminobenzoic acid (PABA); this reaction is catalyzed by dihydropteroate synthase. Glutamate and dihydropteroic acid condense to form dihydrofolate (DHF). DHF is reduced to tetrahydrofolate (THF) by dihydrofolate reductase (DHFR). THF and its congeners (not shown) serve as one-carbon donors in numerous reactions necessary for the formation of DNA, RNA, and proteins. In each such reaction, the reduced folate (THF) becomes oxidized to DHF, and the THF must then be regenerated via reduction by DHFR. Inhibitors of folate metabolism target three steps in the folate pathway. Sulfonamides inhibit dihydropteroate synthase; trimethoprim, methotrexate, and pyrimethamine inhibit DHFR; 5-fluorouracil (5-FU) and flucytosine inhibit thymidylate synthase. Note that bacteria synthesize folate de novo from pteridine and PABA, whereas humans require dietary folate.

OBJECTIVES

- Understand how antimicrobial and antineoplastic agents achieve selectivity in their pharmacologic actions.

- Understand how the selectivity of agents impacts their therapeutic utility and adverse effects.

◼ CASE 1

The country is Germany, and the year is 1935. Hildegard, daughter of Dr. Gerhard Domagk, is near death with a streptococcal infection from a pinprick. She has failed to respond to any treatments. In desperation, Hildegard's father injects her with prontosil, a red dye with which he has been experimenting in his laboratory. Miraculously, she makes a complete recovery.

QUESTIONS

1. What is the antibacterial mechanism of action of prontosil?
   A. Its metabolite causes polymerization of folate, resulting in bacterial toxicity.
   B. Its metabolite prevents the incorporation of folate into the bacterial cell wall.
   C. Its metabolite prevents the bacterial uptake of folate.
   D. Its metabolite inhibits the synthesis of folate by bacteria.
   E. Its metabolite binds to folate and enhances its elimination from the body.

This story actually begins 3 years earlier, when Dr. Domagk observed that prontosil protects mice and rabbits from lethal doses of staphylococci and streptococci. He discovered this

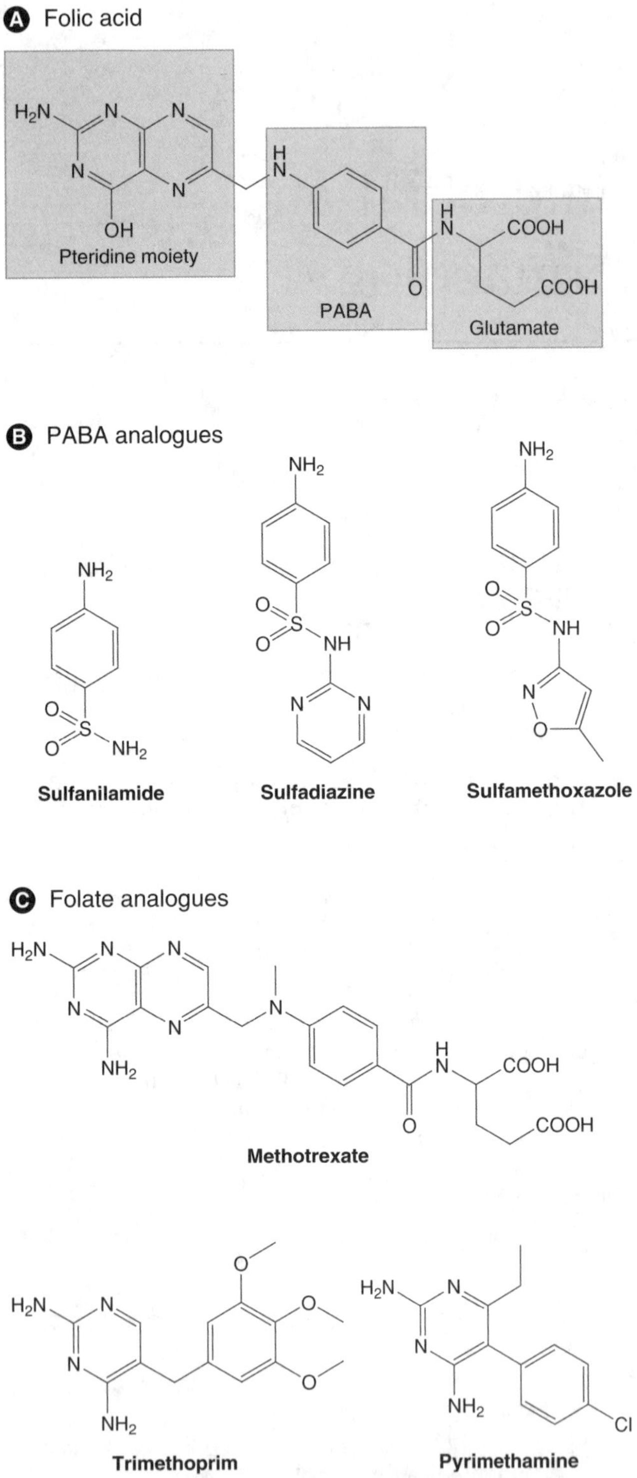

A Folic acid

Pteridine moiety

PABA

Glutamate

B PABA analogues

Sulfanilamide

Sulfadiazine

Sulfamethoxazole

C Folate analogues

Methotrexate

Trimethoprim

Pyrimethamine

Figure 31-2. Structures of Folic Acid, Para-Aminobenzoic Acid (PABA) Analogues (Sulfonamides), and Folate Analogues (Dihydrofolate Reductase Inhibitors). A. Folic acid is formed by the condensation of pteridine, PABA, and glutamate. Folate is the deprotonated form of folic acid. **B.** PABA analogues (sulfonamides) structurally resemble PABA. These drugs inhibit dihydropteroate synthase, the enzyme that catalyzes the formation of dihydropteroic acid from PABA and pteridine. **C.** Folate analogues (dihydrofolate reductase inhibitors) structurally resemble folic acid. These drugs inhibit dihydrofolate reductase, the enzyme that converts dihydrofolate to tetrahydrofolate.

by screening thousands of dyes (which are, in actuality, simply chemicals that bind to proteins) for antibacterial activity. When his daughter became ill, however, Domagk was not sure whether prontosil's antibacterial efficacy in mice would carry over to infections in humans. He kept his emergency test of the drug a secret until data from other physicians indicated that the drug had been successful in curing other patients of their infections. In 1939, Gerhard Domagk was awarded the Nobel Prize in Physiology or Medicine for his discovery of the therapeutic benefit of prontosil.

2. Why does prontosil kill bacteria but not human cells?

   A. Mammalian cells do not take up folate.

   B. Mammalian cells do not express dihydrofolate reductase.

   C. Mammalian cells do not express dihydropteroate synthase.

   D. Mammalian cells do not express para-aminobenzoic acid (PABA).

   E. Mammalian cells do not take up sulfa drugs.

3. What has caused the utility of sulfonamides (prontosil being an early agent with a similar mechanism) to decline over the past 70 years?

   A. Safer drugs have been developed that do not require metabolism to active metabolites.

   B. Drugs with greater selectivity for dihydropteroate synthase have been developed.

   C. Drugs with greater selectivity for dihydrofolate reductase have been developed.

   D. The incidence of sulfonamide-associated kernicterus has increased substantially.

   E. The incidence of sulfonamide resistance in bacteria has increased substantially.

4. Why are drugs of the same class as prontosil now used in combination with other antibacterial agents?
   A. This combination allows for the inhibition of bacterial folate synthesis, while "rescuing" mammalian cells, which require folate.
   B. This combination allows for the synergistic inhibition of bacterial folate synthesis.
   C. This combination prevents bacterial resistance to dihydropteroate reductase inhibitors.
   D. This combination enhances the selectivity of the sulfonamides for dihydropteroate synthase.
   E. This combination prevents the development of kernicterus in newborns who require sulfonamide therapy.

5. Despite the selectivity of sulfonamides for the enzyme dihydropteroate synthase, bacteria do develop resistance to these agents. How does this occur?
   A. Bacteria become able to scavenge pre-formed folate.
   B. Bacteria develop a mutation in dihydrofolate reductase, resulting in reduced binding of sulfonamides.
   C. Bacteria develop new folate synthetic pathways that do not require PABA.
   D. Bacteria overproduce PABA and continue folate synthesis despite the presence of sulfonamides.
   E. Bacteria develop a reduced permeability to the PABA–sulfonamide complex.

■ CASE 2

Sasha M. is a 37-year-old woman who is thrilled to learn that she is pregnant after 18 months of infertility treatment with clomiphene citrate (a selective estrogen receptor modulator [SERM] that is used to induce ovulation) and intrauterine insemination. She and her husband are cautiously optimistic and await their 10-week appointment with an obstetrician. At about 6.5 weeks' gestation, Ms. M. notes some nagging left lower quadrant abdominal discomfort, which she attributes to constipation from her prenatal vitamins with iron. However, the discomfort persists, and she makes an appointment with her fertility gynecologist. Her doctor, Dr. Caseman, notes Ms. M.'s examination to be normal except for tenderness in the left lower quadrant of the abdomen, as well as left adnexal tenderness on bimanual pelvic examination.

She orders laboratory studies and a pelvic ultrasound to evaluate the status of Ms. M's pregnancy. Much to Ms. M's dismay, the serum concentration of quantitative β-hCG (human chorionic gonadotropin, the hormone indicative of pregnancy) is no longer appropriately rising at a rate consistent with the gestation of her pregnancy. The pelvic ultrasound shows no gestational sac, yolk sac, or embryo within the uterus and a 2 × 3 cm complex mass within her left salpinx. Dr. Caseman explains to Mr. and Ms. M that the findings are consistent with an ectopic pregnancy in her left fallopian tube. She explains to Ms. M. and her husband the potential treatment options for the ectopic pregnancy, given that she is hemo-dynamically stable. After discussion of the risks of medical versus surgical therapy and the potential effects on her future fertility, Ms. M decides to undergo methotrexate and leucovorin therapy. She and her husband receive counseling on the risks and potential adverse effects of the drugs. A social worker from the reproductive clinic joins them while they await the medication.

QUESTIONS

1. What is the mechanism of action of methotrexate?
   A. Methotrexate arrests cell division during M phase.
   B. Methotrexate is a folate analogue that inhibits the action of dihydropteroate synthase.
   C. Methotrexate is a PABA analogue that inhibits the action of dihydrofolate reductase.
   D. Methotrexate is a folate analogue that inhibits the normal cellular uptake of folate.
   E. Methotrexate is a folate analogue that inhibits the action of dihydrofolate reductase.

2. Considering its mechanism of action, what will be the ultimate effect of methotrexate therapy on a developing embryo?
   A. Methotrexate will reduce the blood supply to the embryo.
   B. Methotrexate will induce potentially teratogenic mutations in the embryo.
   C. Methotrexate will slow the growth of the embryo.
   D. Methotrexate will induce migration of the embryo to the uterine cavity.
   E. Methotrexate will cause the death of the embryo.

3. Considering its mechanism of action, which of the following is a common potential adverse effect of methotrexate?
   A. peripheral neuropathy
   B. diarrhea
   C. hepatitis
   D. headache
   E. osteoporosis

4. What is the purpose of administering leucovorin with methotrexate?

   A. Leucovorin provides folinic acid for DNA synthesis in normal cells.

   B. Leucovorin is a folate analogue that restores the activity of dihydrofolate reductase.

   C. Leucovorin selectively inhibits the action of methotrexate in normal cells.

   D. Leucovorin is metabolized to purines, which are used for DNA synthesis by normal cells.

   E. Leucovorin blocks the uptake of methotrexate by normal cells.

5. Which of the following statements regarding the selectivity of antimicrobial and antineoplastic agents is correct?

   A. Methotrexate is a selective chemotherapeutic agent.

   B. Selectivity is achieved when an antimicrobial agent targets an enzyme that is shared by a bacterium and a human cell.

   C. Selectivity is achieved when an antimicrobial agent targets an enzyme that is unique to a bacterium.

   D. A highly selective antimicrobial agent has a small therapeutic index.

   E. Methotrexate has a large therapeutic index because of its selectivity.

32

Pharmacology of Bacterial Infections: DNA Replication, Transcription, and Translation

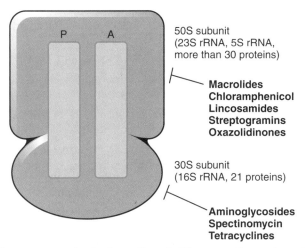

70S ribosome

P   A

50S subunit
(23S rRNA, 5S rRNA,
more than 30 proteins)

**Macrolides
Chloramphenicol
Lincosamides
Streptogramins
Oxazolidinones**

30S subunit
(16S rRNA, 21 proteins)

**Aminoglycosides
Spectinomycin
Tetracyclines**

Figure 32-1. The Prokaryotic 70S Ribosome. The prokaryotic 70S ribosome consists of a 30S subunit and a 50S subunit. Each subunit is composed of ribosomal RNA (rRNA) and numerous proteins. The rRNAs are responsible for most of the important activities of the ribosome and are the targets of antibiotic drugs that inhibit translation. Aminoglycosides, spectinomycin, and tetracyclines bind to and inhibit the activity of 16S rRNA in the 30S subunit. Macrolides, chloramphenicol, lincosamides, streptogramins, and oxazolidinones bind to and inhibit the activity of 23S rRNA in the 50S subunit. *A,* aminoacyl site (site of binding of aminoacyl tRNA); *P,* peptidyl site (site of binding of tRNA that is covalently joined to the elongating peptide chain).

Understand the indications for and adverse effects of these agents based on their mechanisms of action.

■ CASE 1

It is the summer of 1976. Participants returning from an American Legion convention in Philadelphia are falling severely ill with a mysterious type of pneumonia. The outbreak centers on the Bellevue Stratford Hotel, where 150 hotel occupants and 32 passers-by contract ''Legionnaires' disease.'' Twenty-nine victims ultimately die. Conventional sputum stains, cultures, and even autopsy material show no consistent pathogens. The terror of an unknown epidemic disease sparks rumors and news reports of poison gases, tainted water supplies, terrorists, and deadly viruses.

Several months later, laboratory and field investigation teams from the Centers for Disease Control and Prevention (CDC) identify the causative aerobic gram-negative bacterium, and name it *Legionella pneumophila.* It is observed that affected individuals treated with erythromycin and tetracycline have better outcomes than those treated with other agents. Today, erythromycin and the other macrolides, clarithromycin and azithromycin, are often used for treating Legionnaires' disease, as well as many chlamydial, streptococcal, and staphylococcal infections.

OBJECTIVES

Understand the mechanism by which antimicrobial agents affect bacterial DNA replication, transcription, and translation.

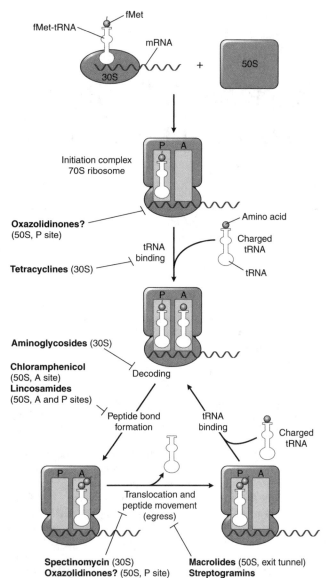

fMet
fMet-tRNA
mRNA
30S + 50S

Initiation complex
70S ribosome

Oxazolidinones?
(50S, P site)

Tetracyclines (30S)

tRNA
binding

Amino acid
Charged
tRNA
tRNA

Aminoglycosides (30S)

Chloramphenicol
(50S, A site)
Lincosamides
(50S, A and P sites)

Decoding

Peptide bond
formation

tRNA
binding

Charged
tRNA

Translocation and
peptide movement
(egress)

Spectinomycin (30S)
Oxazolidinones? (50S, P site)

Macrolides (50S, exit tunnel)
Streptogramins

Figure 32-2. Prokaryotic Translation. Prokaryotic translation begins with the assembly of a complex containing a 30S ribosomal subunit, mRNA, formyl-methionine-linked tRNA (fMet-tRNA), and a 50S ribosomal subunit. This assembly step is dependent on the binding of fMet-tRNA to an initiator codon in the mRNA. The assembled 70S ribosome contains two binding sites, referred to as the aminoacyl *(A)* and peptidyl *(P)* sites. The A site accepts incoming triplet codons of mRNA and allows the corresponding amino acid-linked tRNA (i.e., charged tRNA) to bind to its corresponding triplet. The decoding function of 16S rRNA helps ensure that the mRNA codon binds to the correct tRNA. Once a charged tRNA has entered the A site, the peptidyl transferase activity of the 23S rRNA catalyzes the formation of a peptide bond between the amino acid occupying the A site and the carboxy-terminus of the nascent peptide residing in the P site. Once the peptide bond has formed, the tRNA–mRNA complex translocates from the A site to the P site, the tRNA molecule that had occupied the P site dissociates from the P site, and the elongating polypeptide chain moves out through the exit tunnel. The A site is now empty, and introduction of the next charged tRNA molecule into the A site completes the cycle. Translation continues until a stop codon is encountered in the mRNA, at which point the newly synthesized protein is released from the ribosome.

Pharmacologic agents that inhibit translation interfere with the activities of the prokaryotic ribosome. Aminoglycosides bind to rRNA

QUESTIONS

1. Which steps in translation are blocked by tetracyclines?
   A. Tetracyclines bind and inhibit the action of RNA polymerase.
   B. Tetracyclines inhibit the termination of translation by topoisomerase IV.
   C. Tetracyclines target the 30S ribosomal subunit and cause a misreading of mRNA.
   D. Tetracyclines target the 30S ribosomal subunit and prevent elongation of the peptide chain.
   E. Tetracyclines target the 50S ribosomal subunit and prevent termination of peptide synthesis.

2. Which steps in translation are blocked by macrolides?
   A. Macrolides prevent the separation and decoding of supercoiled mRNA.
   B. Macrolides target the 50S ribosomal subunit and block the translocation of the growing peptide chain.
   C. Macrolides target the 50S ribosomal subunit and inhibit peptide bond formation between aminoacyl tRNA and the growing peptide chain.
   D. Macrolides target the 30S ribosomal subunit and prevent termination of peptide synthesis.
   E. Macrolides prevent the attachment of mRNA with the 30S ribosomal subunit.

3. How do bacteria develop resistance to these drugs and to other inhibitors of transcription and translation?
   A. Bacteria can sequester calcium salts, which bind to, and inactivate these drugs.
   B. Bacteria can alter normal gastrointestinal flora, which degrade these drugs before their absorption.
   C. Bacteria can develop methods of enhancing drug efflux from the bacterial cell.
   D. Bacteria can develop mutations in DNA, which prevent drug binding.
   E. Bacteria can acquire new DNA strands, which do not require repetitive transcription and translation.

4. Why are macrolides bacteriostatic, while some antibiotics, such as quinolones and aminoglycosides, are bactericidal?
   A. Macrolides inhibit normal protein synthesis, while quinolones promote cell wall destruction and cell death.

in the 30S subunit and enable the binding of incorrect tRNAs to mRNA; tetracyclines block aminoacyl-tRNA binding to the A site; chloramphenicol and lincosamides inhibit the peptidyl transferase activity of the 50S subunit. Spectinomycin, macrolides, and streptogramins inhibit peptide translocation. The mechanism(s) of action of the oxazolidinones are uncertain, but some possible sites of action are indicated. Adapted with permission from PharmAid (copyright 2003, Jeffrey T. Joseph and David E. Golan).

B. Macrolides cause the synthesis of abnormally functioning proteins, which can be compensated for by a bacterium.

C. Macrolides inhibit protein synthesis, but this is insufficient to kill a bacterium.

D. Macrolides only inhibit protein synthesis in growing cells, while aminoglycosides completely inhibit all protein synthesis at high concentrations.

E. Macrolides can be pumped out of bacterial cells, limiting their effectiveness, while quinolones and aminoglycosides can not.

5. Why are macrolides an effective treatment for Legionnaires' disease?

A. Macrolides can be administered orally, increasing patient compliance with therapy.

B. Macrolides inhibit the P450-assisted growth of *Legionella* spp. in the liver.

C. Macrolides are bactericidal when used to treat infection with *Legionella* spp.

D. Macrolides prevent the development of resistant strains of *Legionella* spp.

E. Macrolides have intracellular activity against *Legionella* spp.

■ CASE 2

You are working on the infectious disease consultation team in your hospital. As part of today's consultation, you are asked to evaluate and make recommendations for antimicrobial therapy on a patient. The patient, Danny L., is a 47-year-old man with a history of a low cervical spinal cord injury, as a result of a diving accident at the age of 17. He is a paraplegic and has a chronic indwelling Foley catheter, which drains urine from his bladder. As a result, he has developed recurrent urinary tract infections over the past 10 years. He was readmitted to the hospital with a high fever and presumed pyelonephritis yesterday. The preliminary results of his admission urine culture have returned this morning and show greater than 100,000 colonies of a Gram-negative bacillus, confirming a urinary tract infection. You review Mr. L.'s urine analyses from prior admissions and find multiple infections with Gram-negative species that were resistant to ciprofloxacin, levofloxacin, sulfonamides, tetracycline, doxycycline, and chloramphenicol.

QUESTIONS

1. You will be expected to make a recommendation regarding empiric therapy for Mr. L.'s pyelonephritis. Given your review of the case, which of the following agents would you recommend?

A. minocycline

B. amikacin

C. erythromycin

D. vancomycin

E. ofloxacin

2. Which of the following is a potential toxicity associated with the appropriate drug that you have recommended to treat this patient?

A. hypothermia, lethargy, flaccidity, vomiting, respiratory distress

B. colitis

C. cholestatic hepatitis

D. discolored teeth

E. ototoxicity

3. Multi-drug antimicrobial therapy is often necessary to treat complex infections. However, certain combinations of antibiotics such as aminoglycosides and penicillins are synergistic in their actions, while erythromycin and penicillins have a negative effect on each other's actions. What is an explanation for this?

A. Erythromycin inhibits the P450 enzyme activation of penicillins.

B. Erythromycin inhibits the synthesis of proteins that are necessary for penicillins to destroy the cell wall.

C. Penicillins inhibit cell wall synthesis and facilitate the entry of aminoglycosides into the bacterial cell.

D. Aminoglycosides cause a misreading of mRNA, which would normally code for protective proteins to make the cell wall resistant to the action of penicillins.

E. Penicillins inhibit cell wall synthesis and destroy the normal binding sites of erythromycin.

4. Many antimicrobials exert their action at sites or within processes, which are unique to the DNA replication of prokaryotic cells. This confers a degree of selectivity to these agents, which should limit potential adverse effects in humans. Which of the following statements regarding the selectivity of an antimicrobial drug and its adverse effects is correct?

A. Bacterial topoisomerases are structurally different from eukaryotic topoisomerases, contributing to the lack of adverse effects from fluoroquinolones.

B. The bacterial RNA polymerase is identical to eukaryotic RNA polymerase, contributing to the high rate of adverse effects associated with rifampin.

C. Chloramphenicol specifically inhibits bacterial protein synthesis and has a low rate of adverse effects.

D. Tetracyclines inhibit both bacterial and mammalian protein synthesis and have a high rate of adverse effects.

E. Chloramphenicol inhibits mitochondrial protein synthesis, accounting for its selectivity as an antimicrobial agent.

5. Which of the following antimicrobial agents is bactericidal?

A. spectinomycin

B. azithromycin

C. doxycycline

D. levofloxacin

E. chloramphenicol

33

Pharmacology of Bacterial Infections: Cell Wall Synthesis

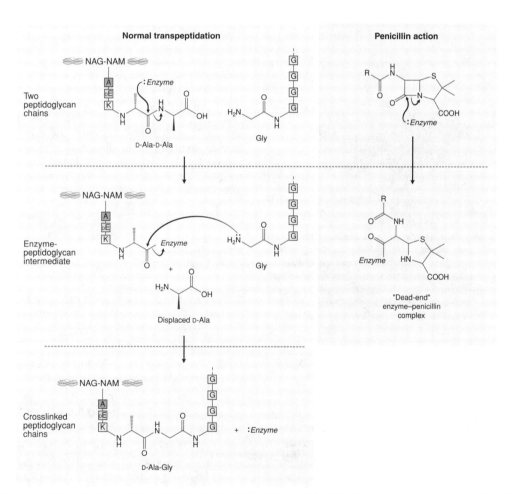

Figure 33-1. Transpeptidase Action and Its Inhibition by Penicillin. The left side of the figure shows the mechanism by which transpeptidases catalyze transpeptidation, a reaction that occurs in bacteria but not in mammalian cells. A nucleophilic group on the transpeptidase (enzyme) attacks the peptide bond between the two D-Ala residues at the terminus of a pentapeptide moiety on one peptidoglycan chain (top panel). The terminal D-alanine residue is displaced from the peptidoglycan chain, and an enzyme-D-alanine-peptidoglycan intermediate is formed. This intermediate is then attacked by the amino terminus of a polyglycine pentapeptide linked at its carboxy terminus to L-lysine or diaminopimelic acid on an adjacent peptidoglycan chain (middle panel). As the enzyme is liberated from the intermediate, a new peptide bond (crosslink) is formed between the terminal glycine residue on one peptidoglycan chain and the enzyme-activated D-alanine residue on the adjacent peptidoglycan chain. The free enzyme can then catalyze another transpeptidation reaction (bottom panel). The right side of the figure shows the mechanism by which penicillin interferes with transpeptidation, leading to the formation of a penicilloyl-enzyme "dead-end complex." In this form, the enzyme is incapable of catalyzing further transpeptidation (crosslinking) reactions.

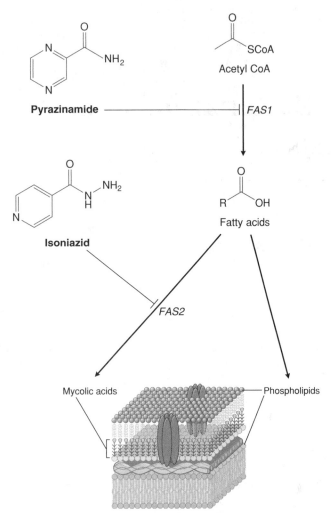

Figure 33-2. Mycolic Acid Synthesis and Antimycobacterial Drug Action. Mycolic acids are produced by the crosslinking of fatty acid chains derived from acetyl coenzyme A (acetyl CoA). Each of the arrows in this simplified representation denotes multiple synthetic steps; the focus is on the fatty acid synthetases (FAS1 and FAS2) because of their importance as drug targets. Specifically, FAS1 is inhibited by pyrazinamide, and FAS2 is inhibited by isoniazid.

OBJECTIVES

■ Understand the pharmacology of, indications for, adverse effects, and limitations of antibacterial agents that exert their action through their effects on the synthesis of the bacterial cell wall.

■ CASE 1

It is April 1953. The Korean War has reached an uneasy stalemate. In the general hospital in Tokyo, Dr. Alan Pierce's ward has just received a new casualty from the front. Three days earlier, 22-year-old Private Morgan H. had been caught by sniper fire while on reconnaissance and had been hit just

above the left knee. At the MASH unit, the wound had been debrided and dressed, and Pvt. H. had been started immediately on a course of high-dose penicillin.

QUESTIONS

1. Penicillin belongs to the most widely prescribed class of antibiotics acting on the bacterial cell wall. What is the mechanism of action of penicillin?
   A. Penicillin provides a suicide substrate for bactoprenol, subsequently preventing polymer transport into the periplasmic space for cross-linking.
   B. The β-lactam ring destroys the Park peptide, causing insufficient polymer for cross-linking.
   C. The β-lactam ring binds transpeptidase and prevents polymer cross-linking.
   D. The β-lactam ring binds to transglycosylase and prevents polymer cross-linking.
   E. Penicillin activates autolysins, which subsequently destroy the cell wall.

Nevertheless, by the time he reaches Tokyo, Pvt. H. has grown faint and delirious and has developed a fever to 103°F. On initial inspection, Dr. Pierce notices a sickly sweet odor about Pvt. H.' leg. When he removes the dressing, he finds the leg bloated below the knee and the wound soaked in putrid, bloody pus. His diagnosis is gangrene, an infection caused by the Gram-positive bacterium *Clostridium perfringens*. Dr. Pierce orders immediate amputation in hopes of saving the young private's life.

Dr. Pierce is troubled by the case. In the past year, he has seen any number of wounds worse than that of Pvt. H., but they have always responded well to aggressive treatment with penicillin.

2. What is the most common mechanism for the development of bacterial resistance to penicillin?
   A. Mutations in bacterial pores prevent penicillin crossing the outer membrane.
   B. An acquired plasmid for a β-lactamase protein gives bacteria the ability to destroy the β-lactam ring.
   C. A chromosomal mutation of bacterial transpeptidase prevents its binding to the β-lactam ring.
   D. An acquired plasmid for resistant transpeptidases prevents their binding to the β-lactam ring.
   E. A chromosomal mutation in bacterial outer membrane lipopolysaccharides prevents β-lactam adherence to the cell.

3. The most common potential adverse effect of β-lactam therapy is:
   A. a disulfiram-like reaction when ethanol is concurrently ingested
   B. autoantibodies to hematopoietic cells and bone marrow suppression

C. the development of *Clostridium difficile* colitis

D. urticarial drug rash and fever

E. seizures at high doses

As he is thinking this over, Dr. Pierce receives word of more incoming patients—eight men, rumored to be suffering from tuberculosis, who have just been released as part of the Operation Little Switch prisoner exchange. Dr. Pierce knows he has streptomycin on hand but decides to see what he can do about getting a 6-month supply of the new antituberculosis drug, isoniazid, from the States.

4. What is the primary reason Dr. Pierce requested a supply of isoniazid from the States?

A. A high rate of mycobacterial resistance to antimycobacterial agents necessitates multi-drug therapy.

B. Multi-drug therapy with antimycobacterial agents prevents the drug toxicity associated with the administration of any one drug.

C. Mycobacteria from Korea have plasmid-acquired resistance to streptomycin.

D. Multi-drug therapy completely cures tuberculosis more rapidly than that associated with single-drug therapy.

E. Antimycobacterial agents induce their own metabolism, necessitating multi-drug therapy with ever-increasing dosages.

5. The development of antibacterial resistance is a growing concern in the management of bacterial infections. This prompts the judicious use of appropriate antibacterial agents by clinicians, and the ongoing search for new antibacterial agents by pharmacology researchers. Which of the following combinations (drug : method of bacterial resistance to drug) is correct?

A. ampicillin : plasmid acquired β-lactamase inhibitor destroys the drug

B. bacitracin : overexpression of alanine racemase allows monomer formation to proceed despite the enzyme inhibition caused by bacitracin

C. vancomycin : plasmid acquired β-lactamase activity destroys the drug

D. fosfomycin and fosmidomycin : mutation in cell transporters prevents intracellular drug entry

E. aminoglycosides : inhibition of protein synthesis and monomer formation at the 30S ribosomal subunit

■ CASE 2

Your cousin, Matt, has returned from 2 years working in the Peace Corps. He recently developed a persistent cough and has lost 10 pounds. He had a skin test performed at his doctor's office to determine if he has had exposure to tuberculosis. He has tested "PPD positive." (PPD is an abbrevia-

tion for purified protein derivative, an extract of mycobacterial antigens, that is injected intradermally as the tuberculin or Mantoux test. If someone has been exposed to the bacterium and developed sensitivity to its antigens, he or she will develop a delayed hypersensitivity reaction to the injection, which manifests as a raised, slightly hard, red area in the injection site.) Matt is started on multi-drug therapy including pyrazinamide, rifampin, and isoniazid with pyridoxine supplementation. He is being followed closely for hepatitis and wants to know what might put him at risk for isoniazid-associated hepatitis.

QUESTIONS

1. The risk of isoniazid-associated hepatitis is increased in patients with:

A. concomitant use of drugs that inhibit the hepatic P450 enzyme system

B. concomitant use of drugs that inhibit renal excretion of isoniazid

C. pyridoxine deficiency

D. hyperuricemia

E. older age

2. What is the mechanism of action of isoniazid in affecting the mycobacterial cell wall?

A. Isoniazid inhibits FAS2 linkage of saturated hydrocarbon chains to make mycolic acid.

B. Isoniazid prevents the formation of arabinogalactans.

C. Isoniazid inhibits FAS1 synthesis of saturated hydrocarbon chain precursors of mycolic acid.

D. Isoniazid inhibits the formation of pores in the mycobacterial outer membrane.

E. Isoniazid prevents the addition of mycolic acid to arabinogalactan on the cell wall.

Your cousin wants to know why he is also being treated with pyridoxine, a vitamin. He asks why he can't take a multi-vitamin instead.

3. What is the role of pyridoxine as a concurrent therapy with isoniazid?

A. Pyridoxine supplementation allows isoniazid to overcome mycobacterial resistance caused by mutations in the catalase-peroxidase enzyme.

B. Pyridoxine supplementation protects the liver from isoniazid-induced hepatitis.

C. Pyridoxine supplementation replaces isoniazid-induced depletion of pyridoxine.

D. Pyridoxine supplementation prevents the development of acute gout associated with isoniazid.

E. Pyridoxine supplementation prevents neuro-ophthalmologic isoniazid toxicity.

4. Your cousin also has a seizure disorder, and since starting his isoniazid therapy, his antiepileptic phenytoin levels have been elevated. What is the relationship between isoniazid and phenytoin metabolism?

   A. Isoniazid blocks the renal elimination of phenytoin.

   B. Isoniazid inhibits the transport of phenytoin across the blood–brain barrier.

   C. Isoniazid inhibits the metabolism of phenytoin by the hepatic P450 enzyme system.

   D. Isoniazid competes with, and reduces the protein binding of phenytoin.

   E. Isoniazid enhances hepatic activation of phenytoin to its active metabolite.

5. Bacteria are initially rapidly identified and classified as Gram positive or Gram negative based on their color appearance after being exposed to gentian violet as a component of the Gram's stain. What portion of the bacterial cell wall retains the purple color of gentian violet after the staining process?

   A. the mycolic acid residues

   B. the murein coat

   C. the lipid bilayer

   D. the lipopolysaccharides of the outer membrane

   E. the porins

34

Pharmacology of Fungal Infections

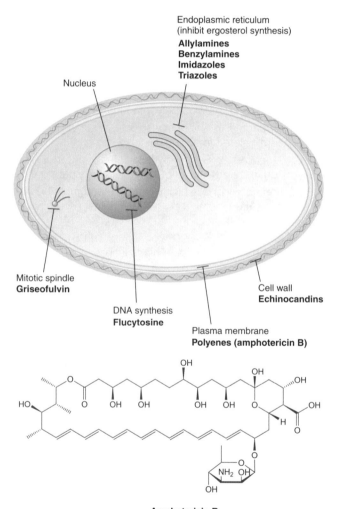

Amphotericin B

Figure 34-1. Cellular Targets of Antifungal Drugs. The currently available antifungal agents act on distinct molecular targets. Flucytosine inhibits fungal DNA synthesis. Griseofulvin inhibits fungal mitosis by disrupting mitotic spindles. Allylamines, benzylamines, imidazoles, and triazoles inhibit the ergosterol synthesis pathway in the endoplasmic reticulum. Polyenes bind to ergosterol in the fungal membrane and thereby disrupt plasma membrane integrity. Amphotericin B is a representative polyene. Echinocandins inhibit fungal cell wall synthesis.

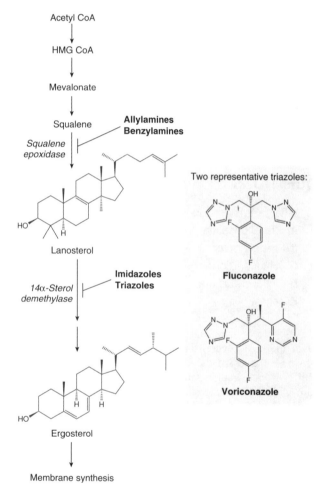

Figure 34-2. Ergosterol Synthesis Pathway. Ergosterol is synthesized within fungal cells from acetyl CoA building blocks. One of the intermediates, squalene, is converted to lanosterol by the action of squalene epoxidase. Allylamines and benzylamines inhibit the action of squalene epoxidase. 14α-Sterol demethylase, a cytochrome P450 enzyme not expressed in mammalian cells, catalyzes the first step in the conversion of lanosterol to the unique fungal sterol ergosterol. Imidazoles and triazoles inhibit 14α-sterol demethylase and thereby prevent the synthesis of ergosterol, which is the principal sterol in fungal membranes. Fluconazole and voriconazole are two representative triazoles.

OBJECTIVES

 Understand the mechanisms by which antifungal agents affect fungal cell growth, replication, and cell wall maintenance.

 Understand the indications for and adverse effects of these agents based on their mechanisms of action.

CASE 1

James F., a 31-year-old HIV-positive man, presents to his physician with a 3-week history of fever, cough, and chest pain after touring southern California. His history is notable for past intravenous drug use. Clinical evaluation and chest x-ray reveal a left lower lobe infiltrate and left paratracheal adenopathy. Sputum cultures are positive for *Coccidioides immitis*, and blood tests are notable for an elevated titer of antibodies directed against this fungal pathogen. The physician makes a preliminary diagnosis of pulmonary coccidioidomycosis and prescribes a course of amphotericin B.

QUESTIONS

1. What factors predisposed Mr. F. to fungal infection?
  A. travel in southern California
  B. male gender
  C. HIV infection
  D. intravenous drug use
  E. chest pain

Over the next several days, however, Mr. F. does not improve. He goes to the emergency department with fever, chills, sweats, cough, fatigue, and headaches. His temperature is 100°F, but he shows no evidence of meningitis or peripheral adenopathy. Lung examination reveals diffuse wheezing over the left lung fields, noted on both inspiration and expiration. Bronchoscopy shows narrowing of the tracheal lumen by numerous mucosal granulomas from the left main-stem bronchus to the level of the midtrachea. Fungal culture grows *C. immitis*, a definitive diagnosis of chronic pulmonary coccidioidomycosis is made, the granulomas are bronchoscopically removed, and amphotericin B is continued. One week later, Mr. F.'s symptoms begin to subside, amphotericin B is discontinued, and a course of fluconazole is initiated.

2. What is the mechanism of action of amphotericin B?
  A. Amphotericin B prevents the formation of cholesterol from lanosterol.
  B. Amphotericin B binds lanosterol and prevents its incorporation into the fungal cell wall.

  C. Amphotericin B prevents the formation of ergosterol from lanosterol.
  D. Amphotericin B binds ergosterol and prevents its incorporation into the fungal cell wall.
  E. Amphotericin B binds ergosterol and creates pores in the fungal cell wall.

3. What are the potential adverse effects that Mr. F. may experience as a consequence of treatment with amphotericin B?
  A. fever and hypotension
  B. acute liver failure
  C. hypercholesterolemia
  D. gastric hyperacidity
  E. bone marrow suppression

4. How do the pharmacokinetics of amphotericin B affect its administration?
  A. Amphotericin B is poorly soluble unless converted to a salt in the acidic environment of the stomach.
  B. Amphotericin B is poorly soluble and must be orally administered in a colloidal suspension.
  C. Amphotericin B is highly lipid soluble and must be administered intravenously in a lipid suspension.
  D. Amphotericin B is highly insoluble and must be administered intrathecally to treat central nervous system fungal infections.
  E. Amphotericin B is 90% protein bound and does not distribute well to tissue binding sites.

5. What is the mechanism of action of fluconazole?
  A. Fluconazole inhibits fungal DNA synthesis.
  B. Fluconazole inhibits the formation of lanosterol from squalene.
  C. Fluconazole inhibits the formation of ergosterol from lanosterol.
  D. Fluconazole binds to lanosterol and prevents its incorporation into the fungal cell wall.
  E. Fluconazole binds to ergosterol and prevents its incorporation into the fungal cell wall.

CASE 2

Jessica H., a 23-year-old mother, brings her 5-year-old son, Jason, to their family practitioner for an evaluation of a rash on his scalp. A round, dry, somewhat scaly patch of skin has been growing very slowly on the back of Jason's scalp for the past 6 weeks. Despite applying creams and moisturizers to the area, Ms. H. says it is not improving. In fact, the scaly patch seems to be slightly larger than when it first appeared. She is concerned because the hair in the area seems to be breaking and falling out. Jason says the rash is slightly itchy. The family doctor finds Jason to be well appearing with a 2-cm, round, scaly patch on the occipital region of his scalp. There is minimal hair growth in the area, and what hair that is present is broken short at the level of the scalp. Jason has no other skin rashes. The doctor diagnoses Jason with ''ringworm'' of the scalp and hair, a fungal infection likely caused by *Trichophyton* spp. He prescribes a course of oral griseofulvin.

QUESTIONS

1. What is the mechanism of action of griseofulvin?
   A. Griseofulvin is an antimetabolite that inhibits DNA synthesis.
   B. Griseofulvin disrupts microtubules and cell mitosis.
   C. Griseofulvin inhibits squalene epoxidase formation of lanosterol.
   D. Griseofulvin inhibits 14α-sterol demethylase formation of ergosterol.
   E. Griseofulvin inhibits ergosterol incorporation into the fungal cell membrane.

2. What laboratory tests should be monitored while Jason is taking griseofulvin?
   A. creatinine
   B. calcium
   C. liver function tests
   D. chloride
   E. bicarbonate

As they are leaving the office, Ms. H. asks if she might be able to take a few doses of the griseofulvin herself: she thinks she has a vaginal yeast infection, which is not responding to an over-the-counter preparation of clotrimazole.

3. Clotrimazole is a member of the imidazole antifungal class. Which of the following statements regarding this class of antifungal agents is correct?

A. Ms. H. could apply topical clotrimazole to Jason's scalp to treat his infection.
B. These antifungal agents inhibit the action of squalene epoxidase.
C. A potential serious adverse effect of these agents is acute renal failure.
D. Drug resistance can develop as a result of mutations in the fungal P450 enzymes.
E. Nystatin is a prototypic drug of the azole class.

Ms. H.'s family practitioner examines her and confirms that she does have a vaginal yeast infection, probably caused by *Candida* spp. infection. After reviewing any and all current medications that she might be taking, including oral contraceptives, the physician offers Ms. H. single-dose therapy with oral fluconazole.

4. Why did Ms. H.'s family practitioner review her medication list before administering fluconazole?
   A. Drugs that alter the gastric acidity will decrease the absorption of fluconazole.
   B. Fluconazole concentrations rapidly increase when taken with other drugs that compete for renal elimination.
   C. The metabolism of fluconazole can be affected by drugs that inhibit or induce the P450 enzymes.
   D. Fluconazole inactivates oral contraceptive agents.
   E. Fluconazole can cause hypersensitivity in patients taking sulfites.

5. Which of the following is a potential adverse effect associated with the use of ketoconazole?
   A. achlorhydria
   B. aseptic meningitis
   C. inhibition of estrogen synthesis
   D. adrenal insufficiency
   E. seborrheic dermatitis

35

Pharmacology of Parasitic Infections

OBJECTIVES

■ Understand the pharmacology of antiparasitic agents, as it relates to the pathophysiology of parasitic infections.

■ CASE 1

Binata, a 3-year-old girl living in Senegal, is in good health when, one day, she begins to feel hot, has sweats and shaking chills, stops eating, and becomes intermittently listless and lethargic. Several days later, these symptoms climax in a seizure and coma, prompting Binata's parents to rush her to the local health care clinic. In the clinic, the unconscious child's neck is supple, but she is febrile to 103°F. Her lungs are clear to auscultation, and there is no rash. A smear of Binata's peripheral blood discloses *Plasmodium falciparum* ring trophozoites in approximately 10% of her erythrocytes. Binata is given the only antimalarial medicines available at the clinic, chloroquine and pyrimethamine–sulfadoxine; however, the child does not improve, and she dies within 24 hours.

QUESTIONS

1. What are the causes of morbidity in patients with *P. falciparum* infection?
   A. Sporozoites can migrate through subcutaneous tissues, causing itching and rashes.
   B. Tissue schizonts can cause liver abscesses.
   C. Blood schizonts are transported to the cornea and cause blindness.
   D. Blood schizonts infect erythrocytes and cause hemolysis.
   E. Blood schizonts migrate from erythrocytes and cause local endothelial damage.

2. What is the mechanism of action of chloroquine in the treatment of malaria?

A. Chloroquine prevents the entry of parasites into the erythrocyte.
B. Chloroquine prevents the breakdown of hemoglobin and "starves" the parasite.
C. Chloroquine causes an accumulation of a toxic heme metabolite, which poisons the parasite.
D. Chloroquine prevents erythrocyte glycolysis and adenosine triphosphate (ATP) generation, which inhibits parasite growth.
E. Chloroquine prevents DNA synthesis in the parasite.

3. What is a rationale for combination therapy with chloroquine and pyrimethamine–sulfadoxine?
   A. Chloroquine and pyrimethamine–sulfadoxine have different mechanisms of action in treating malaria.
   B. Chloroquine treats hepatic schizonts, and pyrimethamine–sulfadoxine treats blood schizonts.
   C. Chloroquine resistance is growing, while pyrimethamine–sulfadoxine sensitivity is still widespread, making it a good second-line agent.
   D. Chloroquine and pyrimethamine–sulfadoxine have low toxicity when given in a high-dose combination.
   E. Chloroquine and pyrimethamine–sulfadoxine compete for metabolism, prolonging their half-lives and reducing the frequency of administration.

4. Why did Binata not improve after receiving antimalarial drugs?
   A. The *P. falciparum* was resistant to the combination therapy.
   B. Cerebral malaria has an 80% fatality rate.
   C. Binata had only a partial immune response to the infection.
   D. *P. falciparum* continued to be released from Binata's liver.
   E. Binata developed toxic levels of ferriprotoporphyrin IX.

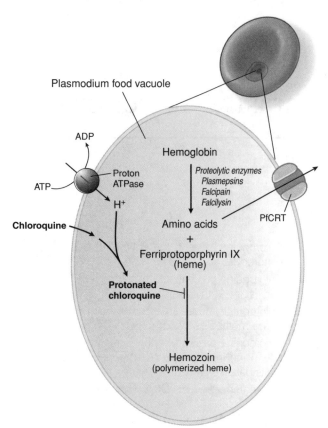

Plasmodium food vacuole

ADP

ATP

Proton
ATPase

H⁺

Chloroquine

Hemoglobin

Proteolytic enzymes
Plasmepsins
Falcipain
Falcilysin

Amino acids
+
Ferriprotoporphyrin IX
(heme)

**Protonated
chloroquine**

Hemozoin
(polymerized heme)

PfCRT

Figure 35-1. Proposed Mechanisms of Heme Metabolism in the Plasmodial Food Vacuole. Malarial plasmodia possess a specialized food vacuole that maintains an acidic intravacuolar environment by the action of a proton ATPase in the vacuolar membrane. Within the vacuole, human hemoglobin is used as a food source. Hemoglobin is proteolyzed to amino acids by several plasmodial-derived proteolytic enzymes, including plasmepsins, falcipain, and falcilysin. Protonated amino acids are then removed from the food vacuole through the PfCRT transporter. Degradation of hemoglobin also releases heme (ferriprotoporphyrin IX). Free ferriprotoporphyrin IX can react with oxygen to produce superoxide (O_2^-); oxidant defense enzymes, which may include plasmodial-derived superoxide dismutase and catalase, convert the potentially cytotoxic superoxide to H_2O (not shown). Plasmodia polymerize ferriprotoporphyrin IX into the nontoxic derivative hemozoin; evidence suggests that polymerization requires the activity of positively charged histidine-rich proteins (not shown). The iron moiety in ferriprotoporphyrin IX can also be oxidized from the ferrous (Fe^{2+}) to the ferric (Fe^{3+}) state, with concomitant production of hydrogen peroxide (H_2O_2). Many antimalarial agents are thought to disrupt the process of malarial heme metabolism; proposed mechanisms of drug action include inhibition of heme polymerization, enhancement of oxidant production, and reaction with heme to form cytotoxic metabolites. The inhibition of ferriprotoporphyrin IX polymerization by protonated chloroquine is shown. ADP = adenosine diphosphate; ATP = adenosine triphosphate.

 CASE 2

Mr. G. is a 36 year-old married software engineer who was born and raised in India. He comes to the United States and is completely well for 6 months. He then begins to experience episodes of fever, headache, and body aches. One week later, he goes to his physician, who examines a smear of Mr. G.'s blood, diagnoses malaria, and prescribes chloroquine for treatment. Therapy with chloroquine resolves his symptoms completely. However, Mr. G. notes recurrence of fevers and the other symptoms 3 months later and returns to his doctor's office.

QUESTIONS

1. What is the most likely explanation for the return of Mr. G.'s fever?
   A. Mr. G. did not complete his course of chloroquine.
   B. Mr. G. had dormant cerebral forms of plasmodia that released new merozoites into his circulation.
   C. Mr. G. had a delayed hypersensitivity reaction to chloroquine.
   D. Mr. G. had a drug-resistant form of plasmodia infection.
   E. Mr. G. had dormant hepatic forms of plasmodia that released new merozoites into his circulation.

2. After treating Mr. G. for his blood stream infection, how can he be treated so that his illness will not return?
   A. Mr. G. requires only a second course of chloroquine.
   B. Mr. G. requires treatment with another agent, such as primaquine.
   C. Mr. G. requires treatment with another quinoline compound, such as mefloquine.
   D. Mr. G. requires treatment with another nonquinoline compound, such as artemisinin.
   E. Mr. G. requires chloroquine-pyrimethamine-sulfadoxine combination therapy to prevent his plasmodium infection from returning.

3. Which of the following antimalarial drugs can be used as prophylaxis against infection?
   A. quinine
   B. mefloquine
   C. quinidine
   D. artemisinin
   E. sulfonamide–pyrimethamine

 CASE 3

Mr. S., a 29-year-old American journalist, returns from a trip to Southeast Asia. He feels fine for 5 weeks but then begins to experience mild diarrhea, abdominal pain, and malaise. He does not attribute his symptoms to the trip because

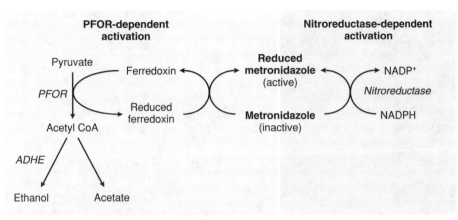

Figure 35-2. Fermentation Enzymes of Anaerobic Organisms and Mechanisms of Metronidazole Activation. Anaerobic organisms metabolize pyruvate to acetyl coenzyme A (CoA); this conversion is catalyzed by the enzyme pyruvate:ferredoxin oxidoreductase (PFOR). Acetyl CoA is then either hydrolyzed to acetate or oxidized to ethanol by alcohol dehydrogenase E (ADHE). Metronidazole is a prodrug; it contains a nitro group that must be reduced for the drug to become active. Reduced metronidazole is highly effective against anaerobic organisms, probably because of the formation of cytotoxic intermediates that cause DNA, protein, and membrane damage. Two aspects of anaerobic metabolism provide opportunities for selective reduction of the nitro group. First, the reaction catalyzed by PFOR results in the reduction of ferredoxin; reduced ferredoxin can then transfer its electrons to metronidazole, resulting in reduced (active) metronidazole and reoxidized ferredoxin. Second, many anaerobic organisms express nitroreductase enzymes that selectively reduce metronidazole and, in the process, convert reduced nicotinamide adenine dinucleotide phosphate (NADPH) to oxidized nicotinamide adenine dinucleotide phosphate (NADP$^+$).

they developed well after he returned home. Furthermore, Mr. S.'s wife shared the same food and water during the trip, and she remains well. As a result, Mr. S. ignores the symptoms for a week, but he eventually goes to his physician when the symptoms do not abate spontaneously. Physical examination reveals tenderness in the right upper quadrant of the abdomen. Blood tests are notable for elevated liver enzymes, and a computed tomography scan reveals a liver abscess. Stool examination is positive for heme and for *Entamoeba histolytica* cysts.

QUESTIONS

1. Why is Mr. S.'s wife asymptomatic?
   A. Mrs. S. had prior immunity to *E. histolytica*.
   B. Mrs. S. was infected with *Entamoeba dispar*.
   C. Mrs. S. may never develop symptoms of entamoeba infection.
   D. Mrs. S. ingested inactive cysts and not active trophozoites.
   E. *E. histolytica* is more likely to cause invasive disease in males because of protective estrogen-associated gastrointestinal factors.

2. What are the potential complications if Mr. S.'s condition is left untreated?
   A. abscess rupture and sepsis
   B. migration of trophozoites into the cornea and blindness
   C. release of sporozoites into the circulation and hemolysis
   D. migration of trophozoites into the subcutaneous tissues with subsequent rash
   E. liver failure

3. *E. histolytica* and other luminal parasites depend on novel fermentation enzymes to perform electron transfer under anaerobic conditions. Pyruvate:ferredoxin oxidoreductase (PFOR) is one of these enzymes. What is the relationship between protozoal PFOR and potential therapies for these infections?
   A. Intraluminal iodoquinol kills amoeba with PFOR.
   B. Pentamidine inhibits the activity of protozoal PFOR.
   C. Metronidazole can cause human toxicity because of its activation of mammalian PFOR.
   D. Metronidazole activation is dependent on the presence of reduced ferredoxin, produced by PFOR.
   E. Metronidazole inhibits the activity of protozoal PFOR in abscesses.

 CASE 4

Thumbi is a boy who enjoys fishing in a river near his village in the Democratic Republic of Congo. At the age of 13, he emigrates with his family to the United States. Shortly thereafter, he begins to scratch his arms and legs vigorously. Six months later, his mother brings him to a dermatologist. Physical examination reveals a macular and papular rash with excoriations on the arms and legs, as well as a few subcutaneous nodules. Examination of peripheral blood discloses high-level eosinophilia. A nodule is excised and examined by a pathologist, leading to a diagnosis. Thumbi begins treatment with ivermectin but returns the next day feverish and feeling more itchy than before.

QUESTIONS

1. What did the pathologist see in the subcutaneous nodule?
   A. *Simulium* spp. cysts
   B. *Onchocerca volvulus* larvae
   C. *O. volvulus* adult filarial worms
   D. *O. volvulus* microfilariae
   E. *O. volvulus* cysts

2. Why did Thumbi feel worse immediately after treatment with ivermectin?
   A. Thumbi developed neurotoxicity from ivermectin in the central nervous system.
   B. Thumbi experienced a hypersensitivity reaction because of the drug-induced migration of adult filariae.
   C. Thumbi developed systemic glutamate activation as a result of ivermectin.
   D. Thumbi developed an allergic response to the presence of dying microfilariae.
   E. Thumbi was infected with a resistant strain of *O. volvulus.*

3. Which of the following statements regarding antihelminthic agents is correct?
   A. Because ivermectin kills microfilariae, it is a curative agent for *O. volvulus* infection.
   B. Ivermectin potentiates glutamate and gamma-aminobutyric acid (GABA) transmission and kills microfilariae by causing paralysis.
   C. Ivermectin is effective against strongyloidiasis, schistosomiasis, and scabies.
   D. Praziquantel acts by inhibiting tubulin polymerization and disrupting nematodal motility and DNA replication.
   E. Diethylcarbamazine must be administered every 6 months in the treatment of filariol onchocerciasis.

36

Pharmacology of Viral Infections

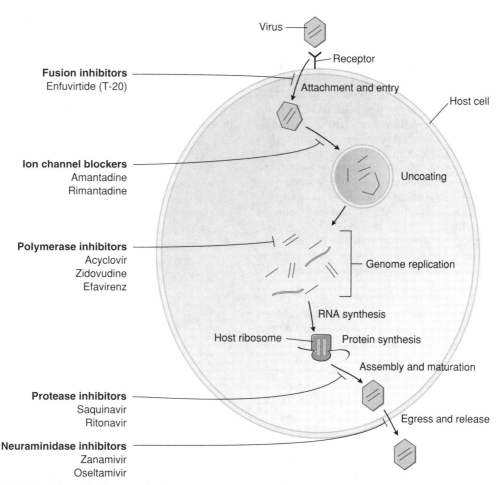

Figure 36-1. Viral Life Cycle and Pharmacologic Intervention. The viral life cycle can be divided into a sequence of individual steps, each of which is a potential site for pharmacologic intervention. Shown is a generic replication cycle of viruses in cells, alongside which are listed the names of drug classes and examples of individual agents that block each step. The majority of the currently approved antiviral agents are nucleoside analogues that target genome replication, typically by inhibiting viral DNA polymerase or reverse transcriptase. Several other drug classes target other steps in the viral life cycle, including attachment and entry, uncoating, assembly and maturation, and egress and release. It should be noted that the details of viral replication differ for each type of virus, often presenting unique targets for pharmacologic intervention and drug development. For example, the life cycle of HIV (and other retroviruses) includes additional steps such as integration.

OBJECTIVES

■ Understand the mechanisms by which antiviral agents inhibit viral infection and replication.

■ Understand the indications for, and adverse effects of these agents based on their mechanisms of action.

■ CASE 1

The year is 1993. Mr. M., a 26-year-old man, complains to Dr. Rose, his primary care physician, of a sore throat, fever, and tiredness for the past several weeks. On physical examination, Dr. Rose notes bilateral cervical lymphadenopathy consistent with the patient's "flu-like symptoms." Dr. Rose thinks it likely that Mr. M. has an infection, possibly a simple "cold," the "flu," or strep throat. Because of Mr. M.'s mononucleosis-like symptoms, Dr. Rose also includes cytomegalovirus (CMV), Epstein-Barr virus (EBV), toxoplasmosis, and HIV in her differential diagnosis. Laboratory test results for *Streptococcus* spp, CMV, EBV, and toxoplasmosis, and HIV are negative. Mr. M. is concerned about the possibility of HIV infection, although he denies any unprotected sexual activity, intravenous drug use, and other potential exposure risks. Dr. Rose tells Mr. M. that his symptoms will soon resolve with rest but that he should return for follow-up within 6 months. She explains to Mr. M. that, if he has recently contracted HIV, his body would not yet have produced sufficient antibodies to show up on an anti-HIV antibody test.

Five years later, Mr. M. returns to Dr. Rose's office. He has not seen any physician in the interim and now presents with a number of new symptoms. There are multiple open lesions on his lips and in his mouth, and he confides that he has similar lesions in his genital area. An enzyme-linked immunosorbent assay (ELISA) test is positive for anti-HIV antibodies, and a viral load measurement shows high levels of HIV RNA in his blood. Mr. M.'s CD4 count is 100 per mm^3 (normal range, 800–1200 per mm^3). Dr. Rose immediately prescribes a drug regimen of zidovudine (AZT), lamivudine (3TC), and ritonavir, explaining to Mr. M. that a combination of anti-HIV drugs is his best option for reducing the viral load and forestalling more serious disease. In addition, Dr. Rose prescribes oral acyclovir to treat Mr. M.'s oral and genital herpes.

QUESTIONS

1. What are the mechanisms of action of the three anti-HIV drugs prescribed by Dr. Rose?
   A. AZT and 3TC are nucleoside analogues, and ritonavir inhibits viral neuraminidase-associated viral release from the host cell.
   B. AZT and 3TC inhibit viral attachment and entry, and ritonavir is a nucleoside analogue.
   C. AZT inhibits viral attachment and entry, 3TC inhibits viral uncoating, and ritonavir is a viral protease inhibitor.
   D. AZT and 3TC are nucleoside analogues, and ritonavir is a viral protease inhibitor.
   E. AZT and 3TC inhibit viral uncoating and ritonavir inhibits viral neuraminidase-associated viral release from the host cell.

2. What is the mechanism of action of acyclovir?
   A. Acyclovir inhibits the herpes virus protease.
   B. Acyclovir is a nucleoside analogue.
   C. Acyclovir prevents uncoating of the herpes virus.
   D. Acyclovir inhibits the herpes virus reverse transcriptase.
   E. Acyclovir inhibits the herpes virus RNA polymerase.

Over the next 3 years, Mr. M.'s HIV viral load falls to undetectable levels, and his condition improves. The herpes infections are also kept in check. Today, Mr. M. appears in good health and, although it takes considerable effort, he takes his medications diligently.

3. Acyclovir is used to treat herpes simplex virus (HSV) and varicella zoster virus (VZV) infection. It has a high therapeutic index. Why does acyclovir not cause significant toxicity in humans?
   A. HSV and VZV enzymes do not phosphorylate mammalian nucleosides as efficiently as they do acyclovir.
   B. Acyclovir specifically inhibits HSV and VZV RNA polymerase, which is structurally unique and unlike mammalian RNA polymerase.
   C. Acyclovir is a nucleoside analogue that is specific to HSV and VZV DNA.
   D. Mammalian enzymes degrade acyclovir, while HSV and VZV activate it for use in viral DNA synthesis.
   E. Mammalian enzymes do not phosphorylate acyclovir as efficiently as do HSV and VZV.

4. What is a reason for prescribing three anti-HIV drugs (AZT, 3TC, and ritonavir) and just one antiherpesvirus drug (acyclovir) for Mr. M.?
   A. AZT, 3TC, and ritonavir inhibit each other's metabolism, increasing their plasma levels and efficacy.
   B. Acyclovir is highly toxic and cannot be administered with other herpes antiviral agents.
   C. Administering AZT, 3TC, and ritonavir in combination decreases the risk of toxicity associated with any one of the agents.
   D. The herpes virus will be completely eradicated by acyclovir, but the HIV virus requires multi-drug therapy to decrease the viral load.
   E. Multi-drug therapy is necessary to completely eradicate HIV infection.

5. Which of the following antiviral agents has activity against latent HSV and latent HIV?

A. enfuvirtide

B. amantadine

C. valacyclovir

D. ritonavir

E. none of the above

CASE 2

In 2000, a fixed-dose combination of HIV protease inhibitors was approved by the Food and Drug Administration. This drug combination, which consisted of 133.3 mg of lopinavir and 33.3 mg of ritonavir in a soft gelatin capsule, had increased clinical efficacy compared with regimens that included only a single protease inhibitor. The plasma levels of lopinavir obtained using this combination were significantly increased compared with the levels achieved using lopinavir as a single agent. Using the combination, lopinavir plasma levels exceeded the inhibitory concentrations for many HIV strains, including some strains that were resistant to other protease inhibitors.

The package insert for the lopinavir/ritonavir combination recommended against giving lovastatin (an HMG CoA reductase inhibitor), midazolam (a benzodiazepine), or flecainide (an antiarrhythmic agent) concurrently to patients receiving this two-drug combination.

The following list provides examples of drugs that are metabolized by two of the major P450 enzymes in the human liver:

CYP2D6: clozapine, codeine, encainide, flecainide, fluoxetine, metoprolol, ritonavir, timolol

CYP3A4: diazepam, diltiazem, erythromycin, ethinyl estradiol, indinavir, lopinavir, lovastatin, midazolam, progesterone, ritonavir, saquinavir, tamoxifen, triazolam

QUESTIONS

1. When lopinavir and ritonavir are used in combination, the plasma levels of lopinavir are significantly increased compared with those achieved when lopinavir is used as single therapy. What might be an explanation for this finding when these two protease inhibitors are administered in combination?

A. Ritonavir prevents the development of viral resistance to lopinavir.

B. Lopinavir inhibits its own metabolism.

C. Lopinavir inhibits the metabolism of ritonavir.

D. Ritonavir inhibits the metabolism of lopinavir.

E. Ritonavir enhances the gastrointestinal absorption of lopinavir.

2. What effect might the use of this combination have on

patients who are taking medications for the treatment of an anxiety disorder?

A. bradycardia

B. seizures

C. drowsiness

D. vomiting

E. hepatic failure

3. Rifampin (an antibiotic) is known to induce several P450 enzymes, including CYP2C9, CYP2C19, and CYP3A4. What effect would concurrent administration of rifampin have on plasma levels of lopinavir and ritonavir?

A. The plasma levels of lopinavir will be increased, but levels of ritonavir will be reduced.

B. The plasma levels of both drugs will be increased.

C. The plasma levels of lopinavir will be increased.

D. The plasma levels of lopinavir will be reduced.

E. The plasma levels of ritonavir will be increased.

4. What is the basis for the recommendation not to administer lovastatin, midazolam, or flecainide concurrently with the lopinavir–ritonavir combination?

A. Lovastatin, midazolam, and flecainide metabolism may be inhibited, resulting in elevated plasma concentrations and clinical toxicity.

B. These drugs induce the metabolism of the lopinavir–ritonavir combination, reducing their efficacy.

C. These drugs inhibit the metabolism of the lopinavir–ritonavir combination, resulting in a metabolic acidosis.

D. When used in combination, lovastatin, midazolam, and flecainide reverse the protease inhibition caused by lopinavir and ritonavir.

E. Lovastatin, midazolam, and flecainide metabolism may be induced, resulting in elevated plasma concentrations and reduced efficacy.

5. What is the role of interferons in the treatment of viral infections?

A. Interferons are used to actively immunize people against specific viral antigens.

B. Interferons induce the expression of innate immune system proteins with antiviral effects.

C. Interferon α is approved for the treatment of HIV.

D. Interferon administration can induce an antibody response and serum sickness.

E. Inhaled interferon is an effective treatment of respiratory syncytial virus (RSV) in children.

37

Pharmacology of Cancer: Genome Synthesis, Stability, and Maintenance

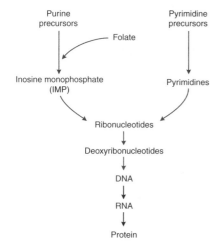

■ Understand how various cancer chemotherapeutic agents exert their therapeutic and toxic effects through their modification of genome synthesis, stability, and maintenance.

■ CASE 1

One day, J.L., a 23-year-old graduate student who had previously been in good health, noticed a hard lump in his left testis while showering. Concerned by the finding, J.L.'s physician ordered an ultrasound examination, which showed a solid mass suggestive of cancer. The testis was removed surgically; pathologic review confirmed the diagnosis of testicular cancer. A chest x-ray revealed several lung nodules

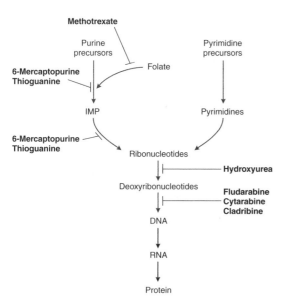

Figure 37-1. Overview of de Novo Nucleotide Biosynthesis. A. Folate is an essential cofactor in the synthesis of inosine monophosphate (IMP), from which all purine nucleotides are derived. Pyrimidine synthesis does not require folate, although folate is required for the methylation of deoxyuridylate (dUMP) to deoxythymidylate (dTMP). Ribonucleotides contain one of the purine or pyrimidine bases linked to ribose phosphate. Subsequent reduction of the ribose at the 2′ position produces deoxyribonucleotides. Whereas deoxyribonucleotides are polymerized into DNA, ribonucleotides are used to form RNA (not shown). The central dogma of molecular biology states that the DNA code determines the sequence of RNA (transcription) and that RNA is then translated into protein. **B.** Methotrexate inhibits dihydrofolate reductase (DHFR) and thereby prevents the utilization of folate in purine nucleotide and dTMP synthesis. 6-Mercaptopurine and thioguanine inhibit the formation of purine nucleotides. Hydroxyurea inhibits the enzyme that converts ribonucleotides to deoxyribonucleotides. Fludarabine, cytarabine, and cladribine are purine and pyrimidine analogues that inhibit DNA synthesis. 5-Fluorouracil inhibits the enzyme that converts dUMP to dTMP (not shown).

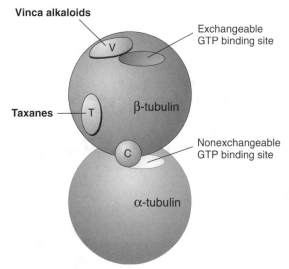

Vinca alkaloids

V

Exchangeable
GTP binding site

Taxanes

T

β-tubulin

Nonexchangeable
GTP binding site

C

α-tubulin

Figure 37-2. Tubulin Binding Sites of Microtubule-Inhibiting Drugs. The tubulin heterodimer is composed of α-tubulin and β-tubulin. α-Tubulin and β-tubulin both bind GTP. The GTP on α-tubulin is not hydrolyzed; for this reason, the GTP binding site on α-tubulin is referred to as the nonexchangeable GTP binding site. β-Tubulin hydrolyzes GTP to GDP; for this reason, the GTP binding site on β-tubulin is referred to as the exchangeable GTP binding site. The two classes of antineoplastic microtubule inhibitors bind to distinct sites on the tubulin heterodimer. Vinca alkaloids, which inhibit microtubule polymerization, bind to a site on β-tubulin located near the exchangeable GTP binding site (V). Vinca alkaloids associate preferentially at the (+) end of microtubules and thereby inhibit the addition of new tubulin subunits to the microtubule. Taxanes, which stabilize polymerized microtubules, bind to a different site on β-tubulin (T). Taxanes may stabilize either the interactions between tubulin subunits or the shape of microtubule protofilaments. Colchicine binds to a site located at the interface between α-tubulin and β-tubulin (C). Colchicine is not used in cancer chemotherapy but is used in the treatment of gout (see Chapter 47). Adapted with permission from Downing KH. Structural basis for the interaction of tubulin with proteins and drugs that affect microtubule dynamics. Ann Rev Cell Dev Biol 2000;16:89–111, Figure 9.

that were thought to represent metastatic spread of the cancer. J.L. was treated with several cycles of combination chemotherapy, including bleomycin, etoposide, and cisplatin. The lung nodules disappeared completely.

QUESTIONS

1. What is the molecular target of each of the drugs in J.L.'s combination chemotherapy regimen?
   A. Bleomycin targets ribonucleotide reductase and prevents the conversion of nucleotides to deoxynucleotides, and subsequent DNA synthesis.
   B. Bleomycin targets guanine residues and causes intra-strand DNA crosslinks.
   C. Etoposide targets topoisomerase I and stabilizes DNA single strand nicking.

   D. Etoposide targets topoisomerase II and stabilizes double-stranded DNA breaks.
   E. Cisplatin binds DNA and chelates iron to cause free radical–induced DNA strand breaks.

2. By what mechanisms could etoposide, bleomycin, and cisplatin act synergistically against J.L.'s testicular cancer?
   A. Cisplatin and bleomycin damage DNA, and etoposide inhibits DNA repair.
   B. Cisplatin delays the renal elimination of bleomycin and etoposide, and prolongs their effects.
   C. All three agents can be given in combination to limit the toxicity associated with any one agent.
   D. Etoposide administration limits the likelihood of cancer cell resistance to cisplatin and bleomycin.
   E. Bleomycin enhances the DNA binding of cisplatin and etoposide.

One year later, J.L. was able to resume his studies, and there were no signs of recurrence of the cancer. Nonetheless, at every subsequent follow-up visit, J.L.'s physician asks him whether he is developing shortness of breath.

3. Why does J.L.'s physician inquire about shortness of breath at each follow-up visit?
   A. He is looking for evidence of recurrent pulmonary metastases.
   B. He is looking for evidence of bleomycin-induced heart failure.
   C. He is looking for evidence of bleomycin-induced pulmonary fibrosis.
   D. He is looking for evidence of cisplatin-induced pulmonary fibrosis.
   E. He is looking for evidence of cisplatin-induced heart failure.

4. How did serendipity lead to the discovery of cisplatin, the most efficacious drug against testicular cancer?
   A. Sailors exposed to cisplatin during World War II were noted not to develop testicular cancer.
   B. Experiments on the effects of electricity in bacteria noted that cisplatin inhibited DNA synthesis.
   C. Botany experiments with the periwinkle plant noted that plant cells exposed to cisplatin were unable to divide during the M phase of mitosis.
   D. Experiments with protozoa noted that cisplatin prevented the repair of DNA double-strand breaks.
   E. Veterans with gouty arthritis treated with allopurinol and cisplatin were noted to be protected from testicular cancer.

TABLE 37-1

Drug	Mechanism of Action	Major Toxicity	MW (Daltons)	Lipophilicity
A	DNA alkylation	Bone marrow suppression	743	++
B	Inhibition of microtubule polymerization	Peripheral neurologic toxicity	882	+
C	Purine analog	Bone marrow suppression	697	+
D	Topoisomerase inhibition	Mucous membrane ulceration	876	++++
E	DNA repair inhibition	Bladder irritation	922	++

5. Some antimetabolites act as nucleotide analogues. These analogues can participate in nucleotide synthesis pathways and be incorporated into DNA, where they disrupt its structure, cause chain termination, and induce strand breakage. Which of the following is a pyrimidine analogue?

A. thioguanine

B. fludarabine phosphate

C. cladribine

D. cytarabine

E. telomerase

 CASE 2

As the director of developmental therapeutics at a major cancer center, you are asked to review data on five new drugs generated by your investigators. They present you with the following table summarizing the information generated on the new agents.

QUESTIONS

1. One of the investigators proposes using compounds A and C in combination in a clinical trial. What are the potential benefits or drawbacks of using this combination, as opposed to using the drugs as single agents?

A. A potential benefit is that adverse effects will be limited to one organ system.

B. A potential benefit is that both agents cause DNA damage and may be synergistic in their ability to kill cells.

C. A potential benefit is that these agents will easily cross the blood–brain barrier to treat central nervous system (CNS) malignancies.

D. A potential drawback is that these agents do not inhibit cell mitosis.

E. A potential drawback is that this combination must be administered frequently.

2. Patients given drug B in a phase I clinical trial develop numbness and tingling of their fingers and toes. Why does drug B cause this toxicity?

A. Drug B inhibits microtubule polymerization and the normal cellular turnover of sensitive skin cells in the tips of the digits.

B. Drug B inhibits microtubule polymerization and the microtubule-dependent process of trafficking along long peripheral nerves.

C. Drug B exhibits low lipophilicity and accumulates in peripheral nervous tissue.

D. Drug B exhibits high lipophilicity and accumulates in peripheral nervous tissue.

E. Drug B has the same molecular weight as sodium ions and blocks peripheral nerve cell sodium channels and action potential generation.

3. Intravenous administration of which of these drugs is most likely to be capable of treating tumor cells in the CNS, and why?

A. Drug A: It alkylates DNA and will be able to cause cell damage in slowly dividing brain cells.

B. Drug B: It damages nerve tissues and will be able to penetrate the blood–brain barrier.

C. Drug C: It has the lowest molecular weight and will be able to diffuse across the blood–brain barrier.

D. Drug D: It has the highest lipophilicity and will be able to diffuse across the blood–brain barrier.

E. Drug E: It has the highest molecular weight and will become concentrated in the CNS.

4. Allopurinol is frequently given to patients to ameliorate the hyperuricemia that results from the destruction of cancer cells by chemotherapeutic agents, the "tumor lysis syndrome." When allopurinol is used in conjunction with one of these drugs, excessive toxicity is seen. With which of the new agents would this drug–drug interaction be most likely to occur, and why?

A. Drug A: Allopurinol enhances the movement of this alkylating agent into the bone marrow.

B. Drug B: Allopurinol causes the precipitation of damaged microtubules in the renal tubules.

C. Drug C: Allopurinol inhibits the metabolism of this purine analogue.

D. Drug D: Allopurinol prevents the diffusion of this drug into the CNS.

E. Drug E: Allopurinol exacerbates bladder irritation and may cause hemorrhage.

5. Folic acid is an essential cofactor in the synthesis of purine ribonucleotides and deoxythymidylate. It is therefore a site of action of some chemotherapeutic agents. Which of the following statements regarding folic acid is correct?

A. Tetrahydrofolate catalyzes 1-carbon transfers in the synthesis of inosinate (IMP) in purine synthesis.

B. Tetrahydrofolate catalyzes 1-carbon transfers in the synthesis of uridylate (UMP) in pyrimidine synthesis.

C. Agents that inhibit the activity of dihydrofolate reductase prevent the formation of dihydrofolate.

D. 5-Fluorouracil inhibits thymidylate synthesis by forming a covalent bond with, and inactivating dihydrofolate.

E. Leucovorin (folinic acid) administration repletes tetrahydrofolate and diminishes the effectiveness of 5-fluorouracil.

38

Pharmacology of Cancer: Signal Transduction

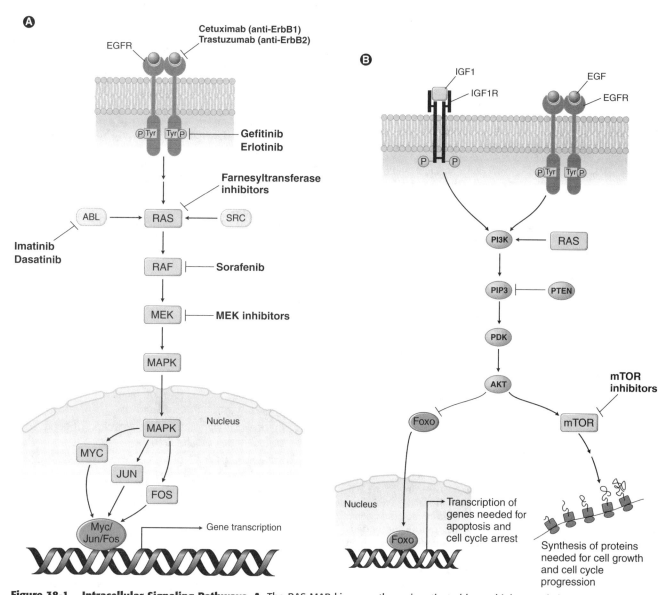

Figure 38-1. Intracellular Signaling Pathways. A. The RAS-MAP kinase pathway is activated by multiple growth factor receptors (here exemplified by the EGF receptor, EGFR) as well as several intracellular tyrosine kinases such as SRC and ABL. RAS is recruited to the plasma membrane by farnesylation and activated by binding to GTP. Activated RAS stimulates a sequence of phosphorylation events mediated by

(continues)

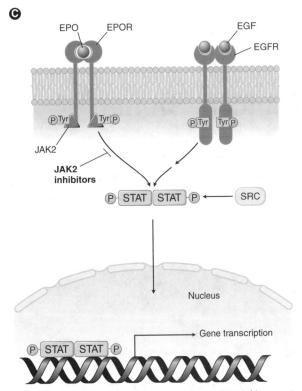

Figure 38-1. *(continued)* RAF, MEK, and ERK (MAP) kinases. Activated MAP kinase (MAPK) translocates to the nucleus and activates proteins such as MYC, JUN, and FOS that promote the transcription of genes involved in cell-cycle progression. Cetuximab and trastuzumab act as antagonists at the EGF receptor (ErbB1) and HER-2 receptor (ErbB2), respectively. Gefitinib and erlotinib inhibit the receptor tyrosine kinase. Farnesyltransferase inhibitors prevent RAS activation. Imatinib and dasatinib inhibit ABL kinase; sorafenib inhibits RAF kinase; and several agents under development inhibit MEK kinase. **B.** The PI3 kinase (PI3K) pathway is activated by RAS and by a number of growth factor receptors (here exemplified by the insulin-like growth factor receptor 1 [IGF1R] and the epidermal growth factor receptor [EGFR]). Activated PI3K generates phosphatidylinositol-3,4,5-triphosphate (PIP3), which activates phosphoinositide dependent kinase-1 (PDK). In turn, PDK phosphorylates AKT. PTEN is an endogenous inhibitor of AKT activation. Phosphorylated AKT transduces multiple downstream signals, including activation of the mammalian target of rapamycin (mTOR) and inhibition of the FOXO family of transcription factors. mTOR activation promotes the synthesis of proteins required for cell growth and cell-cycle progression. Because the FOXO family of transcription factors activates the expression of genes involved in cell-cycle arrest, stress resistance, and apoptosis, inhibition of FOXO promotes cell proliferation and resistance to apoptosis. Rapamycin (sirolimus) and its derivatives are mTOR inhibitors that inhibit cell-cycle progression and promote apoptosis. **C.** The STAT pathway is activated by SRC and by a number of growth factor receptors (here exemplified by the erythropoietin receptor [EPOR], which signals to STAT proteins through JAK2 kinase, and by the EGF receptor [EGFR], which signals to STAT proteins indirectly). Phosphorylation of STAT induces SH2 domain-mediated homodimerization, and phosphorylated STAT homodimers translocate to the nucleus and activate transcription. JAK2 inhibitors are under development for the treatment of polycythemia vera and other myeloproliferative disorders, many of which share a common activating mutation in JAK2 (V617F).

OBJECTIVES

■ Understand the biochemical pathways that regulate normal cell growth.

■ Understand how pharmacologic agents that target regulatory pathways in cell growth can be used as cancer therapies.

■ CASE 1

M.W. is a 65-year-old woman with metastatic non–small cell lung cancer. She has never smoked, and her primary tumor is an adenocarcinoma with bronchioalveolar features. She is initially treated with cisplatin and paclitaxel, but her tumor progresses. After discussion with her oncologist, M.W. is treated with the oral epidermal growth factor receptor (EGFR) inhibitor erlotinib. She develops a skin rash and diarrhea but otherwise tolerates this medication well. Restaging computed tomography scans are performed 2 months after starting treatment with erlotinib. The scans reveal a dramatic reduction in her tumor burden, and after 6 months, there is no residual evidence of cancer. Sequencing of the EGFR gene from her primary tumor reveals a mutation in the kinase domain at codon 858, resulting in substitution of arginine for leucine (L858R). Unfortunately, M.W. subsequently develops resistance to erlotinib with recurrence of her disease. A repeat biopsy reveals a new mutation in the EGFR kinase domain in codon 790 (T790M). She decides to participate in a clinical trial of HKI-272, an irreversible EGFR inhibitor that has shown activity *in vitro* against lung cancer cells with this mutation.

QUESTIONS

1. How does signaling through the epidermal growth factor receptor promote cell growth and survival?

   A. Intracellular signals promote the translocation of growth factors to the cell surface.

   B. Intracellular signals promote activation of genes involved in protein degradation.

   C. Intracellular signals promote activation of genes involved in cell proliferation.

   D. Intracellular signals promote expression of genes involved in cell cycle arrest.

   E. Intracellular signals promote adherence to new blood vessels.

2. Inhibition of EGFR-initiated signals can inhibit cancer cell growth. By what molecular mechanism does erlotinib inhibit the activity of the epidermal growth factor receptor?

   A. Erlotinib modifies the EGFR tyrosine kinase domain so that it is unable to bind effector molecules.

B. Erlotinib promotes the intracellular endocytosis of the EGFR.

C. Erlotinib covalently binds to and destroys the binding site at the EGFR tyrosine kinase domain.

D. Erlotinib competes for binding of ATP at the EGFR tyrosine kinase domain.

E. Erlotinib promotes autoantibody destruction of cells expressing EGFR on their plasma membranes.

3. How might subsets of patients be selected for effective targeted therapy?

A. All tumors with bronchioalveolar histology are sensitive to targeted therapy.

B. All tumors in female, nonsmoking, Asian women are sensitive to targeted therapy.

C. Tumors can be screened for the presence of mutations that make EGFR resistant to degradation by EGFR antagonists.

D. Tumors can be screened for the presence of mutations that promote the presence of EGFR.

E. Tumors can be screened for the presence of mutations that activate EGFR and make them more sensitive to EGFR antagonists.

4. Although M.W. initially responded well to therapy with erlotinib, she eventually developed resistance to its effects and recurrence of her lung cancer. What mechanisms are responsible for resistance to targeted therapy with EGFR antagonists?

A. Secondary mutations in phospholipase expression make some cancer cells resistant to the effects of EGFR antagonists.

B. Secondary mutations in the kinase domain of EGFR make some cancer cells resistant to the effects of EGFR antagonists.

C. Secondary mutations in genes coding for other ErbB receptors allow growth signals to bypass the EGFR and make some cancer cells resistant to the effects of EGFR antagonists.

D. Deletions in the gene encoding EGFR make it unable to bind EGFR antagonists.

E. Point mutations in the binding site of EGFR make it resistant to degradation by EGFR antagonists.

5. Bortezomib is a proteasome inhibitor that has been shown to induce growth inhibition and apoptosis of tumor cells. Which of the following statements regarding the function of the ubiquitin–proteasome pathway is correct?

A. The ubiquitin–proteasome pathway is an intracellular signaling pathway that regulates gene transcription for cell mitosis.

B. The specificity of the polyubiquitin chain for targeted proteins is determined by the E3 ubiquitin ligase component.

C. Proteins that are targeted by the ubiquitin pathway amplify signals for cell growth and immortalization.

D. Proteasome activation by bortezomib leads to gene transcription for protein synthesis.

E. Bortezomib targets the E3 ubiquitin ligase and promotes its attachment to tumor cells.

 CASE 2

In November, 1971, the *New England Journal of Medicine* published a five-page article called ''Tumor Angiogenesis: Therapeutic Implications.'' The author, Judah Folkman, MD, a pediatric surgeon at Children's Hospital in Boston, suggested that tumor growth was dependent on a supply of new blood vessels delivering oxygen and nutrients to growing tumor cells. Moreover, tumors had the ability to elaborate factors, which could initiate or suppress the process of angiogenesis.

QUESTIONS

1. How does angiogenesis occur?

A. Binding of vascular endothelial growth factor (VEGF) to its endothelial receptor triggers the division, replication and metostasis of endothelial cells.

B. Binding of VEGF to its endothelial receptor triggers the proliferation of endothelial cells.

C. Binding of VEGF to its endothelial receptor triggers the formation of inter-endothelial tight junctions that promote new endothelial cell adherence.

D. Binding of VEGF to metalloproteinases promotes the destruction of abnormal endothelial cells to allow new endothelial cell growth.

E. Binding of VEGF to its endothelial receptor causes tyrosine residues to become phosphorylated, allowing inter-endothelial junctions to open, facilitating intercellular communication.

2. VEGF proteins and receptors are key regulators of angiogenesis. How do growing tumors interact with VEGF to promote angiogenesis?

A. Tumors that experience hypoxia produce excessive amounts of von Hippel Lindau protein, which subsequently activates VEGF.

B. Tumors with certain activated oncogenes are able to produce VEGF.

C. Tumors that have genes encoding hypoxia inducible factor (HIFα) produce an abnormal variant of VEGF.

D. Tumors that are targeted by EGFR antagonists become resistant by stimulating VEGF release.

E. Tumors that elaborate inflammatory cytokines produce VEGF.

Dr. Folkman's hypothesis regarding tumor growth and metastasis opened up new areas of research in the field of oncology, and prompted decades of research on the molecular mechanisms of angiogenesis. In 1994, the first natural angiogenesis inhibitor was isolated by Michael O'Reilly, MD, a research fellow in Dr. Folkman's laboratory. This substance, called angiostatin, inhibited tumor growth in mice. Subsequently, endostatin, a second angiogenesis inhibitor, was isolated by Dr. O'Reilly in 1997. Today angiogenesis inhibitors have been approved for use in the United States and in 28 other countries.

3. By what mechanism might an angiogenesis inhibitor control the growth of tumors?

- **A.** Inhibition of VEGF activity allows the disorganized growth of abnormal vessels, with subsequent tumor hemorrhage and involution.
- **B.** Inhibition of VEGF activity promotes increased permeability of new vessels, subsequently damaging high interstitial fluid pressures within tumors.
- **C.** Inhibition of VEGF activity "starves" tumors of oxygen and nutrients.
- **D.** Inhibition of VEGFR activation promotes normal regulatory intercellular communication, and limits abnormal tumor growth.
- **E.** Inhibition of VEGFR limits tumor cell growth by preventing its division in M phase.

4. Thalidomide use in pregnant women in the 1950s led to teratogenic effects, including stunted limb development, or phocomelia. How could the molecular effects of thalidomide relate to its current investigational use as a cancer therapy?

- **A.** Thalidomide promotes the production of basic fibroblast growth factor, which is necessary for activation of tumor growth signals and normal limb development.
- **B.** Thalidomide inhibits the activation of the glutamate receptor, stimulating negative feedback of tumor growth and necessary neuronal development in limbs.
- **C.** Thalidomide promotes the synthesis of TNF-α necessary for tumor migration and normal bone and cartilage elongation.
- **D.** Thalidomide inhibits angiogenesis necessary for tumor growth and normal limb development.
- **E.** Thalidomide inhibits the migration of fibroblasts necessary for limb development and tumor metastasis.

5. Monoclonal antibodies that target lymphocytic leukemic cells have which of the following potential adverse effects?

- **A.** alopecia
- **B.** cardiomyopathy
- **C.** neovascularization of bone marrow
- **D.** sludging of cells and thrombosis
- **E.** immunosuppression

39

Principles of Combination Chemotherapy

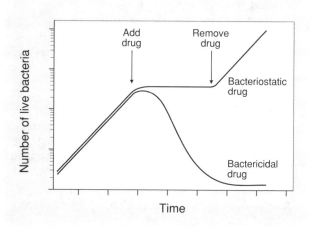

Figure 39-1. Comparison of the Effects of Bacteriostatic and Bactericidal Drugs on Bacterial Growth Kinetics. In the absence of drug, bacteria grow with exponential (first-order) kinetics. A bactericidal drug kills the target organism, as demonstrated by the time-dependent decrease in the number of live bacteria. A bacteriostatic drug prevents microbial growth without killing the bacteria. Removal of a bacteriostatic drug is followed by an exponential increase in bacterial number as the previously inhibited bacteria resume growth. Bacteriostatic drugs eradicate infections by limiting the growth of the infecting organism for a long enough period of time to allow the host immune system to kill the bacteria.

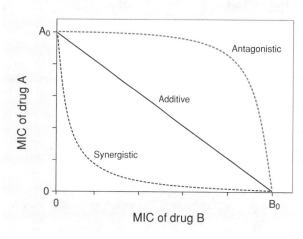

Figure 39-2. Quantification of Additive, Synergistic, and Antagonistic Drug Interactions. Drug combinations can exhibit additive, synergistic, or antagonistic effects. The nature of this interaction can be depicted graphically by observing the effect that each drug has on the other's minimum inhibitory concentration (MIC). If two drugs have an additive interaction, then the addition of increasing amounts of Drug B to Drug A results in a linear decrease in the MIC of Drug A; in this case, each of the two drugs can be thought of as interchangeable. If two drugs have a synergistic interaction, then the addition of Drug B to Drug A results in a significantly lower MIC for Drug A (i.e., there is an increase in the potency of Drug A). If two drugs have an antagonistic interaction, then the addition of Drug B to Drug A does not significantly lower the MIC of Drug A; in some cases *(not shown),* much higher doses of each drug must be administered to achieve the same effect as that of each drug used alone. A_0 and B_0 are the MICs of Drugs A and B, respectively, when used as single agents.

OBJECTIVES

■ Understand the principles of combination chemotherapy as they apply to antimicrobial and antineoplastic agents.

CASE 1

Mr. M. is a 27-year-old man from rural Haiti who presents to a clinic with a chronic cough. He could not afford treatment at a private clinic, so he went to a drug store and asked the pharmacist for some appropriate medicines. The pharmacist thought that Mr. M. may have tuberculosis and sold Mr. M. a 2-week supply of isoniazid and rifampin. Mr. M. took both drugs for a couple of days, but they made him nauseated, so he decided to take just the isoniazid for 2 weeks. His symptoms resolved.

Three months later, Mr. M.'s cough returned. This time, he noticed blood in his sputum, and he had night sweats. He took the remainder of the 2-week supply of rifampin and experienced a brief lull in his symptoms. Within a few days, however, his cough, bloody sputum, and night sweats returned.

QUESTIONS

1. Why were Mr. M.'s initial efforts at treatment unsuccessful?

   A. It was necessary to take both isoniazid and rifampin concurrently for 2 weeks in order to eradicate tuberculosis.

   B. Mr. M. probably had multi-drug resistant tuberculosis when he presented to his pharmacist.

   C. Mr. M. probably already had 10^8 to 10^9 resistant bacteria in his tuberculous cavities at the time he started therapy.

   D. Mr. M.'s use of single therapy probably killed susceptible mycobacteria, but selected for isoniazid- and rifampin-resistant mycobacteria.

   E. Mycobacteria in Haiti are resistant to isoniazid.

Because he did not have enough money to buy additional drugs, Mr. M. traveled to the nearest government hospital to seek free care and medications. The government doctor took three sputum samples, all of which were positive for acid-fast bacilli. The doctor also sent sputum to the laboratory for culture, but because the causative agent of tuberculosis, *Mycobacterium tuberculosis*, is slow-growing, he also started Mr. M. on a drug regimen consisting of isoniazid, rifampin, pyrazinamide, and ethambutol for 2 months, followed by isoniazid and rifampin for 4 months.

2. What is the primary reason that the government doctor prescribed four different drugs for Mr. M.?

   A. Multi-drug therapy is cheaper than single-dose therapy.

   B. Multi-drug therapy is necessary to kill isoniazid-resistant mycobacteria.

   C. Multi-drug therapy will kill resistant strains of mycobacteria.

   D. Multi-drug therapy is necessary to treat tuberculosis in areas of rural Haiti.

   E. Multi-drug therapy is necessary to treat intracellular forms of mycobacteria.

After several weeks, however, the culture revealed that Mr. M.'s tuberculosis is not susceptible to either isoniazid or rifampin. He is now seeking a new recommendation for treatment.

3. How is resistance transferred from one generation of tubercle bacilli to the next?

   A. Resistance develops through plasmid-acquired mutations that are amplified throughout the mycobacterial population of a tubercle.

   B. Resistance develops through chromosomal mutations that are passed on to daughter cells.

   C. Resistance develops through point mutations in T lymphocytes, making them unable to take up the drug.

   D. Resistance develops through mycobacterial-associated hypersensitivity reactions and antibody-mediated drug degradation.

   E. Resistance develops through point mutations in T lymphocytes, making them more efficient at pumping out the drug.

4. Mr. M.'s sputum culture results returned several weeks after his visit to the government doctor, revealing that his tuberculosis was not susceptible to either isoniazid or rifampin. Given these results, what drugs should comprise his therapy?

   A. streptomycin, levofloxacin, rifabutin, ethionamide, and clofazimine

   B. isoniazid, rifampin, pyrazinamide, and ethambutol

   C. isoniazid, rifabutin, pyrazinamide, and ethionamide

   D. isoniazid, rifampin, streptomycin, and ethambutol

   E. streptomycin, rifampin, ethambutol, and ethionamide

5. Antimicrobial agents are characterized by their minimum inhibitory concentration (MIC) and their minimum bactericidal concentration (MBC). Which of the following statements regarding the relationship of MIC and MBC to an agent's antimicrobial action is correct?

   A. Drugs with synergistic actions when used in combination have a MIC_A/MIC_B ratio of 1.0.

   B. Drugs with a low MBC tend to have significant human toxicity.

   C. Cidal drugs tend to have a MIC that is much lower than their MBC.

   D. Static drugs tend to have a MIC that is much greater than their MBC.

   E. The MIC for a drug may differ when it is applied to a Gram-positive coccus compared to a Gram-negative bacillus.

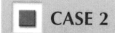
CASE 2

You receive a call from your great aunt Amelia late one night, with the news that her 37-year-old stepson has been diagnosed with ''Hodgkin's lymphoma, stage three.'' She tells you that he has been admitted to a local hospital for treatment with doxorubicin cancer chemotherapy. She knows that you are studying medical pharmacology and wants to know your opinion of this treatment.

QUESTIONS

1. You do some research for your great aunt on the therapy of stage III Hodgkin's lymphoma. Which of the following facts do you find regarding chemotherapy for this disease?
   A. Doxorubicin is given as a single agent to prevent cardiac toxicity before intensification of chemotherapy.
   B. Doxorubicin is curative in stage III Hodgkin's lymphoma when combined with radiation therapy.
   C. Doxorubicin is a component of combination chemotherapy in stage III Hodgkin's lymphoma.
   D. Doxorubicin is a component of a combination of antineoplastic agents, all intended to arrest malignant cell growth in S phase.
   E. The toxicity associated with the doxorubicin/bleomycin/vinblastine/dacarbazine (ABVD) combination has been reduced since the introduction of MOPP (Mechlorethamine, vincristine, procarbazine, prednisone).

Great Aunt Amelia calls you the next day. She also has done some online research on the treatment of this disease and confirms your information. However, she does not understand why her stepson must undergo chemotherapy in 4-week cycles over the course of the next 3 months. She asks,: ''Why can't he get all of the medication in the beginning and kill the cancer right from the start?''

2. What can't Great Aunt Amelia's stepson receive his chemotherapy all at once?
   A. Slowly growing tumors require intermittent dosing of chemotherapy.
   B. Intermittent dosing of chemotherapy may decrease the growth fraction of tumors over sequential cycles.
   C. Intermittent dosing of chemotherapy allows normal cells and tissues time to recover from chemotherapy-induced toxicity.
   D. Anti-neoplastic agents exert their cytotoxic effects in a time-dependent manner.
   E. High-dose chemotherapy administered continuously promotes rapid growth and resistance in tumor cells.

3. What is the relationship between the percentage of actively dividing cells in a tumor (the growth fraction) and the effectiveness of anti-neoplastic chemotherapy?
   A. The actively dividing fraction of cells is resistant to chemotherapy.
   B. The actively dividing fraction of cells is affected by chemotherapeutic agents that target the G_0 phase.
   C. The growth fraction of the tumor may decrease with subsequent cycles of chemotherapy.
   D. The actively dividing fraction of cells includes the cells that are most susceptible to the toxic effects of ABVD therapy.
   E. Large tumors have a high growth fraction, and are highly sensitive to the effects of combination chemotherapy.

4. Anti-neoplastic therapy usually follows first-order kinetics in cell killing. What does this mean?
   A. A constant number of tumor cells is killed with each cycle of chemotherapy.
   B. An increasing number of tumor cells is killed with each cycle of chemotherapy.
   C. A time-dependent fraction of tumor cells is killed, proportional to the time over which chemotherapy is being administered.
   D. A constant fraction of tumor cells is killed with each cycle of chemotherapy.
   E. A logarithmic proportion of tumor cells is killed with each cycle of chemotherapy.

5. When two drugs (A and B) are used in combination and the effect of their actions, yields a linear relationship on an MIC_A versus MIC_B plot, the drugs are said to be:
   A. additive
   B. synergistic
   C. antagonistic
   D. concentration dependent
   E. time dependent

ANSWERS TO SECTION V

CHAPTER 31 ANSWERS

CASE 1

1. **The answer is D. Its metabolite inhibits the synthesis of folate by bacteria.** Prontosil is a sulfonamide pro-drug, although it is not currently used as an antibiotic. The molecular structure of the sulfonamides is similar to that of PABA, one of the precursors used in bacterial folate synthesis. This structural similarity allows sulfonamides to competitively bind and inhibit the activity of dihydropteroate synthase. This prevents bacterial folate synthesis, and thereby inhibits bacterial synthesis of purines, pyrimidines, and amino acids. Folate is not a component of the bacterial cell wall.

2. **The answer is C. Mammalian cells do not express dihydropteroate synthase**, the bacterial enzyme used for folate synthesis. By targeting dihydropteroate synthase, bacteria are selectively affected by the inhibitory effects of sulfonamides. In contrast, mammalian cells, which do not synthesize folate, are not affected by dihydropteroate synthase inhibition.

3. **The answer is E. The incidence of sulfonamide resistance in bacteria has increased substantially**, limiting the effectiveness of these antibacterial agents as single therapy. Because of their high selectivity, sulfonamides have a very low incidence of toxicity. In addition, newer antibacterial agents with better therapeutic indices have been developed. Kernicterus is a condition characterized by elevated concentrations of unconjugated bilirubin in neonates; sulfonamides can exacerbate kernicterus due to the competition between sulfonamides and bilirubin for albumin-binding sites.

4. **The answer is B. This combination allows for the synergistic inhibition of bacterial folate synthesis.** Sulfonamides limit the synthesis of folate thereby increasing the effectiveness of dihydrofolate reductase inhibitors, such as trimethoprim. Trimethoprim, a folate analogue, is better able to compete with the reduced concentration of dihydrofolate for dihydrofolate re-

ductase. This combination blocks sequential steps in the synthesis of tetrahydrofolate, also termed *sequential blockade*. In addition, this combination of drugs can be effective in treating bacteria that have become resistant to dihydrofolate reductase inhibitors used as single agents.

5. **The answer is D. Bacteria overproduce PABA and continue folate synthesis despite the presence of sulfonamides.** This allows bacteria to overwhelm the capacity of sulfonamides to inhibit dihydropteroate synthase. Alternatively, bacteria may develop a mutation in the PABA-binding site of dihydropteroate synthase, reducing its binding affinity for sulfonamides. Finally, some bacteria develop a decreased permeability of the bacterial membrane to sulfonamides through the acquisition of a resistance plasmid.

CASE 2

1. **The answer is E. Methotrexate is a folate analogue that inhibits the action of dihydrofolate reductase.** Inhibition of this enzyme prevents the formation of tetrahydrofolate from dihydrofolate. The shortage of tetrahydrofolate prevents de novo purine and thymidylate synthesis, and subsequent DNA and RNA synthesis. Cell division is arrested in the S phase of the cell cycle.

2. **The answer is E. Methotrexate will cause the death of the embryo.** Because embryonic cells are rapidly growing and dividing, folate is essential for their proper growth and differentiation. Methotrexate is therefore extremely toxic to a developing pregnancy. It is now used to treat certain early ectopic pregnancies. As cancer chemotherapy, methotrexate is used to treat patients with carcinomas of the breast, lung, and head and neck, acute lymphoblastic leukemia, and choriocarcinoma.

3. **The answer is B. Diarrhea** is a common potential adverse effect of methotrexate therapy. Because methotrexate acts on rapidly dividing cells, it can damage the gastrointestinal mucosa as well as the bone marrow.

4. **The answer is A. Leucovorin provides folinic acid for DNA synthesis in normal cells.** It is used as a "rescue" therapy with high-dose methotrexate chemotherapy. Leucovorin (N-5 formyltetrahydrofolate) repletes folinic acid, which is concentrated in normal cells. This may protect normal cells from the toxic effects of methotrexate. It may also allow normal cells to resume cell growth and division after methotrexate therapy.

5. **The answer is C. Selectivity is achieved when an antimicrobial agent targets an enzyme that is unique to a bacterium.** In other words, the more unique the target of an agent, the less likely it is to cause adverse effects in humans, the greater its margin of safety, and the larger its therapeutic index. Penicillin and the sulfonamides are examples of highly selective antimicrobial agents. In contrast, methotrexate is a non-selective chemotherapeutic agent that affects the use of folate by both normal and malignant cells. It has a high incidence of adverse effects and a small therapeutic index.

CHAPTER 32 ANSWERS

CASE 1

1. **The answer is D. Tetracyclines target the 30S ribosomal subunit and prevent elongation of the peptide chain.** Specifically, tetracyclines bind to the 16S rRNA of the 30S subunit and block the binding of aminoacyl tRNA, and the addition of further amino acids to the growing peptide chain. Aminoglycosides target the 30S ribosomal subunit and cause a misreading of mRNA, and the formation of proteins containing incorrect amino acids. Topoisomerases and RNA polymerase are involved in the replication and transcription of DNA.

2. **The answer is B. Macrolides target the 50S ribosomal subunit and block the translocation of the growing peptide chain.** Specifically, macrolides target the 23S rRNA of the 50S subunit and block the exit tunnel of the ribosome from which the nascent peptide should emerge. Chloramphenicol targets the 23S rRNA of the 50S ribosomal subunit and inhibits peptide bond formation between an incoming aminoacyl tRNA and the growing peptide chain. Quinolones inhibit the action of type II topoisomerases in nicking, uncoiling, and religating DNA. They also convert these enzymes into DNA-damaging agents.

3. **The answer is C. Bacteria can develop methods of enhancing drug efflux from the bacterial cell.** For example, alteration or elimination of porins, or the acquisition of plasmid-encoded efflux pumps, can decrease the permeability of the bacterial cell membrane to these drugs. Mutational modification of drug binding sites, such as the RNA polymerase, and the ribosomal subunits, can also limit drug binding and effectiveness. Fi-

nally, some bacteria develop or acquire enzymatic means of inactivating these drugs by adenylation, acetylation, phosphorylation, or hydrolysis.

4. **The answer is C. Macrolides inhibit protein synthesis, but this is insufficient to kill a bacterium.** Bacteria are able to become dormant during a period of growth inhibition. Thus, they may be able to survive complete inhibition of protein synthesis. In contrast to other protein synthesis inhibitors, aminoglycosides, which adversely affect proper mRNA decoding, can be bactericidal at high doses. This may be a result of dose-dependent damage to the cell membrane caused by aminoglycosides and the abnormal proteins that result from their effects on mRNA. Quinolones are bactericidal because of their promotion of topoisomerase-induced DNA damage.

5. **The answer is E. Macrolides have intracellular activity against *Legionella* spp.** They also have excellent lung tissue penetration and are therefore used to treat many pulmonary infections, including Legionnaires' disease.

CASE 2

1. **The answer is B. Amikacin**, an aminoglycoside, might be a preferred choice based on the preliminary culture results of a Gram-negative bacterium, and the patient's prior resistant infections. Based on prior infections resistant to fluoroquinolones and tetracyclines, the current bacteria may also be resistant to ofloxacin and minocycline, respectively. Erythromycin and vancomycin are more effective in treating Gram-positive infections, and less effective than aminoglycosides in treating Gram-negative infections.

2. **The answer is E. Ototoxicity** is the single most important toxicity limiting the use of aminoglycosides. It is caused by aminoglycoside accumulation within the perilymph and endolymph of the inner ear, causing damage to hair cells at high concentrations. Other toxicities associated with aminoglycosides include acute renal failure, and a nondepolarizing neuromuscular blockade at very high doses. Hypothermia, lethargy, flaccidity, vomiting, respiratory distress, and gray discoloration are hallmarks of gray baby syndrome, which is caused by chloramphenicol use in newborns. Pseudomembranous colitis from *Clostridium difficile* toxin is most commonly associated with clindamycin use. Cholestatic hepatitis has been associated with erythromycin use. Discolored teeth can occur in children who are administered tetracyclines.

3. **The answer is C. Penicillins inhibit cell wall synthesis and facilitate the entry of aminoglycosides into the bacterial cell.** A high concentration of aminoglycosides entering the cell completely inhibits protein synthesis and is bactericidal. In addition, penicillin inhibits the growth and repair of the cell wall of actively growing bacteria. Because erythromycin inhibits bacterial protein synthesis, it inhibits bacterial growth. This negates the antimicrobial effect of penicillins.

4. **The answer is A. Bacterial topoisomerases are structurally different from eukaryotic topoisomerases, contributing to the lack of adverse effects from fluoroquinolones.** The quinolone antibiotics inhibit DNA gyrase and topoisomerase IV, both prokaryotic type II topoisomerases. Although bacterial RNA polymerases are similar to mammalian RNA polymerases, mammalian RNA polymerases are inhibited by only very high concentrations of rifampin, so the incidence of adverse effects is low. Chloramphenicol inhibits both bacterial and mitochondrial protein synthesis and has a high rate of adverse effects. Tetracyclines inhibit both bacterial protein synthesis and mammalian protein synthesis in vitro. However, they are actively concentrated in bacterial cells by an energy-dependent process and have limited effects on mammalian cells. Therefore, they have a rather low rate of adverse effects.

5. **The answer is D. Levofloxacin**, a fluoroquinolone, is bactericidal.

CHAPTER 33 ANSWERS

CASE 1

1. **The answer is C. The β-lactam ring binds transpeptidase and prevents polymer crosslinking.** This ring portion of the penicillin molecule is an analogue of the terminal D-Ala-D-Ala dipeptide of the Park peptide. When the β-lactam binds transpeptidase, it creates a "dead-end" complex that prevents further crosslinking to the adjacent peptide. In this way, penicillin, as do all β-lactams, prevents cell wall synthesis in actively dividing bacteria. This allows the normal action of bacterial autolysins to cause autolysis and cell death. Bactoprenol transports the murein monomer across the cell membrane. Transglycosylases add murein units to the growing peptidoglycan polymer chain before crosslinking occurs.

2. **The answer is B. An acquired plasmid for a β-lactamase protein gives bacteria the ability to destroy the β-lactam ring.** This is the most common means through which bacteria develop β-lactam resistance. Extended-spectrum β-lactamases confer resistance to most β-lactam antibiotics. A less common means of developing resistance to β-lactams is through a chromosomal mutation of bacterial transpeptidase, which prevents its binding to the β-lactam ring. Pores and lipopolysaccharides are components of the outer membrane of Gram-negative bacteria.

3. **The answer is D.** The most common potential adverse effect of β-lactam therapy is a hypersensitivity reaction, which commonly manifests as an **urticarial drug rash and fever**. Anaphylaxis and drug-induced autoimmune hemolytic anemia are potentially life-threatening hyper-

sensitivity reactions to the β-lactams. Less common adverse effects of these agents include the development of *C. difficile* colitis associated with antistaphylococcal β-lactams, and a disulfiram-like reaction when ethanol is concurrently ingested with cefotetan or cefoperazone, both fourth-generation cephalosporins. Seizures can occur at high doses of intravenous penicillin, imipenem, and meropenem.

4. **The answer is A. A high rate of mycobacterial resistance to antimycobacterial agents necessitates multidrug therapy.** Based on the local prevalence of isoniazid resistance, patients are treated with three to four drugs simultaneously. Resistance to antimycobacterial agents occurs through chromosomal mutations, the frequency of which to any single agent is about one in 10^6 bacteria. Multidrug therapy with antimycobacterial agents limits the toxicity associated with the administration of any one drug.

5. **The answer is D. Fosfomycin and fosmidomycin : mutation in cell transporters prevents intracellular drug entry.** Both of these agents inhibit intracellular murein monomer synthesis. Their action depends on their transport into the cytoplasm. Therefore, mutations in the glycerophosphate or glucose-6-phosphate transporters prevent entry of these drugs into the cell. Ampicillin resistance occurs through plasmid-acquired β-lactamase. Overexpression of alanine racemase allows murein monomer formation to proceed despite the presence of the alanine racemase inhibitor cycloserine. Vancomycin resistance occurs through mutations for enzymes that encode D-Ala-D-lactate, which is not bound by vancomycin. Aminoglycosides are bactericidal drugs that inhibit protein synthesis at the 30S ribosomal subunit.

CASE 2

1. **The answer is E. Older age**, underlying liver disease, and concomitant use of drugs that induce the hepatic P450 enzyme system, all predispose patients on isoniazid to a risk of hepatitis. In addition, ethanol use and genetic factors in liver enzyme acetylation also influence the risk of isoniazid-associated hepatitis. Isoniazid is hepatically metabolized. Hepatitis associated with this drug is caused by reactive intermediates formed during isoniazid metabolism. These intermediates bind to hepatocytes and cause cell death. Asymptomatic hyperuricemia is associated with pyrazinamide use.

2. **The answer is A. Isoniazid inhibits FAS2 linkage of saturated hydrocarbon chains in the synthesis of mycolic acid.** Pyrazinamide also inhibits mycolic acid synthesis by inhibiting the FAS1 synthesis of saturated hydrocarbon chain precursors of mycolic acid. Mycolic acid is normally added to the arabinogalactan chain and forms the inner half of the mycobacterial outer membrane. Ethambutol decreases the synthesis of arabinogalactans. The mycobacterial outer membrane does not contain pores.

3. **The answer is C. Pyridoxine supplementation replaces isoniazid-induced depletion of pyridoxine.** Isoniazid and its metabolites competitively inhibit the activation of pyridoxine to its active form, pyridoxal-5-phosphate, and enhance the elimination of pyridoxal-5-phosphate. Depletion of pyridoxine can cause peripheral neuropathy. Pyridoxine is also a cofactor in the synthesis of gamma-aminobutyric acid (GABA), the major inhibitory neurotransmitter in the brain. Without pyridoxine, GABA concentrations become depleted and seizures can occur. Optic neuritis and blindness are toxicities of ethambutol, not isoniazid.

4. **The answer is C. Isoniazid inhibits the metabolism of phenytoin by the hepatic P450 enzyme system.** Isoniazid affects the metabolism of a number of drugs, including rifampin, carbamazepine, and azole antifungal agents.

5. **The answer is B. The murein coat** retains the purple color of gentian violet applied during the process of Gram's staining. Gram-positive bacteria have a thick murein coat and no lipid bilayer outer membrane, thus facilitating the passage of hydrophilic molecules.

CHAPTER 34 ANSWERS

CASE 1

1. **The answer is C. HIV infection** and resulting immune compromise were the likely factors contributing to Mr. F.'s infection with *Coccidioides* spp, which is prevalent in the soil of southern California. Other patient populations with immune compromise who are susceptible to mycotic infections include organ transplant recipients and patients being treated with cancer chemotherapy or other immunosuppressive agents. Fungal infections also occur in susceptible intensive care unit patients and patients with prostheses.

2. **The answer is E.** Amphotericin B **binds ergosterol and creates pores in the fungal cell wall** that alter fungal membrane permeability and allow the leakage of essential cellular components. This disruption of fungal membrane stability ultimately leads to cell death. Amphotericin B is also oxidized, generating toxic free radicals that also contribute to instability of the fungal cell membrane.

3. **The answer is A. Fever and hypotension** can occur within several hours of amphotericin B administration. These clinical signs are a result of the "cytokine storm" caused by amphotericin B when it elicits the release of tumor necrosis factor-α (TNF-α) and interleukin-1 (IL-1). Dose-dependent bone marrow suppression can result from flucytosine.

4. **The answer is D. Amphotericin B is highly insoluble and must be administered intrathecally to treat central nervous system fungal infections** as it does not cross the blood–brain barrier. It is poorly absorbed from the gastrointestinal tract and must be administered intravenously in a colloidal suspension. After it is administered, more than 90% of the drug binds to tissue sites.

5. **The answer is C.** Fluconazole, a triazole, **inhibits the formation of ergosterol from lanosterol** by 14α-sterol demethylase, a microsomal cytochrome P450 enzyme. The lack of ergosterol ultimately disrupts the fungal cell membrane. Flucytosine inhibits fungal DNA synthesis. Terbinafine, naftifine, and butenafine inhibit the formation of lanosterol from squalene.

CASE 2

1. **The answer is B. Griseofulvin disrupts microtubules and cell mitosis.** It binds to tubulin and disrupts the formation of the mitotic spindle and arrests cell division in M phase. It also inhibits fungal RNA and DNA synthesis. Flucytosine is metabolized to 5-fluorouracil, an antimetabolite that inhibits DNA synthesis. Terbinafine, naftifine, and butenafine inhibit squalene epoxidase formation of lanosterol. The azoles inhibit 14α-sterol demethylase formation of ergosterol.

2. **The answer is C. Liver function tests** should be monitored for evidence of hepatotoxicity, which has a low incidence of occurrence. Hematologic parameters may show leucopenia, neutropenia, and monocytosis during the first month of griseofulvin therapy. Albuminuria can occur in the absence of renal insufficiency.

3. **The answer is D. Drug resistance can develop as a result of mutations in the fungal P450 enzymes**, as well as the expression of membrane efflux transporter proteins, which limit cellular drug accumulation. *Candida* spp are the most notable to develop resistance to these agents. The azoles inhibit the action of 14α-sterol demethylase. Ketoconazole is a prototypic drug of the imidazole class. Ms. H. could apply clotrimazole to Jason's scalp, but topical azoles are not effective in treating fungal infections of the hair or nails. These infections, usually due to *Trichophyton*, can be treated with griseofulvin, terbinafine, or itraconazole.

4. **The answer is C. The metabolism of fluconazole can be affected by drugs that inhibit or induce the P450 enzymes.** In addition, fluconazole can inhibit the P450 enzyme metabolism of other drugs. Drugs that reduce gastric acidity decrease the absorption of oral ketoconazole, which is dependent on the conversion of the drug to its salt in the acidic environment of the stomach. However, the gastrointestinal absorption of fluconazole is not influenced by the gastric pH. It is 100% bioavailable after oral administration. A topical ketoconazole cream contains sulfites and can cause a hypersensitivity reaction in sulfite-sensitive patients.

5. **The answer is D. Adrenal insufficiency** can occur as a result of ketoconazole antagonism of P450-dependent enzymes responsible for steroid hormone synthesis in the adrenal gland. High-dose ketoconazole can also inhibit androgen synthesis, resulting in gynecomastia and impotence. Topical ketoconazole is used in the treatment of patients with seborrheic dermatitis.

CHAPTER 35 ANSWERS

CASE 1

1. **The answer is D. Blood schizonts infect erythrocytes and cause hemolysis.** When the infected erythrocyte ruptures, another generation of merozoites is released into the circulation, causing recurrent high fever. Sporozoites are the form of *Plasmodia* spp with which humans are infected by *Anopheles* spp mosquitos. They migrate to the liver, forming tissue schizonts. Merozoites are subsequently released from the hepatocytes to infect erythrocytes. Erythrocytes infected with *P. falciparum* malaria express surface proteins, which allow them to attach to endothelial surfaces. This "sludging" of erythrocytes in the microvasculature can cause organ hypoxia, necrosis, and hemorrhage.

2. **The answer is C. Chloroquine causes an accumulation of a toxic heme metabolite, which poisons the parasite.** *Plasmodia* spp are dependent on the breakdown of erythrocyte hemoglobin for amino acids. Degradation of hemoglobin produces ferriprotoporphyrin IX, a toxic metabolite, which must be detoxified by polymerization. Chloroquine diffuses into the parasite's food vacuole, becomes protonated, and binds to ferriprotoporphyrin IX, preventing its polymerization and detoxification.

3. **The answer is A. Chloroquine and pyrimethamine–sulfadoxine have different mechanisms of action in treating malaria:** Chloroquine acts through the accumulation of ferriprotoporphyrin IX, and pyrimethamine-sulfadoxine acts through the inhibition of parasite folate synthesis. These agents are inexpensive and widely available, but resistance to both is growing in many developing areas of the world. Neither agent treats the hepatic forms of *Plasmodia* spp infection. Chloroquine is associated with significant toxicity at high doses. Hypersensitivity reactions can occur to the sulfonamide component of pyrimethamine-sulfadoxine.

4. **The answer is A. The *P. falciparum* was likely resistant to the combination therapy,** a growing health problem in areas of the world such as Senegal. The combination of chloroquine and pyrimethamine–sulfadoxine is often ineffective, particularly in nonimmune patients such as young children. Worldwide, a child dies of malaria every 20 seconds. More than 90% of these deaths occur in children in sub-Sa-

haran Africa as a result of *P. falciparum* infection. Cerebral malaria has a 20% fatality rate, even with effective antimalarial therapy.

CASE 2

1. **The answer is E. Mr. G. had dormant hepatic forms of plasmodia that released new merozoites into his circulation.** Chloroquine does not eliminate the dormant hepatic forms of *Plasmodium vivax* and *Plasmodium ovale*.

2. **The answer is B. Mr. G. will require treatment with another agent, such as primaquine.** Primaquine is the only standard agent effective against the hepatic forms of *P. vivax* and *P. ovale* infection. It is used to prevent recrudescence of these infections. Its mechanism of action is through the inhibition of electron transport in the parasite. Primaquine also causes nonspecific oxidative damage and cannot be used in pregnant patients or in patients with G6PD deficiency because of the risk of massive hemolysis.

3. **The answer is B. Mefloquine,** chloroquine, primaquine, atovaquone, proguanil, and doxycycline can all be used as components of a prophylactic regimen against plasmodia infection.

CASE 3

1. **The answer is C. Mrs. S. may never develop symptoms of entamoeba infection.** Although *E. histolytica* can cause invasive colitis and metastatic infections with abscess formation, some infected persons may excrete the protozoa asymptomatically as carriers, and never develop clinical disease. Infection occurs as a result of the ingestion of inactive cysts. Activate trophozoites invade the intestinal mucosa and spread locally, or through the portal circulation. *E. dispar* does not cause invasive disease.

2. **The answer is A. Abscess rupture and sepsis** are potential complications of untreated invasive *Entamoeba* spp infection. Colonic perforation and peritonitis are also possible complications of this infection.

3. **The answer is D. Metronidazole activation is dependent on the presence of reduced ferredoxin, produced by PFOR.** Activated metronidazole forms reduced cytotoxic compounds that bind to proteins, membranes, and DNA, causing protozoal damage. Because PFOR does not have a mammalian analogue, metronidazole is selectively toxic to amoeba and other anaerobic organisms. Metronidazole is well absorbed from the upper gastrointestinal tract and is therefore used to treat invasive amebiasis. In contrast, iodoquinol and paromomycin are poorly absorbed, and are used to kill intraluminal parasites. Nitazoxanide inhibits PFOR activity. Pentamidine inhibits DNA, RNA, protein, and phospholipid synthesis.

CASE 5

1. **The answer is C. *Onchocerca volvulus* adult filarial worms** develop and rest in subcutaneous tissues of patients infected with *O. volvulus* nematodes. Gravid female worms then release millions of *O. volvulus* microfilariae, which migrate through the skin and cornea. The initial infection occurs when the person is bitten by the *Simulium* spp blackfly and inoculated with *O. volvulus* larvae.

2. **The answer is D. Thumbi developed an allergic response to the presence of dying microfilariae.** This inflammatory or allergic response, a "Mazzotti-type reaction," includes headache, dizziness, weakness, rash, pruritus, abdominal pain, fever, and hypotension. Ivermectin does not cross the blood–brain barrier into the central nervous system, and does not affect adult filariae.

3. **The answer is B. Ivermectin potentiates glutamate and GABA transmission and kills microfilariae by causing paralysis.** Hyperpolarization of the neuromuscular cells and peripheral nerves of the nematode results in a blockade of neuromuscular transmission and paralysis. Because ivermectin kills microfilariae and not adult worms, it is not a curative agent for *O. volvulus* infection, and it must be administered every 6 months in order to reduce the burden of microfilariae and microfilaria-mediated ocular damage. In contrast, diethylcarbamazine kills adult filarial worms and is curative for certain filarial infections. Similar to ivermectin, it can also precipitate a "Mazzotti reaction." Ivermectin is effective against nematode infections, including strongyloidiasis and cutaneous larva migrans, and the ectoparasitic infection, scabies. It is not effective against cestode or trematode infections. Albendazole, mebendazole, and thiabendazole inhibit tubulin polymerization and disrupt nematodal motility and DNA replication, as well as cestodal larval growth. Praziquantel is the drug of choice for infection with adult cestode and trematode infections.

CHAPTER 36 ANSWERS

CASE 1

1. **The answer is D. AZT and 3TC are nucleoside analogues, and ritonavir is a viral protease inhibitor.** Both AZT and 3TC are sequentially phosphorylated and become substrates for viral reverse transcriptase. When they are incorporated into the growing DNA chain as abnormal nucleosides, they act as obligatory chain-terminators, and they inhibit DNA synthesis. Ritonavir inhibits the maturation phase of immature HIV by preventing the normal cleavage of viral proteins by the viral protease. Enfuvirtide is an anti-HIV peptide that inhibits viral entry into the host cell by targeting a viral protein that is necessary for fusion of the virus with the host cell membrane. Amantadine and rimantadine inhibit influenza A viral uncoating. Zanamivir and oseltamivir inhibit viral neuraminidase-associated influenza virus release from the host cell.

2. **The answer is B. Acyclovir is a nucleoside analogue.** It consists of a guanine base attached to an incomplete sugar ring. After sequential phosphorylation, acyclovir triphosphate acts as a substrate for, and an inhibitor of, the herpesvirus DNA polymerase. When incorporated into the growing DNA chain, it acts as a chain terminator, and inhibits viral DNA synthesis. The herpesvirus is a DNA virus and does not utilize a reverse transcriptase.

3. **The answer is E. Mammalian enzymes do not phosphorylate acyclovir as efficiently as do HSV and VZV,** which encode a viral thymidine kinase. As a result, HSV- and VZV-infected cells tend to accumulate much more phosphorylated acyclovir than do noninfected cells. Phosphorylated acyclovir also inhibits viral DNA replication more than it does cellular processes. These factors account for the relative selectivity of acyclovir for infected cells and the low incidence of adverse effects of the drug.

4. **The answer is C. Administering AZT, 3TC, and ritonavir in combination decreases the risk of toxicity associated with any one of the agents.** AZT and 3TC can be phosphorylated by cellular kinases and become substrates for cellular and mitochondrial DNA polymerases. This increases their potential toxicity. When used in combination, the toxicity associated with each agent is limited. In addition, viral resistance to AZT and 3TC can develop rapidly. When used in combination, the emergence of resistance is reduced. Finally, combination anti-HIV therapy (highly active antiretroviral therapy, or HAART) has been shown to significantly reduce the HIV viral load. In contrast, acyclovir is highly selective for the herpesvirus DNA polymerase and exhibits relatively little toxicity.

5. **The answer is E. None of the above** antiviral agents is effective in treating latent viral infections, whether caused by HSV, VZV, or HIV. No currently available antiviral drug attacks viruses during latency, but acts only on actively replicating viruses.

CASE 2

1. **The answer is D. Ritonavir inhibits the metabolism of lopinavir** by the CYP3A4 enzymes. In the presence of ritonavir, the hepatic metabolism of lopinavir is slowed and plasma levels of lopinavir become elevated, with a resultant increase in efficacy. The resultant plasma levels of lopinavir are not achievable in the absence of ritonavir. In combination, lopinavir levels may exceed the EC_{90} for most clinical strains of HIV. (Ritonavir also inhibits CYP2D6 to a lesser extent, so it may inhibit its own metabolism.)

2. **The answer is C. Drowsiness** may occur in patients who are taking diazepam, a benzodiazepine, for anxiety. Diazepam is metabolized by CYP3A4, the activity of which is inhibited in the presence of ritonavir.

3. **The answer is D. The plasma levels of lopinavir will be reduced.** Rifampin, an inducer of CYP3A4, will enhance the metabolism of lopinavir and reduce its plasma levels, and resultant efficacy.

4. **The answer is A. Lovastatin, midazolam, and flecainide metabolism may be inhibited, resulting in elevated plasma concentrations and clinical toxicity.** Many of the protease inhibitors affect P450 enzymes. Inhibition of CYP3A4 and CYP2D6 by a protease inhibitor combination can reduce the hepatic metabolism of a number of drugs, leading to potential toxicity.

5. **The answer is B. Interferons induce the expression of innate immune system proteins with antiviral effects.** These effects may include turning off protein synthesis in viral infected cells. Active and passive immunization provides antibodies against viral envelope proteins, which prevent the attachment and entry of virus into human cells. Interferon α is approved for the treatment of patients with hepatitis C virus, hepatitis B virus, *condyloma accuminata* caused by some human papilloma viruses, and Kaposi's sarcoma. Aerosolized ribavirin is approved for the treatment of respiratory syncytial virus infection in children.

CHAPTER 37 ANSWERS

CASE 1

1. **The answer is D. Etoposide targets topoisomerase II and stabilizes double-stranded DNA breaks.** Both etoposide and teniposide are derivatives of the plant *Podophyllum*. They bind topoisomerase II and DNA, and inhibit topoisomerase II-mediated religation of double-stranded DNA breaks. Camptothecins, extracts of *Camptotheca* plants, target topoisomerase I and stabilize DNA single-strand nicking. Bleomycin binds DNA and chelates iron to cause free radical-induced DNA strand breaks. Cisplatin targets guanine residues and causes intrastrand DNA crosslinks between adjacent guanine residues, and subsequent DNA damage. Hydroxyurea targets ribonucleotide reductase and prevents the conversion of nucleotides to deoxynucleotides, and subsequent DNA synthesis.

2. **The answer is A. Cisplatin and bleomycin damage DNA, while etoposide inhibits DNA repair.** In combination, all three drug classes induce sufficient DNA damage to trigger cancer cell apoptosis.

3. **The answer is C. He is looking for evidence of bleomycin-induced pulmonary fibrosis.** Bleomycin's alkylation of DNA creates reactive intermediates in the presence of oxygen. Because of this reactivity with oxygen, bleomycin can cause cumulative and irreversible pulmonary fibrosis. Cisplatin is associated with nephrotoxicity.

4. **The answer is B. Experiments on the effects of electricity in bacteria noted that cisplatin inhibited DNA synthesis.** Cisplatin was produced by, and isolated from the platinum electrode used in these experiments.

5. **The answer is D. Cytarabine** (araC) is a cytidine analogue. Thioguanine, fludarabine phosphate, and cladribine are purine analogues. Telomerase is an enzyme that synthesizes telomeres at the capping end of DNA strands. Activation of telomerase allows cells to restore telomere length and to continue dividing indefinitely. The activation of this enzyme is associated with the immortalization process of tumor formation.

CASE 2

1. **The answer is B. A potential benefit is that both agents cause DNA damage and may be synergistic in their ability to kill cells.** Their mechanisms of action on DNA are different, leading to a potentially synergistic damaging effect. Using multiple drugs also decreases the likelihood of the emergence of tumor cell resistance. However, the adverse effects of both drugs involve the same organ system. This is a potential downside. Generally, the use of drugs with different dose-limiting toxicities is preferable. Neither drug is very lipophilic, so neither will cross the blood–brain barrier very easily.

2. **The answer is B. Drug B inhibits microtubule polymerization and the microtubule-dependent process of trafficking along long peripheral nerves.** Agents that inhibit microtubule polymerization and extension include the vinca alkaloids, vinblastine and vincristine. In contrast, the taxanes, paclitaxel and docetaxel, inhibit microtubule depolymerization. This stabilizes the microtubules and arrests the cell in mitosis.

3. **The answer is D. Drug D: It has the highest lipophilicity and will be able to diffuse across the blood–brain barrier.** This will make it most able to kill tumor cells in the central nervous system.

4. **The answer is C. Drug C: Allopurinol will inhibit the metabolism of this purine analogue.** Allopurinol inhibits xanthine oxidase in the catabolism of purines. As a purine analogue, drug C's metabolism would also be inhibited by the coadministration of allopurinol. Drug C's toxicity would subsequently be potentiated.

5. **The answer is A. Tetrahydrofolate catalyzes 1-carbon transfers in the synthesis of inosinate (IMP) in purine synthesis.** This is one of the first steps in the synthesis of the purines, adenine and guanine. Therefore, a lack of tetrahydrofolate limits purine synthesis. In the process of thymidylate synthesis, methylenetetrahydrofolate donates a methyl group in the formation of dTMP from dUMP. Agents that inhibit the activity of dihydrofolate reductase prevent the formation of tetrahydrofolate from dihydrofolate, and limit its recycling for

further dTMP synthesis. 5-Fluorouracil is converted to a metabolite that inhibits thymidylate synthesis by forming a covalent bond with thymidylate synthase and methylenetetrahydrofolate. Leucovorin (folinic acid) administration repletes methylenetetrahydrofolate and enhances the effectiveness of 5-fluorouracil.

CHAPTER 38 ANSWERS

CASE 1

1. **The answer is C. Intracellular signals promote activation of genes involved in cell proliferation.** When an EGFR is activated several intracellular pathways are activated. Two important categories of intracellular pathways are activated by the receptor tyrosine kinases: the RAS-MAP kinase pathway promotes activation of genes involved in proliferation. The PI3K lipid kinase pathway activates AKT, resulting in promotion of translation and cell growth, as well as inhibition of genes involved in cell cycle arrest, stress resistance, and apoptosis.

2. **The answer is D. Erlotinib competes for binding at the EGFR tyrosine kinase domain.** Similar to gefitinib, erlotinib antagonizes the activation of the EGFR and prevents the subsequent activation of intracellular signaling pathways.

3. **The answer is E. Tumors can be screened for the presence of mutations that activate EGFR, and make them more sensitive to EGFR antagonists.** For example, activating mutations in the kinase domain enhance tyrosine kinase activity in response to EGF, and increase the sensitivity of these tumors to EGFR antagonists.

4. **The answer is B. Secondary mutations in the kinase domain of EGFR make some cancer cells resistant to the effects of EGFR antagonists.** The effects of this mutation, T790M, can be overcome through the use of experimental irreversible EGFR inhibitors such as HKI-272, which crosslink the receptor binding site. Lapatanib is a new inhibitor of both EGFR and ErbB.

5. **The answer is B. The specificity of the polyubiquitin chain for targeted proteins is determined by the E3 ubiquitin ligase component.** The ubiquitin–proteasome pathway is an intracellular signaling pathway that regulates cell cycle progression and apoptosis through targeted protein degradation. The E3 ubiquitin ligase regulates the transfer of the polyubiquitin chain to targeted proteins. Targeted proteins are then degraded by the 26S proteasome. Bortezomib targets the 20S catalytic subunit of the proteasome.

CASE 2

1. **The answer is B. Binding of VEGF to its endothelial receptor triggers the proliferation of endothelial cells.** The VEGF proteins regulate angiogenesis by their binding to receptors on endothelial cells. Binding to VEGFR2, a tyrosine kinase receptor, promotes the proliferation of endothelial cells and the promotion of endothelial cell survival. VEGF also stimulates vascular permeability through the formation of transendothelial cell vesicular organelles, and the opening of interendothelial junctions. Invasion and migration of endothelial cells is promoted by matrix metalloproteinases.

2. **The answer is B. Tumors with certain activated oncogenes are able to produce VEGF.** Activation of *RAS*, *SRC*, and *BCR-ABL* genes, or inactivation of tumor suppressor genes such as p53, can result in the production of VEGF and the promotion of angiogenesis. Angiogenesis also occurs as a result of tissue hypoxia under conditions in which von Hippel Lindau protein is unable to degrade hypoxia inducible factor (HIFα), which signals the transcription of hypoxia-inducible genes and VEGF production. Stimulation of EGFRs can cause VEGF expression. Finally, cytokines such as interleukin-1, interleukin-6, and prostaglandins stimulate the production of VEGF.

3. **The answer is C. Inhibition of VEGF activity "starves" tumors of oxygen and nutrients.** Bevacizumab is a recombinant humanized mouse monoclonal antibody against VEGF-A. It inhibits the activity of VEGF and prevents angiogenesis. It may also decrease vascular permeability and enhance the delivery of other chemotherapeutic agents to the tumor site. Bevacizumab therefore potentiates the cytotoxic effects of other chemotherapeutic agents. Sutent and sorafenib are inhibitors of the VEGFR, as well as the platelet-derived growth factor receptor.

4. **The answer is D. Thalidomide inhibits angiogenesis, necessary for tumor growth and normal limb development.** It inhibits basic fibroblast growth factor–induced angiogenesis. This may be its mechanism of action responsible for the teratogenic effect of phocomelia. Thalidomide is a synthetic glutamic acid derivative that inhibits the synthesis of TNF-α and costimulates T cells. It is commonly termed an immunomodulatory drug.

5. **The answer is E. Immunosuppression** and opportunistic infections are potential adverse effects of tumor specific antibodies that target lymphocytic leukemic cells. This is due to the destruction of both T and B cells.

CHAPTER 39 ANSWERS

CASE 1

1. **The answer is D. Mr. M.'s use of single therapy probably killed susceptible mycobacteria but selected for isoniazid- and rifampin-resistant mycobacteria.** Each tuberculous cavity contains approximately 10^8 to 10^9 mycobacteria. The frequency of mutants resistant to any single drug is about 1 in 10^6. However, treatment with only one drug causes selection for bacilli that are resistant to that drug. Therefore, Mr. M.'s use of single therapy with isoniazid, followed by rifampin, selected for strains of mycobacteria that are resistant to these agents. Combination therapy for only two weeks would be insufficient to eradicate tuberculosis.

2. **The answer is C. Multidrug therapy will kill resistant strains of mycobacteria.** This is one of the rationales for combination chemotherapy. By giving four antituberculous drugs, resistant strains are more likely to be killed, while minimizing the potential toxicity associated with any one of the agents. In addition, some agents may exhibit a synergistic effect when administered in combination. Mycobacteria exist primarily as intracellular forms within macrophages.

3. **The answer is B. Resistance develops through chromosomal mutations that are passed on to daughter cells**. The frequency of these mutations is about 1 in 10^6 bacteria. This mechanism of resistance is in contrast to the plasmid-mediated mechanism by which penicillin resistance is often transferred from one generation of bacteria to the next. Usually, penicillin-resistant bacteria acquire DNA from plasmids that typically code for an inactivating β-lactamase.

4. **The answer is A.** Second-line agents, such as **streptomycin, levofloxacin (a fluoroquinolone), rifabutin, ethionamide, and clofazimine**, would likely constitute his new, more complex, and potentially toxic antimycobacterial therapy. Mr. M.'s new regimen should *not* include any of the drugs that he was previously prescribed. Given the culture resistance to isoniazid and rifampin, these should not be included in his combination therapy. Continuing the use of these agents would only further resistance patterns.

5. **The answer is E. The MIC for a drug may differ when it is applied to a Gram-positive coccus compared to a Gram-negative bacillus.** The MIC and MBC refer to a specific drug–microbe pair, and for a particular drug, the values may vary among different pathogens. Cidal drugs tend to have a MBC that is close to their MIC. Static drugs tend to have a MBC that is much greater than their MIC. The MBC does not relate to human toxicity.

CASE 2

1. **The answer is C. Doxorubicin is a component of combination chemotherapy in stage III Hodgkin's lymphoma** (doxorubicin, bleomycin, vinblastine, dacarbazine or ABVD). This combination is used instead of (or, sometimes, in addition to) MOPP (mechlorethamine, vincristine, procarbazine, prednisone), the first successful antineoplastic drug combination. The ABVD combination combines both cell-cycle selective and nonselective agents in order to target both rapidly dividing and resting cells. Although doxorubicin is associated with cardiac toxicity, the ABVD combination is less toxic than MOPP, and includes drugs with different dose-limiting toxicities. Patients with stage I or II Hodgkin's lymphoma receive radiation therapy with or without chemotherapy.

2. **The answer is C. Intermittent dosing of chemotherapy allows normal cells and tissues time to recover from chemotherapy-induced toxicity.** Because most chemotherapeutic agents exert their effects on rapidly dividing cells, gastrointestinal and hematopoietic toxicity are often associated with their administration. Intermittent dosing of chemotherapy may also "pull" some nondividing cells out of the G_0 phase, making them more susceptible to subsequent cycles of chemotherapy. Slowly growing tumors may be amenable to treatment with continuous-dose chemotherapy. Time-dependent killing refers to bactericidal agents that exhibit a constant rate of bacterial killing, independent of drug concentration, as long as the drug concentration is greater than the MBC.

3. **The answer is D. The actively dividing fraction of cells includes the cells that are most susceptible to the toxic effects of ABVD.** These tend to be the rapidly dividing cells on the peripheral margins of a tumor mass. In contrast, the cells in the center of a tumor tend to become hypoxic as their access to the local vasculature decreases. The hypoxic cells enter the G_0 phase, exhibit limited growth and division, and may die as a result of hypoxia and lack of nutrients. As a consequence, the growth fraction of a tumor tends to decrease as the size of the tumor increases.

4. **The answer is D.** First-order kinetics implies that a **constant fraction of tumor cells is killed with each cycle of chemotherapy.** This is in contrast to the zero-order kinetics of many antimicrobial drugs, in which a fixed number of bacteria are killed per unit time.

5. **The answer is A.** If two drugs have an **additive** interaction, then the addition of increasing amounts of one drug will result in a linear decrease in the MIC of the other: the drugs are nearly interchangeable in their antimicrobial effect. If two drugs are synergistic, they potentiate the effects of each other (i.e., they increase the potency of each other's effect). If two drugs are antagonistic, they decrease the effectiveness of each other.

VI

Principles of
Inflammation and
Immune Pharmacology

40

Principles of Inflammation and the Immune System

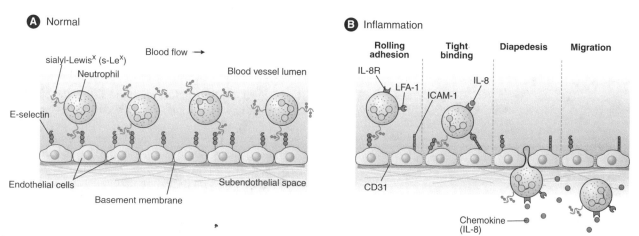

A Normal

sialyl-Lewis^x (s-Le^x)

Neutrophil

Blood flow →

Blood vessel lumen

E-selectin

Endothelial cells

Basement membrane

Subendothelial space

B Inflammation

Rolling adhesion

Tight binding

Diapedesis

Migration

IL-8R

LFA-1

ICAM-1

IL-8

CD31

Chemokine (IL-8)

Figure 40-1. Overview of the inflammatory response. A. Leukocytes circulating in the blood interact with selectins expressed on the surface of vascular endothelial cells. In the absence of inflammation, the interaction between leukocytes and endothelial cells is weak, and leukocytes either flow past or roll along the endothelium. Neutrophil rolling is mediated by the interaction between endothelial cell E-selectin and neutrophil sialyl-Lewis^x (s-Le^x). **B.** During the inflammatory response, endothelial cells up-regulate their expression of intercellular adhesion molecules (ICAMs). ICAM expression increases the potential for strong binding interactions between leukocytes and the activated endothelial cells. For example, ICAM-1 on endothelial cells binds tightly to LFA-1 on neutrophils. The enhanced cell-cell interaction leads to margination of leukocytes onto endothelial cell surfaces and initiates the process of leukocyte diapedesis and transmigration from the vascular space into extravascular tissues. Leukocytes migrate through injured tissue in response to chemokines such as IL-8, which are inflammatory mediators released by injured cells and by other immune cells that have already reached the site of injury. Adapted with permission from Janeway CA, Travers P, Walport M, eds. Immunobiology: The Immune System in Health and Disease, 4th Ed, Figure 10.11, page 378. New York: Garland Publishing, Inc., 1999.

OBJECTIVES

■ Understand the components and normal functions of the inflammatory response and the immune system.

■ Understand how pharmacologic agents can modify inflammatory and immune responses.

■ CASE 1

Mark is stressed—he has to take the United States Medical Licensing Examination (USMLE) in 2 weeks, and he has barely begun to study. Throwing aside any pretense of a balanced lifestyle, Mark travels to the microbiology lab late one night to review techniques for performing a Gram stain. While applying the gentian violet component of the Gram stain, Mark cuts his thumb on the edge of the microscope slide. Fearing the worst but thinking he lacks the time to clean his thumb properly, Mark continues to study furiously that day. Over the next 5 hours, Mark's thumb becomes progressively swollen, warm, red, and tender.

| TABLE 40-1 | Chemical Mediators of the Inflammatory Response |

Response	Mediators
Vasodilation	Prostaglandins (PG) PGI_2, PGE_1, PGE_2, PGD_2 Nitric oxide (NO)
Increased vascular permeability	Histamine C3a, C5a (complement components) Bradykinin Leukotrienes (LT), especially LTC_4, LTD_4, LTE_4 Platelet-activating factor Substance P Calcitonin gene-related peptide (CGRP)
Chemotaxis and leukocyte activation	C5a LTB_4, lipoxins (LX) LXA_4, LXB_4 Bacterial products
Tissue damage	Neutrophil and macrophage lysosomal products Oxygen radicals NO
Fever	Interleukin-1, IL-6, tumor necrosis factor LTB_4, LXA_4, LXB_4
Pain	PGE_2, PGI_2 Bradykinin CGRP

Adapted from Cotran RS, Kumar V, Collins T, eds. Robbins Pathologic Basis of Disease, 6th Ed, Table 3-7. Philadelphia: WB Saunders Company, 1999. With permission from Elsevier.

QUESTIONS

1. Within 5 hours of Mark's cutting his thumb, it becomes swollen, warm, red, and tender. What *initial* changes in the vasculature accounted for the development of the swelling?

   A. Histamine mediated arterial and postcapillary venule dilation and endothelial cell contraction.

   B. Histamine mediated complement activation and endothelial cell contraction by the membrane attack complex.

   C. Tissue-specific macrophages released cytokines, which promoted endothelial cell adhesion and contraction.

   D. Antigen presenting cells presented opsonized bacterial particles to endothelial cells, causing contraction and vasodilation.

   E. Bacteria proliferated in the subcutaneous tissues, causing endothelial damage through the production of pores in endothelial cells.

2. Multiple chemical signals mediated the inflammatory response in Mark's thumb. Ibuprofen is a cyclooxygenase (COX) inhibitor that prevents the metabolism of arachidonic acid. If Mark had taken ibuprofen for his thumb pain, which of the following inflammatory mediators would have been reduced in production?

   A. IL-1

   B. C3b

   C. granzymes

   D. ICAMs

   E. prostaglandins

Mark retains focus and continues to study through the evening. By that night, however, he develops a fever and increased swelling in his thumb.

3. Which of the following mediators contributed to the rise in Mark's temperature?

   A. membrane attack complex

   B. leukotrienes

   C. interleukins

   D. histamine

   E. chemokines

By the third day, pus builds up at the site of the cut. By the fourth day, however, Mark's body seems to have gotten the better of the offending agent. The swelling decreases, the site loses its distinctive angry red appearance, and his fever abruptly subsides. Relieved that he has not become a casualty of his own procrastination, Mark continues studying and performs well on his examination, not the least because his wound has provided him with fundamental insights into immunology.

4. Pharmacologic agents have been, and continue to be developed to interrupt the production of chemical mediators involved in the inflammatory cascade. Which of the following combinations (mediator : effect of its inhibition) is correct?

   A. eicosanoids : inability to opsonize bacterial fragments

   B. histamine : decreased adhesion of leukocytes to vascular endothelium

   C. interleukins : lack of fever

   D. C3a and C5a : inability to produce nitric oxide

   E. major histocompatibility complex : inability to form pores in bacterial membranes

5. When Mark cut his finger, the initial inflammatory response included release of histamine, vasodilation, chemotaxis of neutrophils and macrophages, and phagocytosis of bacteria. This response is an example of:

   A. tolerance

   B. innate immunity

   C. anergy

   D. adaptive immunity

   E. bacterial proliferation

CASE 2

Tom is a 15-year-old boy who has started his own summer business mowing lawns, trimming hedges, and providing general lawn maintenance for his neighbors. Today he was clearing weeds and brush at the edge of his neighbor's lawn, which backs into a wooded area. He was careful to wear thick gloves to protect his hands against cuts, but he wore shorts, and his legs were exposed. Tonight he notes some irritated areas on his calves. Although he sees no cuts in the skin, the skin is slightly pink and raised in some areas and quite itchy. He shows this to his mother, who thinks it might be an allergic reaction to something he may have touched during his work today.

QUESTIONS

1. If Tom's skin reaction was caused by a nonspecific response of the immune system, which of the following cells are primarily responsible for this reaction?
   A. cytotoxic T cells
   B. mast cells
   C. squamous epithelial cells
   D. helper T cells
   E. vascular endothelial cells

Tom's mother gives him a dose of diphenhydramine, an antihistamine, to relieve his itching and applies a cool compress to his irritated skin. He eventually falls asleep, but in the morning, he notes linear, red, raised itchy lesions on his lower calves with areas of vesicle formation along some of the red itchy lines. His mother thinks this looks like poison ivy, which he had once before when he was younger. Tom's legs are too itchy and sore for him to go to work. He spends the day at home with his legs elevated, looking up the symptoms of poison ivy on his laptop computer.

2. Poison ivy (*Toxicodendron radicans*) is one of the most common causes of allergic contact dermatitis in the United States. The allergic component of poison ivy is an urushiol oleoresin, which penetrates the epidermis and acts as an antigen. On reexposure to poison ivy, the action of lymphocytes attempting to eliminate this specific antigen is an example of:
   A. tolerance
   B. complement activation
   C. innate immunity
   D. adaptive immunity
   E. costimulation

Despite cool compresses and diphenhydramine, Tom cannot stop scratching the expanding red welts on his legs. His legs are just too itchy! The vesicles have become bigger and look like blisters. Some have opened and leaked some clear fluid as a result of his constant scratching. His ankles look a little swollen, and his mother says he has a low-grade fever of 99°F when she checks his temperature. She takes him to his adolescent pediatrician.

Tom's pediatrician does not think his legs look infected but agrees that he has a very bad case of poison ivy. She prescribes a short course of prednisone, a corticosteroid, and a higher dose of diphenhydramine for his symptoms of pruritis. After several days, Tom's poison ivy has improved. The open lesions are dry and crusted over, and are no longer red and itchy. He decides to close up his lawn business and signs up to volunteer in the local hospital emergency department.

3. Prednisone, a corticosteroid, has a general antiinflammatory activity. Which of the following effects might result from Tom's use of prednisone?
   A. decreased leukocyte chemotaxis
   B. enhanced histamine release
   C. enhanced prostaglandin synthesis
   D. enhanced lysis of bacteria
   E. decreased tolerance

4. Which of the following statements regarding humoral immunity is correct? Humoral immunity refers to:
   A. the recruitment of basophils to an area where a foreign antigen is present
   B. the phagocytosis of bacterial proteins by macrophages
   C. the presentation of bacterial protein fragments with major histocompatibility complex class II molecules (MHC II) by dendritic cells
   D. the stimulation of angiogenesis through the release of epidermal growth factor
   E. the secretion of specific antibodies by differentiated B cells

5. Clinical signs of the inflammatory response include:
   A. blanching pallor
   B. diminished strength
   C. throbbing pain
   D. lack of light touch sensation
   E. cyanosis

41

Pharmacology of Eicosanoids

OBJECTIVES

■ Understand the physiology of arachidonic acid metabolism.

■ Understand how eicosanoid production contributes to disease.

■ Understand the pharmacology, therapeutic uses, and adverse effects of eicosanoid modulators and inhibitors.

CASE 1

Mrs. D., a 57-year-old Caucasian woman, goes to her physician because of joint pain and chronic fatigue. Her history reveals general joint stiffness and pain, especially in the early morning, and pain in the left metatarsophalangeal joint of 3 weeks' duration. Mrs. D. is advised to take ibuprofen as needed, and this medication provides relief of her pain for some time.

QUESTIONS

1. How did ibuprofen control Mrs. D.'s symptoms of joint stiffness and pain?

    A. Ibuprofen promotes the production of arachidonic acid.

    B. Ibuprofen inhibits the action of cyclooxygenase (COX) and the production of prostaglandins.

    C. Ibuprofen inhibits the action of lipoxygenase (LOX) and the production of lipoxins.

    D. Ibuprofen promotes the action of lipoxygenase (LOX) and the production of leukotrienes.

    E. Ibuprofen promotes the release of phospholipase A_2.

Two years later, Mrs. D. notes indigestion and a few isolated instances of vomiting "coffee-grounds"-like material. Her physician recommends an upper gastrointestinal endoscopic examination, which reveals gastric mucosal erosion and hemorrhage. Based on this finding, Mrs. D. is advised to discontinue ibuprofen therapy.

2. How do nonsteroidal antiinflammatory drugs (NSAIDs) contribute to gastric irritation and bleeding?

    A. Local COX-1 inhibition promotes acid production by gastric cells.

    B. Systemic nonselective COX inhibition reduces blood flow to the gastric lining.

    C. Local COX-1 inhibition prevents the cytoprotective effect of leukotrienes on the gastric lining.

    D. Local COX-1 inhibition prevents the cytoprotective effect of prostaglandins on the gastric lining.

    E. Local COX-2 inhibition decreases the inflammatory response to bacteria along the gastric lining.

Her physician is also concerned about the recent progression in Mrs. D.'s joint stiffness and pain and refers her to a rheumatology clinic. Mrs. D. reports to the rheumatologist that her pain has progressed to include both feet, both hands and wrists, both elbows, her neck, and the left hip. Over the past few months, she has noted difficulties with basic household tasks and has avoided physical activity. The metacarpophalangeal and proximal interphalangeal joints of both hands are found to be swollen, tender, and warm. Skin nodules are apparent on the extensor surface of both forearms. Laboratory tests show high erythrocyte sedimentation rate (ESR), low hematocrit, and positive rheumatoid factor (an immune complex formed from IgM and autoimmune-reactive immunoglobulin G [IgG] produced in joints). Synovial fluid aspirate is notable for leukocytosis.

Because the presentation is consistent with a diagnosis of rheumatoid arthritis, Mrs. D. is started on a course of celecoxib (a COX-2 selective inhibitor), etanercept (a tumor necrosis factor-α [TNF-α] antagonist), and prednisone (a glucocorticoid). Over the next several months, Mrs. D.'s joint pain, swelling, and tenderness decrease noticeably. Joint function in the hands is restored, and Mrs. D. is able to resume some physical activity.

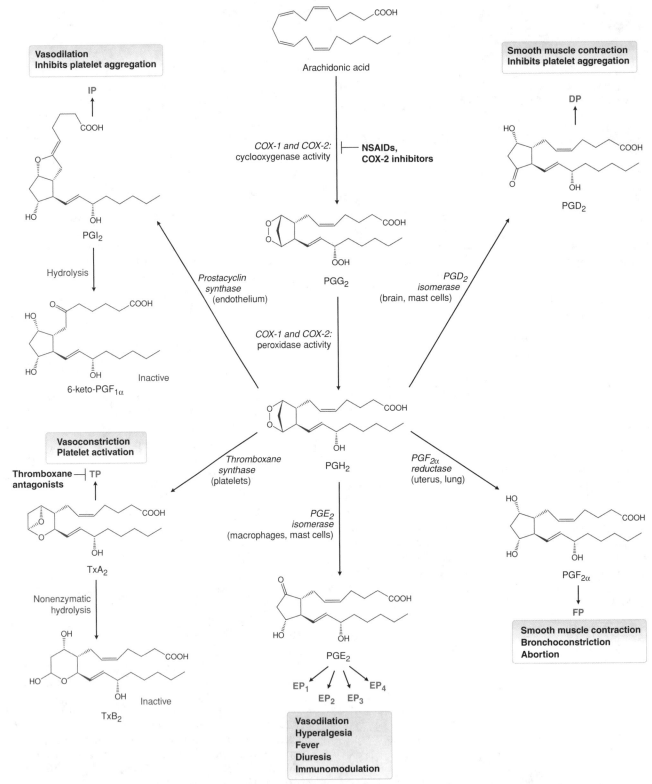

Figure 41-1. Prostaglandin Biosynthesis, Function, and Pharmacologic Inhibition. The biosynthetic pathways from arachidonic acid to prostaglandins (PGs), prostacyclin, and thromboxane (Tx) are shown. Note that tissue-specific enzyme expression determines the tissues in which the various prostaglandin H_2 (PGH$_2$) products are produced. Nonsteroidal antiinflammatory drugs (NSAIDs) and cyclooxygenase-2 (COX-2) inhibitors are the most important classes of drugs that modulate prostaglandin production. Thromboxane antagonists and PGE$_2$ synthase inhibitors are promising pharmacologic strategies that are currently in development. DP = prostaglandin D$_2$ receptor; EP = prostaglandin E$_2$ receptor; FP = prostaglandin F$_{2\alpha}$ receptor; IP = prostaglandin I$_2$ receptor; TP = TxA$_2$ receptor. Adapted with permission from Serhan CS. Eicosanoids. In: Kooperman WJ, ed. Arthritis and Allied Conditions: A Textbook of Rheumatology, 14th Ed, Figure 24.2, page 516. Philadelphia: Lippincott Williams & Wilkins, 1999.

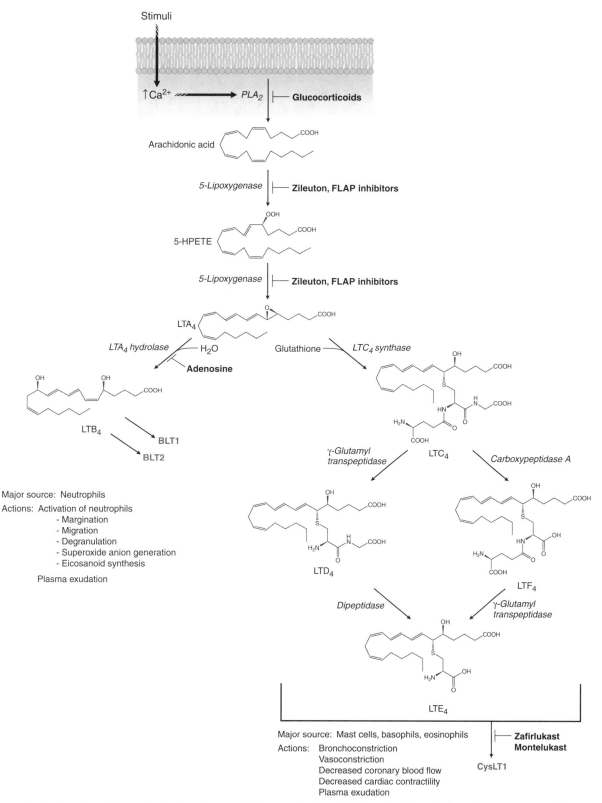

Figure 41-2. Leukotriene Biosynthesis, Function, and Pharmacologic Inhibition. The biosynthetic pathways from arachidonic acid to the leukotrienes are shown. Glucocorticoids decrease phospholipase A_2 (PLA_2) activity, thereby preventing the synthesis of all leukotrienes (LTs). Zileuton and 5-lipoxygenase activating protein (FLAP) inhibitors prevent the conversion of arachidonic acid to 5-hydroperoxyeicosatetraenoic acid (5-HPETE) and LTA_4; zileuton is used in the chronic management of patients with asthma. Adenosine inhibits LTB_4 synthesis in neutrophils but is not used pharmacologically for this purpose. Zafirlukast and montelukast are antagonists at CysLT1, the receptor for all cysteinyl leukotrienes; these drugs are used in the chronic management of asthma. BLT1 and BLT2 are LTB_4 receptors, and CysLT1 is a receptor for LTC_4, LTD_4, LTE_4, and LTF_4. Adapted with permission from Serhan CS. Eicosanoids. In: Kooperman WJ, ed. Arthritis and Allied Conditions: A Textbook of Rheumatology, 14th Ed, Figure 24.6, page 524. Philadelphia: Lippincott Williams & Wilkins, 1999.

3. Mrs. D. was started on etanercept, a TNF-α antagonist, to treat her rheumatoid arthritis symptoms. What is the activity of TNF-α in the setting of this disease?

A. TNF-α is a cytokine that enhances prostaglandin production and upregulates COX-2 activity.

B. TNF-α is a cytokine that contributes to NSAID gastropathy.

C. TNF-α is an isoprostane that enhances platelet aggregation.

D. TNF-α is a lipocortin that amplifies the inflammatory response associated with prostaglandin synthesis.

E. TNF-α is a cytokine that promotes excessive collagen deposition in inflammatory joint disease.

4. Glucocorticoids globally suppress immune and inflammatory responses and are used therapeutically in a number of autoimmune-related diseases. Their beneficial effect is because of the production of:

A. isoprostanes

B. infliximab

C. lipocortins

D. cytokines

E. phospholipase A_2

5. Aspirin is the first and oldest of the NSAIDs. In which of the following ways does aspirin differ from the other NSAIDs?

A. Aspirin is a phospholipase A_2 inhibitor.

B. Aspirin is a selective COX-1 inhibitor.

C. Aspirin is an irreversible COX inhibitor.

D. Aspirin downregulates the activity of COX-2.

E. Aspirin prevents the development of Reye's syndrome.

 CASE 2

In May 1999, Merck & Co. received approval from the Food and Drug Administration (FDA) to market rofecoxib (Vioxx®) for the treatment of arthritis pain and inflammation. The medication was a marketing success for the company, quite effective in treating arthritic symptoms, and very popular with the U.S. public. In November of 2000, the results of the VIGOR (Vioxx Gastrointestinal Outcomes Research) study were published, suggesting an association between the incidence of cardiovascular events and rofecoxib use. In February 2001, the FDA's Arthritis Advisory Committee met to discuss the association between rofecoxib and adverse cardiovascular events. The committee suggested a ''mandatory trial to assess cardiovascular risks or benefits of coxibs.'' In May 2001, Merck issued a press release to reconfirm the favorable cardiovascular safety of Vioxx®, also noting the cardioprotective effects of naproxen in the VIGOR study. Merck had spent more than $100 million annually in direct-to-consumer ads for Vioxx. In April 2002, the FDA instructed Merck to include a cardiovascular risk warning on

the package insert for Vioxx®. In September 2004, Vioxx® was withdrawn from the U.S. market. More than 80 million patients are estimated to have taken the drug. The annual drug sale profits from Vioxx® exceeded $250 billion.

In August 2005, a Texas jury found Merck & Co. liable for the death of a 59-year-old male, who died in 2001 of a malignant arrhythmia. He was a produce manager at a Walmart store, a marathon runner, and an aerobics instructor who had taken Vioxx® for 8 months to treat stiffness in his hands. The jury awarded his widow more than $250 million in punitive and compensatory damages. This case was the first of more than 7000 state and federal Vioxx®-related lawsuits pending across the United States.

QUESTIONS

1. What is the difference between COX-1 and COX-2?

A. COX-1 is expressed in the gastric lining, while COX-2 is expressed in the synovial and renal mesangial cells.

B. COX-1 is expressed in platelets, while COX-2 is expressed in endothelial cells.

C. COX-1 is reversibly inhibited by NSAIDs, while COX-2 is irreversibly inhibited by NSAIDs.

D. COX-1 is constitutively expressed in many tissues, while COX-2 expression is induced under conditions of high glucocorticoid concentration.

E. COX-1 is constitutively expressed in many tissues, while COX-2 expression is induced under conditions of tissue injury or damage.

2. How might COX-2 inhibitors contribute to thrombotic events and cardiovascular toxicity?

A. COX-2 inhibitors prevent endothelial production of PGI_2, but do not prevent platelet production of TXB_2.

B. COX-2 inhibitors prevent endothelial production of PGI_2, but do not prevent platelet production of TXA_2.

C. COX-2 inhibitors prevent endothelial production of TXA_2, but do not prevent platelet production of PGI_2.

D. COX-2 inhibitors permanently prevent endothelial production of PGI_2, but do not permanently prevent platelet production of TXA_2.

E. COX-2 inhibitors are more active in persons with diets rich in fish oils.

3. Leukotriene antagonists are effective in the treatment of antigen-, exercise-, cold-, and aspirin-induced asthma. They reduce:

A. leukotriene-induced bronchoconstriction and mucus production

B. leukotriene-induced utilization of iron

C. leukotriene-induced smooth muscle hypertrophy

D. leukotriene-induced thrombosis in pulmonary capillaries

E. leukotriene-induced vasoconstriction and hypoxia

4. Chronic NSAID use has been associated with a decreased incidence of colorectal cancer. The mechanism of action of NSAIDs that may account for this finding is:

   A. inhibition of COX-1 derived eicosanoids, which downregulate normal cellular differentiation in the colon

   B. inhibition of COX-derived eicosanoids, which regulate excessive blood flow to the colonic mucosa

   C. inhibition of COX-1 derived eicosanoids, which are cytoprotective to the gastrointestinal mucosal cells

   D. inhibition of COX-2 derived eicosanoids, which stimulate cell growth transcription factors

   E. inhibition of COX-2 derived eicosanoids, which transcribe genes for abnormal mucosal cells

5. Acetaminophen is a very weak COX inhibitor that is active primarily at COX-1. It has antipyretic and analgesic, but not antiinflammatory, properties. Overdose of acetaminophen can cause:

   A. bronchoconstriction

   B. gastrointestinal erosion and bleeding

   C. seizures

   D. hepatic toxicity

   E. thrombogenesis and vascular occlusion

42

Histamine Pharmacology

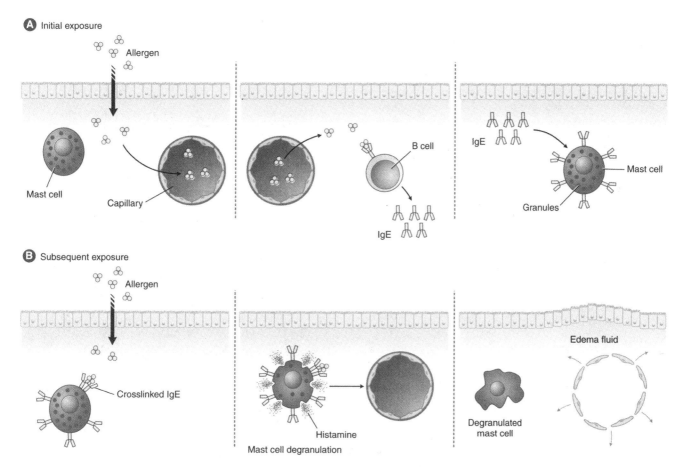

A Initial exposure

Allergen

Mast cell

Capillary

B cell

IgE

IgE

Mast cell

Granules

B Subsequent exposure

Allergen

Crosslinked IgE

Histamine

Mast cell degranulation

Degranulated mast cell

Edema fluid

Figure 42-1. Pathophysiology of the Immunoglobulin E (IgE)–Mediated Hypersensitivity Reaction. Allergen-induced mast cell degranulation requires two separate exposures to the allergen. **A.** On initial exposure, the allergen must penetrate mucosal surfaces so that it can encounter cells of the immune system. Activation of the immune response causes B lymphocytes to secrete allergen-specific IgE antibodies. These IgE molecules bind to Fc receptors on mast cells, leading to sensitization of the mast cells. **B.** On subsequent exposure, the multivalent allergen crosslinks two IgE/Fc receptor complexes on the mast cell surface. Receptor crosslinking causes the mast cell to degranulate. Local histamine release results in an inflammatory response, shown here as edema. Adapted with permission from Janeway CA, Travers P, Walport M, eds. Immunobiology: The Immune System in Health and Disease, 4th Ed, Figure 12.12, page 474. New York: Garland Publishing, Inc., 1999.

OBJECTIVES

■ Understand histamine physiology, including histamine synthesis, release, metabolism, and effects at H1, H2, H3, and H4 receptors.

■ Understand how pharmacologic agents can modify histamine function at the different histamine receptors, resulting in both therapeutic and potentially toxic effects.

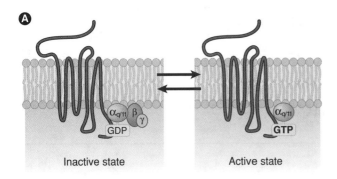

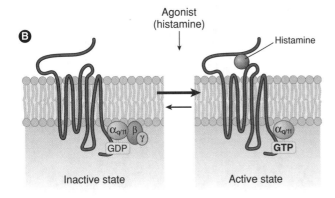

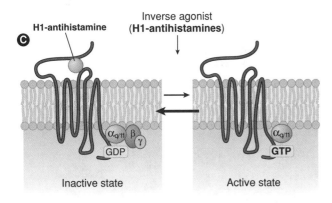

Figure 42-2. Simplified Two-State Model of H1 Receptor. A. H1 receptors coexist in two conformational states—the inactive and active states—that are in conformational equilibrium with one another. **B.** Histamine acts as an agonist for the active conformation of the H1 receptor and shifts the equilibrium toward the active conformation. **C.** Antihistamines act as inverse agonists that bind and stabilize the inactive conformation of the H1 receptor, thereby shifting the equilibrium toward the inactive receptor state. GDP = guanosine diphosphate; GTP = guanosine triphosphate. Adapted with permission from Leurs R, Church MK, Taglialatela M. H1-antihistamines: Inverse agonism, anti-inflammatory actions and cardiac effects. Clin Exp All 2002;32:489–498, Figure 1.

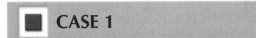

CASE 1

Ellen, a 16-year-old high school student, suffers from allergic rhinitis. Every spring, she develops a runny nose, itchy eyes, and sneezing. To relieve her symptoms, she takes an over-the-counter antihistamine, diphenhydramine. She is an-

noyed by the unpleasant effects that accompany her allergy medication. Every time she takes an antihistamine, Ellen feels drowsy and has a dry mouth. She makes an appointment with her doctor, who, after allergy testing, advises her to take loratadine. After taking her new allergy medication, Ellen's symptoms are relieved, and she experiences no drowsiness or other adverse effects.

QUESTIONS

1. Why does Ellen develop seasonal rhinitis?
   A. Ellen is previously sensitized to environmental allergens.
   B. Ellen has an excessive amount of H1 receptors in her nasal epithelium.
   C. Ellen produces excessive histamine in response to allergens.
   D. Ellen is repeatedly exposed to allergens, which upregulate her H1 receptors.
   E. Ellen overuses diphenhydramine, which upregulates her histamine production.

2. Why does diphenhydramine relieve Ellen's symptoms?
   A. Diphenhydramine competitively antagonizes the H1 receptor.
   B. Diphenhydramine shifts the H1 receptor to the inactivated state.
   C. Diphenhydramine promotes mast cell stabilization.
   D. Diphenhydramine blocks the crosslinking of mast cell IgE/Fc receptors.
   E. Diphenhydramine promotes involution of H1 receptors.

3. Why does diphenhydramine cause drowsiness?
   A. Diphenhydramine antagonizes the effect of histamine reuptake in CNS neurons.
   B. Diphenhydramine crosses the blood–brain barrier and disrupts lipid membranes
   C. Diphenhydramine potentiates the effect of histamine in the CNS.
   D. Diphenhydramine antagonizes the effect of histamine in the CNS.
   E. Diphenhydramine ionizes histamine and prevents its entry into the CNS.

4. Why doesn't loratadine cause drowsiness?
   A. Loratadine is an antagonist at CNS H2 receptors.
   B. Loratadine does not antagonize the CNS H1 receptor.
   C. Loratadine is ionized at physiologic pH and does not cross the blood–brain barrier.
   D. Loratadine acts preferentially at H1 receptors in the nasal mucosa.
   E. Loratadine is highly lipophilic and is trapped in the blood–brain barrier.

5. Cimetidine is a selective H2 receptor antagonist used to inhibit histamine-induced gastric acid secretion. What is a potential adverse effect of this drug?

A. sedation
B. dry mouth
C. prolonged QT interval
D. altered drug metabolism
E. hepatic toxicity

A. ketamine metabolites
B. beer and nuts
C. ingested penicillin tablets
D. ingested ketamine tablets
E. beer laced with penicillin

 CASE 2

You are moonlighting at a medical booth at an outdoor concert when a 16-year-old boy is brought to you for evaluation of weakness and difficulty breathing. Friends admit that they bought white tablets from someone at the concert who was selling ''Special K'' (a street name for ketamine, a dissociative anesthetic). Your patient ingested three tablets with a beer and 20 minutes later began to feel flushed and vomited. Now he says his lips feel ''tingling and swollen,'' and he is having difficulty breathing and swallowing.

On examination, you note his vital signs of a temperature of 99°F, a heart rate of 145 bpm, a respiratory rate of 32 breaths/min., and a blood pressure of 60 mm Hg by palpation only. Your patient is a well developed but weak, anxious male with moderate lip and tongue edema. The posterior oropharynx is not visible on inspection. The tongue is too swollen for you to see anything else in the mouth! His lung examination reveals wheezing, and his heart sounds are tachycardic and regular. His skin is diffusely erythematous, and an urticarial rash is developing on his neck and trunk. Someone calls 911 for emergency services. While you place the patient on a cardiac monitor, establish a peripheral intravenous line, and wonder where the airway equipment is, the patient reports that his only medical history is an allergy to penicillin.

QUESTIONS

1. What is the etiology of anaphylaxis?
   A. a systemic release of histamine
   B. an exaggerated gastric histamine response to an ingested allergen
   C. a hypersensitivity of H1 and H2 receptors to normal environmental antigens
   D. a systemic response to a local histamine release
   E. a migration of mast cells to all areas of the body

2. What is the likely cause of your patient's symptoms?

3. Based on the pathophysiology of anaphylaxis, how might intravenous antihistamines best work in the treatment of this patient?
   A. H1 antihistamines will sedate the patient to facilitate emergent oral intubation for airway protection.
   B. H2 antihistamines will block the action of penicillin at gastric H2 receptors.
   C. H1 antihistamines will reduce the gastric reaction to the ingested penicillin.
   D. H1 antihistamines will reduce the histamine-induced vasodilation, edema, and bronchospasm.
   E. H1 antihistamines will limit gastrointestinal motility and prevent further absorption of penicillin from the gastrointestinal tract.

4. Based on the pathophysiology of anaphylaxis, how might inhaled β_2-receptor agonists work in the treatment of this patient?
   A. Inhaled β_2-receptor agonists will vasoconstrict pulmonary vessels.
   B. Inhaled β_2-receptor agonists will increase heart rate and subsequent blood pressure.
   C. Inhaled β_2-receptor agonists will decrease vascular permeability and tongue edema.
   D. Inhaled β_2-receptor agonists will promote bronchial smooth muscle relaxation.
   E. Inhaled β_2-receptor agonists will counteract histamine binding in the lung.

5. Based on their mechanisms of action, which of the following agents will work the most rapidly to prevent your young patient's death?
   A. inhaled β_2-receptor agonists
   B. oral cromolyn
   C. intravenous epinephrine
   D. intravenous corticosteroids
   E. oral antihistamines

43

Pharmacology of Hematopoiesis and Immunomodulation

OBJECTIVES

■ Understand the physiology of hematopoiesis.

■ Understand how general and specific growth factors can influence hematopoiesis to promote a therapeutic effect.

CASE 1

Fifty-two-year-old Mrs. M. presents with a lump in her left breast. Subsequent mammogram, core biopsy, and lumpectomy lead to the diagnosis of infiltrating ductal carcinoma that is localized but lymph node positive. She begins adjuvant chemotherapy with doxorubicin and cyclophosphamide. Ten days after the first cycle of chemotherapy, her white blood cell count (WBC) drops, as expected; over the next 9 days, her WBC recovers to its normal value. By the third cycle of chemotherapy, Mrs. M. is moderately anemic, with a hematocrit of 28% (normal, 37% to 48%), and she feels quite fatigued. Seven days after the fourth cycle of chemotherapy, her WBC plummets to 800 cells/μL (normal, 4,300–10,800 cells/μL), and her absolute neutrophil count (ANC) is 300 cells/μL. In this setting, she develops shaking chills and a fever to 102°F. She is admitted to the hospital, where she receives parenteral antibiotics, and she remains there for 5 days until her ANC increases to an acceptable level. Mrs. M. completes her doxorubicin and cyclophosphamide chemotherapy, continues chemotherapy with paclitaxel, and receives local radiation therapy.

Mrs. M. is well for 2 years, but then presents with pain in the left leg. Workup reveals that the cancer has metastasized to her left femur and liver. She is again fatigued, and her hematocrit is 27%. She begins chemotherapy with doxorubicin and docetaxel, but again develops severe neutropenia and fever. Thereafter, her chemotherapy is supplemented with recombinant human granulocyte-colony stimulating factor (G-CSF; filgrastim) and recombinant human erythropoietin (epoetin alfa).

QUESTIONS

1. Mrs. M. is supplemented with recombinant human G-CSF when she develops neutropenia as a result of her chemotherapy. What is G-CSF and what is its mechanism of action?
   A. G-CSF is a glycoprotein that stimulates the production of macrophages.
   B. G-CSF is a glycoprotein that stimulates the production of neutrophils.
   C. G-CSF is a glycoprotein that enhances the differentiation of Langerhans cells.
   D. G-CSF is a polypeptide that promotes the differentiation of megakaryocytes.
   E. G-CSF is a hormone that promotes the cytotoxic activity of T cells.

2. Mrs. M. developed anemia associated with her recurrent cancer and chemotherapy. This was treated with recombinant human erythropoietin. What is the mechanism of action of erythropoietin?
   A. Erythropoietin reduces the oxygen binding of hypoxia inducible factor 1α.
   B. Erythropoietin stimulates the differentiation of myeloid cells to reticulocytes.
   C. Erythropoietin stimulates the differentiation of reticulocytes to erythrocytes.
   D. Erythropoietin promotes the oxygen-carrying capacity of myeloid precursors.
   E. Erythropoietin enhances oxygen dissociation from erythrocytes under hypoxic conditions.

Mrs. M.'s neutropenia and fever do not recur, and by 4 weeks after the initiation of erythropoietin therapy, her hematocrit has risen to 34.5%, and she feels less fatigued. The chemo-

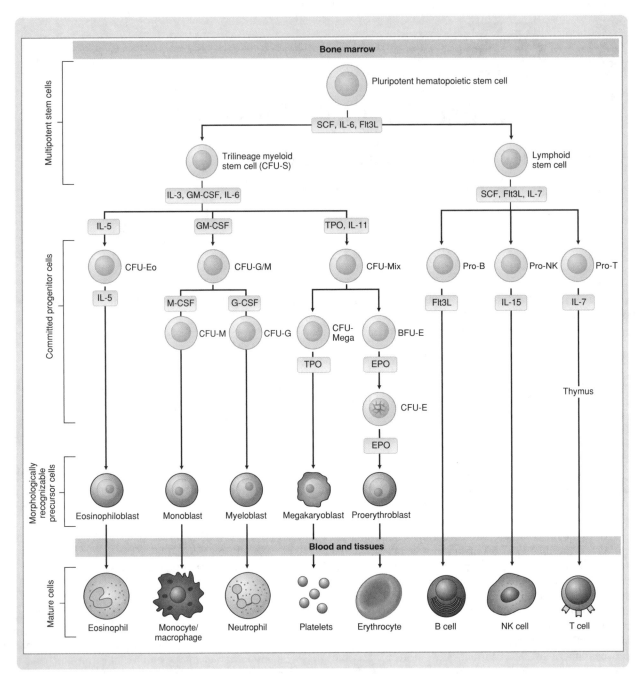

Figure 43-1. Development of Cells of the Hematopoietic System. Mature cells of the hematopoietic system all develop from pluripotent stem cells that reside in the bone marrow. The type of mature cell that develops is dependent on the extracellular milieu and the exposure of stem cells and progenitor cells to specific growth factors. The pluripotent stem cell differentiates into a trilineage myeloid stem cell (CFU-S) or a lymphoid stem cell. Depending on the growth factors that are present, CFU-S cells differentiate into granulocytes (eosinophils, monocyte or macrophages, neutrophils), platelets, or erythrocytes. Lymphoid stem cells differentiate into B cells, NK cells, or T cells. Except for the terminal differentiation of pro-T cells to mature T cells, which takes place in the thymus, the differentiation of all hematopoietic stem cells, progenitor cells, and precursor cells occurs in the bone marrow. Of the growth factors illustrated here, G-CSF, GM-CSF, erythropoietin (EPO), and interleukin-11 (IL-11) are currently used as therapeutic agents. BFU = burst-forming unit; CFU = colony-forming unit; CSF = colony-stimulating factor; SCF = stem cell factor; TPO = thrombopoietin. Adapted from Cotran RS, Kumar V, Collins T, eds. Robbins Pathologic Basis of Disease, 6th Ed, Figure 14-1. Philadelphia: WB Saunders Company, 1999. With permission from Elsevier.

therapy yields excellent palliative results. One years later, she is still in remission and leading an active life.

3. How do recombinant hematopoietic growth factors differ from endogenous "natural" hematopoietic growth factors?

A. Recombinant hematopoietic growth factors bind to the erythropoietin receptor.

B. Recombinant hematopoietic growth factors are proteins.

C. Recombinant hematopoietic growth factors may have modified molecular structures that enhance their metabolism.

D. Recombinant hematopoietic growth factors may have modified molecular structures that enhance their potency.

E. Recombinant hematopoietic growth factors can be administered orally.

4. Recombinant hematopoietic growth factors are associated with some important adverse effects. Which of the following statements regarding hematopoietic growth factors and adverse effects is correct?

A. Recombinant erythropoietin has been associated with axonal degeneration and peripheral neuropathy.

B. Recombinant erythropoietin can cause bone marrow "crowding" of myeloid precursors and subsequent myelosuppression.

C. Recombinant human G-CSF can cause bone pain.

D. Recombinant human G-CSF can contribute to the long-term risk of developing aplastic anemia.

E. Recombinant human IL-11 can stimulate the production of erythrocyte autoantibodies.

5. What might be an indication for the administration of a general growth factor?

A. red cell aplasia

B. acute myelogenous leukemia

C. agranulocytosis

D. pancytopenia

E. metastatic breast cancer

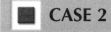 **CASE 2**

Tiernan O. is a 23-year-old man with sickle cell (hemoglobin SS) disease. He comes to his hematologist's office for an urgent appointment. He has been experiencing a painful crisis for the past 2.5 days, and is unable to control the pain with oral analgesics at home. He describes a deep, aching pain in both of his thighs and back. Despite using ibuprofen and oral hydromorphone (a synthetic opioid analgesic), the pain seems to be getting worse. He also feels generally very tired and has no energy. His appetite is decreased, although

he is trying to maintain his oral hydration. He has no abdominal pain, nausea, or vomiting.

On examination, Mr. O. is an alert, thin male who appears very uncomfortable but in no respiratory distress. His vital signs are measured as a temperature of 100.1°F, heart rate of 118 bpm, respiratory rate of 18 breaths/min., and blood pressure of 103/86 mm Hg. His examination is remarkable for moderate scleral icterus and very pale, but moist conjunctivae and mucous membranes. He has tenderness to palpation over his lumbar spine and both thighs.

Mr. O.'s doctor, Dr. Lambreth, reviews his up-to-date medication list and most recent laboratory values. Mr. O.'s medications include folic acid, hydroxyurea, ibuprofen, and hydromorphone for painful crises. Dr. Lambreth orders an intravenous line to be started, laboratory data to be sent, and the administration of intravenous hydromorphone and normal saline infusion.

QUESTIONS

1. How does hydroxyurea work as a therapy for sickle cell disease?

A. Hydroxyurea promotes the expression of HbA-containing erythrocytes

B. Hydroxyurea enhances the oxygen-carrying capacity of HbS-containing erythrocytes

C. Hydroxyurea stimulates the expression of HbB-containing erythrocytes

D. Hydroxyurea prevents the sickling of HbS-containing erythrocytes

E. Hydroxyurea stimulates the expression of HbF-containing erythrocytes

After Mr. O. is more comfortable, Dr. Lambreth questions him closely about other symptoms, including any recent fever, chills, chest pain, cough, or shortness of breath. He also inquires about any diarrheal illness, painful or bloody urination, or skin rashes. Finally, he asks about any recent travel, insect bites, or exposure to ill friends or family members.

2. Why does Dr. Lambreth question Mr. O. closely about potential symptoms of infection?

A. Hydroxyurea is associated with myelosuppression.

B. Hydroxyurea is associated with the development of chronic myelogenous leukemia.

C. Hydroxyurea is associated with bone marrow hyperplasia.

D. Hydroxyurea is associated with a long-term cancer risk.

E. Hydroxyurea is associated with the development of tolerance and physiologic dependence.

Mr. O.'s laboratory studies return, and his hematocrit is measured at 23%. His normal baseline hematocrit is 29%. In light of his profound anemia, Dr. Lambreth recommends that he receive a transfusion of 1 U of packed red blood cells today.

3. Compared with the case of Mrs. M., why is recombinant human erythropoietin not the best treatment for Mr. O.'s anemia?
   A. Erythropoietin stimulates the movement of immature HbS-containing erythrocytes out of the bone marrow and into the circulation.
   B. Erythropoietin stimulates the production of erythrocyte autoantibodies and makes future blood transfusions impossible.
   C. Erythropoietin causes blood hyperviscosity and stroke.
   D. Erythropoietin stimulates erythropoiesis of HbS-containing erythrocytes.
   E. Erythropoietin prevents the induction of HbF-containing erythrocytes.

4. If measured, predict the levels of Mr. O.'s endogenous erythropoietin and reticulocyte count.
   A. erythropoietin reduced; reticulocyte count reduced
   B. erythropoietin reduced; reticulocyte count elevated
   C. erythropoietin elevated; reticulocyte count reduced
   D. erythropoietin elevated; reticulocyte count elevated
   E. erythropoietin elevated; reticulocyte count unchanged from baseline

5. What is the effect of interleukins on hematopoietic cells?
   A. Interleukins control and stimulate white blood cell differentiation.
   B. Interleukins prevent HbS production.
   C. Interleukins limit excess erythrocyte production.
   D. Interleukins protect blood cells from viral infections.
   E. Interleukins stimulate the degradation of thrombopoietin.

44

Pharmacology of Immunosuppression

OBJECTIVES

- Understand the role of the immune system in transplantation and autoimmune diseases.
- Understand the pharmacology of, indications for, and adverse effects of both nonspecific and specific immunosuppressive agents.

 CASE 1

Mrs. W. is 59 years old when she undergoes heart transplantation in the spring of 1990 for heart failure resulting from chronic severe mitral valve regurgitation. Her initial immunosuppressant regimen consists of cyclosporine, glucocorticoids, and azathioprine. Progress during the first 3 months after transplant is excellent, but then Mrs. W. develops anorexia and an echocardiogram shows a significant decrease in her cardiac ejection fraction. The glucocorticoid dose is increased, her ejection fraction improves, and she is discharged from the hospital.

QUESTIONS

1. Mrs. W.'s initial immunosuppressant regimen consists of cyclosporine, glucocorticoids, and azathioprine. What is the mechanism of action of cyclosporine in preventing heart transplant rejection?
   - **A.** Cyclosporine is a preparation of antibodies against thymocytes.
   - **B.** Cyclosporine is a folate analogue that prevents normal immune cell function.
   - **C.** Cyclosporine downregulates the production of inflammatory cytokines, tumor necrosis factor-α (TNF-α), interleukin-1 (IL-1), and interleukin-4 (IL-4).
   - **D.** Cyclosporine prevents IL-2–mediated activation and proliferation of T cells.
   - **E.** Cyclosporine prevents the formation of complement-derived C5 and the formation of the membrane attack complex.

2. Azathioprine is an antimetabolite immunosuppressant drug. Which of the following statements regarding its action is correct?
   - **A.** Azathioprine is a folate analogue that prevents normal lymphocyte function.
   - **B.** Azathioprine is more specific than mycophenolate mofetil in its inhibition of lymphocytes.
   - **C.** Azathioprine inhibits pyrimidine synthesis.
   - **D.** Azathioprine is a metabolite of 6-mercaptopurine.
   - **E.** Azathioprine's effects lack specificity, causing adverse effects.

Four months after surgery, Mrs. W. is admitted to the hospital with dyspnea and fatigue. A right ventricular biopsy demonstrates evidence of moderate acute rejection, with localized areas of lymphocytic infiltration and necrosis. She is treated with a 10-day course of OKT3 (a monoclonal antibody against T cells) that produces adverse effects of fever, myalgias, nausea, and diarrhea. The patient also states, "This OKT3 makes me sleepy."

3. Why does Mrs. W. develop fever, myalgias, nausea, and diarrhea after the administration of OKT3?
   - **A.** She has graft-versus-host disease.
   - **B.** She has developed central tolerance.
   - **C.** She has cytokine release syndrome.
   - **D.** She is undergoing induction therapy.
   - **E.** She has hyperacute transplant rejection.

Mrs. W. is discharged after improvement of her cardiac status. A few months later, however, she returns to the hospital with dyspnea and fatigue. A right ventricular biopsy shows no evidence of rejection, but based on her history and symptoms, rejection is suspected. She is tested for the presence of anti-OKT3 antibodies, but because no neutralizing antibodies are found, a second course of OKT3 is administered, and her symptoms abate.

In December 2000, Mrs. W. arrives at the hospital for her regular annual examination. She is in good health, being maintained on a baseline immunosuppressant regimen of cyclosporine, azathioprine, and glucocorticoids. There has

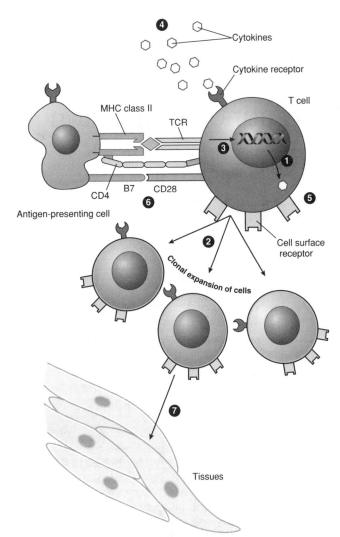

Figure 44-1. Overview of Mechanisms of Pharmacologic Immunosuppression. The molecular mechanisms by which immune cells are activated and function provide eight major points for pharmacologic intervention by immunosuppressive agents. Blockade of T-cell activation can be accomplished by (**1**) inhibition of gene expression, (**2**) selective attack on clonally expanding lymphocyte populations, (**3**) inhibition of intracellular signaling, (**4**) neutralization of cytokines required for T-cell stimulation, (**5**) selective depletion of T cells (or other immune cells), (**6**) inhibition of costimulation by antigen-presenting cells, and (**7**) inhibition of lymphocyte–target cell interactions. Suppression of innate immune cells and complement activation may also block the initiation of immune responses (not shown). MHC = major histocompatibility complex; TCR = T cell receptor.

been no evidence of rejection since 1990. Coronary angiography shows remarkably normal coronary arteries, perhaps the result of aggressive plasma lipid level maintenance by her physicians. However, Mrs. W.'s blood urea nitrogen and creatinine levels are elevated, an indication of damage to her kidneys.

4. What is the likely cause of Mrs. W.'s renal disease?
   A. alloimmunity nephrotoxicity
   B. cyclosporine nephrotoxicity

   C. graft-versus-host disease
   D. atherosclerotic vascular disease
   E. inhibition of renal costimulation

Because of her kidney disease, Mrs. W.'s therapy is adjusted, and she is started on sirolimus. Over the next 2 years, her creatinine level remains stable, and she is able to enjoy time with her grandchildren.

5. What does sirolimus add to Mrs. W.'s immunosuppressant regimen?
   A. Sirolimus prevents opportunistic infection with *Streptomyces hygroscopicus*.
   B. Sirolimus inhibits protein synthesis and T-cell division.
   C. Sirolimus reduces cyclosporine-induced hyperlipidemia.
   D. Sirolimus prevents renal artery stent restenosis in the setting of kidney failure.
   E. Sirolimus is an antibody that binds inflammatory cytokines and downregulates their production.

■ CASE 2

Kerry T. is a 28-year-old woman who was diagnosed with Crohn's disease 2 years ago. She had seen her primary doctor for an evaluation of intermittent episodes of abdominal cramping and diarrhea but was thought to have an "irritable bowel." After a particularly disabling bout of abdominal pain associated with bloody diarrhea and fever, she was admitted to the hospital, where an abdominal computed tomography (CT) scan showed evidence of ileocolitis with distal ileal narrowing. She was treated with bowel rest, hydration, and intravenous antibiotics. A follow-up colonoscopy revealed linear ulcers and a mucosal biopsy was consistent with Crohn's colitis, a chronic inflammatory disease of the gastrointestinal tract. Since then, Ms. T. has been closely followed by Dr. Ravens, her gastroenterologist. Ms. T. is very careful with her diet, gets regular exercise, and has had only one or two mild flares of her symptoms. These have been treated with courses of mesalamine (a salicylate preparation), oral antibiotics, and occasionally, oral corticosteroids.

QUESTIONS

1. Budesonide is a potent oral corticosteroid that is sometimes used in the treatment of moderate to severe active Crohn's disease. It has relatively poor systemic bioavailability because of an extensive first-pass metabolism in the liver, and therefore carries less risk of systemic adverse effects and adrenal suppression. How might an oral corticosteroid be an effective therapy in the treatment of patients with Crohn's disease?
   A. Budesonide will downregulate the expression of inflammatory cytokines and suppress prostaglandin production.
   B. Budesonide will cure Crohn's disease.

C. Budesonide will treat gastrointestinal infection with *Streptomyces* spp.

D. Budesonide will prevent activated T-cell adhesion to the gastrointestinal mucosa through intercellular adhesion molecules (ICAM) binding.

E. Budesonide will enhance the local containment of any inflammatory response.

Ms. T. is seeing Dr. Ravens today for an exacerbation of her Crohn's disease. For the past few weeks, she has noted an increase in diarrhea and more frequent and persistent episodes of abdominal cramping. She has attributed these symptoms to the stress of moving and preparing for a graduate school teaching internship. She restarted her mesalamine and took an oral antibiotic, metronidazole, daily for the past 3 days. However, over the past 2 days, her symptoms have progressed: she has nearly constant aching midabdominal pain, blood in her stools, and a fever to 101°F since last night. Although Ms. T.'s abdomen is mildly and diffusely tender, Dr. Ravens does not appreciate any masses or peritoneal irritation on the abdominal examination. She orders an emergent abdominal CT scan, which is negative for fistula or abscess formation. After some discussion of various therapeutic options, Ms. T. agrees to be admitted to the hospital's observation unit for intravenous fluids and corticosteroids, as well as analgesics. She is continued on metronidazole and started on budesonide and azathioprine. The following day, she is tolerating oral liquids and soft solids, and she feels the pain is sufficiently under control for her to go home and rest, with close follow-up with Dr. Ravens in 2 weeks.

2. What adverse effects should Ms. T. be informed about while taking azathioprine?

A. folate deficiency

B. alopecia

C. weight gain

D. susceptibility to infection

E. renal insufficiency

Despite therapy, Ms. T.'s symptoms do not improve, and over the following week, she loses approximately 7 pounds.

Her temperature remains slightly elevated. She schedules an urgent visit with Dr. Ravens, who considers adding infliximab to the current regimen. Before ordering its intravenous administration, Dr. Ravens questions Ms. T. closely regarding any other infectious symptoms, including sore throat, cough, or dysuria.

3. Why did Ms. T.'s gastroenterologist question her about possible infectious symptoms before administering infliximab?

A. Infliximab will cause fever, the etiology of which may be difficult to discern.

B. Infliximab will cause activation of T cells and increased sensitivity to normally innocuous allergens.

C. Infliximab will undermine normal inflammatory responses to any infectious agents.

D. Infliximab will reactivate any preformed antibodies to prior infectious agents.

E. Infliximab will target and delete any activated T cells, while maintaining normal B-cell function.

4. Which of the following combinations (drug : adverse effect) is correct?

A. glucocorticoids : weight loss

B. cyclophosphamide : interstitial fibrosis and renal insufficiency

C. cyclophosphamide : cardiotoxicity and bladder cancer

D. OKT3 : alopecia

E. abatacept : fever, diarrhea, nausea, drowsiness

5. Of the following agents, which is considered to be a nonspecific immunosuppressant therapy?

A. tacrolimus

B. infliximab

C. methotrexate

D. mycophenolate mofetil

E. OKT3

45

Integrative Inflammation Pharmacology: Peptic Ulcer Disease

OBJECTIVES

■ Understand the physiology of gastric acid secretion and the pathophysiology of peptic ulcer disease.

■ Understand the pharmacology, uses, and adverse effects of agents used in the treatment of peptic ulcer disease.

■ CASE: PART 1

Tom is a 24-year-old graduate student. He is in good health, although he smokes approximately two packs of cigarettes a day, and drinks five cups of coffee a day. He is currently under stress because of the impending deadline for his computer science thesis. He has also been taking two aspirin daily for the past 2 months because of a knee injury he sustained while skiing during winter vacation.

For the past 2 weeks, he has noted a burning pain in his upper abdomen that occurs 1 to 2 hours after eating. In addition, the pain frequently wakens him at approximately 3 AM. His pain is usually relieved by eating and by taking over-the-counter antacids.

When the pain increases in intensity, Tom decides to visit his internist, Dr. Smith, at University Health Services. Dr. Smith notes that the abdominal examination is normal except for epigastric tenderness. Dr. Smith discusses diagnostic options with Tom, including an upper gastrointestinal x-ray series and an endoscopic examination. Tom chooses to undergo the endoscopic examination. During the examination, an ulcer is identified in the proximal portion of the duodenum on the posterior wall. The ulcer is 0.5 cm in diameter. A mucosal biopsy of the gastric antrum is performed for detection of *Helicobacter pylori*.

Tom is diagnosed with a duodenal ulcer. Dr. Smith prescribes omeprazole, a proton pump inhibitor (PPI). The following day, when the pathology report indicates the presence of an *H. pylori* infection, Dr. Smith prescribes bismuth, clarithromycin, and amoxicillin in addition to the PPI. Dr. Smith also advises Tom to stop smoking and drinking coffee and, importantly, to avoid taking aspirin.

QUESTIONS

1. Although Tom is healthy, he has several risk factors for the development of peptic ulcer disease. Which of the following combinations (risk factor : mechanism of ulcer promotion) is correct?

   A. Nonsteroidal anti-inflammatory drug (NSAID) use : decreases prostaglandin-mediated control of pepsin secretion

   B. Antacid use : promotes proliferation of gastrin-secreting G cells

   C. Cigarette use : impairs mucosal blood flow and limits bicarbonate production

   D. *H. pylori* infection : produces inflammatory prostaglandins

   E. Caffeine ingestion : promotes neutrophil activation adjacent to gastric cells

2. *H. pylori* infection is the most common cause of non–NSAID-associated peptic ulcer disease. Which of the following statements regarding *H. pylori* infection and peptic ulcer disease is correct?

   A. *H. pylori* produces and secretes damaging urease, lipase, and proteases.

   B. *H. pylori* infection is associated with the formation of Cushing's ulcers.

   C. *H. pylori* virulence factors limit an inflammatory response to the infection.

   D. *H. pylori* attaches to gastric epithelial cells and limits their gastrin production.

   E. *H. pylori* infection is associated with proliferation of somatostatin-producing D cells.

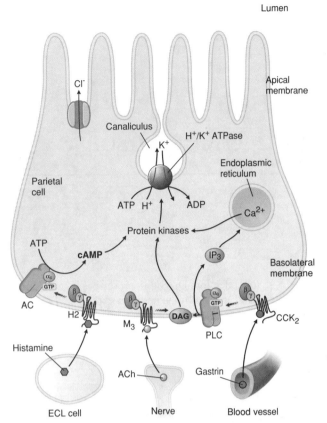

Figure 45-1.   Control of Parietal Cell Acid Secretion. Stimulation of parietal cell acid secretion is modulated by paracrine (histamine), neuroendocrine (acetylcholine [ACh]), and endocrine (gastrin) pathways, which activate their respective receptors (H2, M_3, and CCK_2). H2 receptor activation increases cyclic adenosine monophosphate (cAMP), which activates protein kinases. M_3 and CCK_2 receptor activation stimulate release of Ca^{2+} by the G_q-mediated inositol-1,4,5-trisphosphate (IP3)/diacylglycerol (DAG) pathway; these signals also stimulate protein kinase activity. Protein kinase activation results in phosphorylation and activation of the canalicular membrane H^+/K^+-ATPase, which pumps H^+ ions into the stomach lumen. An apical membrane Cl^- channel couples Cl^- efflux to H^+ efflux, and an apical membrane K^+ channel (not shown) recycles K^+ out of the cell. The net result of this process is the rapid extrusion of HCl into the stomach lumen. AC = adenylyl cyclase; ADP = adenosine diphosphate; ATP = adenosine triphosphate; ECL = enterochromaffin-like cell.

3. Triple therapy is often necessary to eradicate *H. pylori* infection. Why was Tom treated with clarithromycin rather than metronidazole when he was diagnosed?
   A. Clarithromycin permanently eradicates *H. pylori* infection.
   B. *H. pylori* resistance to metronidazole has been reported in the United States.
   C. Metronidazole inhibits the protective effect of bismuth.
   D. Metronidazole is associated with superinfection with *Clostridium difficile*.
   E. Clarithromycin enhances the effectiveness of PPIs.

4. What was the indication for therapy with omeprazole, a

PPI, when Tom was first diagnosed with peptic ulcer disease?
   A. PPIs prevent recurrent hemorrhagic mucosal ulcers.
   B. PPIs are cheap and have no adverse effects.
   C. PPIs produce a protective mucus lining.
   D. PPIs prevent the activity of the Na^+/K^+ ATPase pump.
   E. PPIs irreversibly suppress acid secretion for 18 hours.

5. Many patients try over-the-counter antacids to relieve symptoms of epigastric burning related to gastric irritation and peptic ulcer disease. How do antacids relieve these symptoms?
   A. Aluminum hydroxide binds dietary magnesium, forming protective salts.
   B. Magnesium hydroxide binds phosphate, forming a mucous barrier.
   C. Sodium bicarbonate binds hydrochloric acid, forming a medicinal gas.
   D. Magnesium hydroxide binds bicarbonate ion, forming a water barrier.
   E. Calcium carbonate binds gastric acid, forming calcium chloride and gas.

■ CASE: PART 2

Tom has no medical problems until 10 years after the healing of his duodenal ulcer. At age 34, he develops carpal tunnel syndrome and begins to take several aspirin daily for the pain. One month later, Tom develops a burning pain in his upper abdomen. After vomiting ''coffee grounds'' material and noticing that his bowel movements are black, he decides to visit his internist. Dr. Smith discovers by endoscopy that Tom has a gastric ulcer and that it has recently bled. The doctor explains to Tom that he has a recurrence of his peptic ulcer disease. Tom's breath test is negative for *H. pylori*, and he is told that aspirin is the most likely cause of this recurrence. He is treated with antacids and ranitidine, an H2 receptor antagonist, and is told to stop taking aspirin. Dr. Smith goes over with Tom which pain-relieving medications are considered NSAIDs.

Two weeks pass. Tom informs Dr. Smith that the pain in his wrist has become unbearable and that he must continue taking aspirin to concentrate at work. Dr. Smith tells him that he can take aspirin as long as he switches his antiulcer medication from an H2 antagonist to a PPI.

QUESTIONS

1. What is the mechanism of action of H2 antagonists?
   A. H2 antagonists inhibit histamine binding to parietal cells and subsequent extrusion of hydrogen ions into the gastric lumen.
   B. H2 antagonists inhibit gastrin binding to histamine receptors on parietal cells and subsequent activity of the H^+/K^+ ATPase pump.

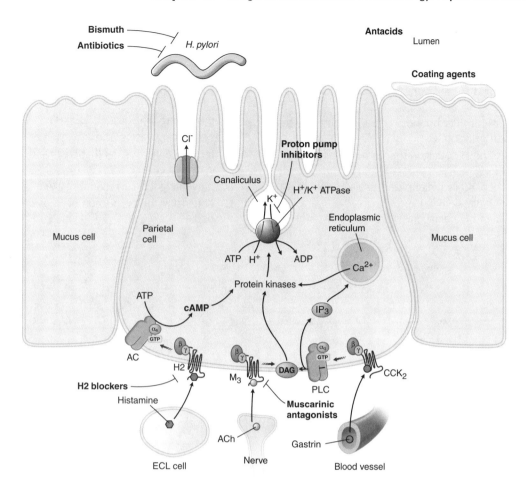

Figure 45-2. Sites of Action of Drugs Used to Treat Peptic Ulcer Disease. H2 receptor antagonists (H2 blockers) inhibit activation of the histamine H2 receptor by endogenous histamine. Muscarinic antagonists inhibit signaling through the M_3 muscarinic acetylcholine (ACh) receptor. Proton pump inhibitors decrease the activity of the H^+/K^+-ATPase on the canalicular membrane of the parietal cell. Antacids neutralize acid in the stomach lumen. Coating agents provide a protective layer on the epithelial surface of the gastric mucosa. Bismuth and antibiotics act to eradicate *H. pylori* from the mucus layer coating the gastric mucosa. *H. pylori* infection is an important contributing factor in the pathogenesis of peptic ulcer disease.

C. H2 antagonists inhibit histamine-mediated prostaglandin destruction and subsequent destruction of the protective mucus lining.

D. H2 antagonists inhibit pepsinogen release and subsequent gastrin extrusion from parietal cells.

E. H2 antagonists inhibit acetylcholine binding to pre-ganglionic receptors and subsequent acetylcholine-mediated bicarbonate sequestration.

2. Potential adverse effects related to the use of H2 antagonists include:

A. Intravenous famotidine use can enhance renal procainamide secretion and exacerbate atrial fibrillation.

B. Ranitidine use in elderly patients can cause ketoconazole toxicity.

C. Cimetidine use in pregnant women can cause gynecomastia.

D. Concurrent use of cimetidine and theophylline can cause tachyarrhythmias.

E. Concurrent use of cimetidine and sulfonamide can cause hepatic failure.

3. NSAIDs contribute to gastrointestinal ulcer formation by inhibiting COX-1–mediated prostaglandin formation, and preventing the cytoprotective effects of prostaglandins on the mucosa. Dr. Smith switches Tom to a PPI while he is taking aspirin. What is the indication for a PPI in this instance?

A. PPIs are synergistic with the protective effects of COX-1 activity, but do not interfere with the antiinflammatory effects of COX-2 inhibition.

B. PPIs prevent *H. pylori* superinfection associated with NSAIDs.

C. PPIs can be administered intravenously to bypass oral NSAID effects on the gastric mucosa.

D. PPIs prevent bleeding caused by NSAIDs.

E. PPIs are superior for healing NSAID-induced ulcers.

4. PPIs and H2 antagonists are important therapies for peptic ulcer disease. Which of the following statements regarding proton pump inhibitors and H2 antagonists is correct?
   A. Both PPIs and H2 antagonists are contraindicated in pregnancy.
   B. Chronic use of PPIs, but not H2 antagonists, is associated with galactorrhea.
   C. Both PPIs and H2 antagonists can be administered intravenously.
   D. PPIs are hepatically metabolized, while H2 antagonists are renally excreted.
   E. Both PPIs and H2 antagonists are associated with the development of gastric carcinoid tumors in rats, but not in humans.

5. Sucralfate alleviates the symptoms of peptic ulcer disease by:
   A. preventing the secretion of gastric acid
   B. neutralizing gastric acid
   C. forming a viscous gel that coats and protects gastric epithelial cells
   D. preventing the secretion of gastrin
   E. enhancing the production of *H. pylori*–directed antibodies

46

Integrative Inflammation Pharmacology: Asthma

OBJECTIVES

- Understand the bronchoconstrictive and inflammatory pathophysiology of asthma.

- Understand the pharmacology, uses, and adverse effects of agents used in the treatment of acute and chronic asthma.

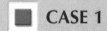

CASE 1

Ahmad, a 14-year-old student in the sixth grade, has a long history of allergic rhinitis. He was first diagnosed with asthma at age 6 years. Ahmad plays soccer during recess but often has to quit early because of difficulty breathing. He has struggled in school because he frequently misses class because of exacerbations of his asthma. When Ahmad was first diagnosed with asthma, his doctor prescribed theophylline, one tablet to be taken twice daily. He has continued on this medicine ever since. Sometimes he also self-administers an inhaled medication containing epinephrine, although afterward he has trouble concentrating because he says he feels "too nervous."

At home, Ahmad frequently awakens with coughing and chest tightness. He develops symptoms when exposed to cats or cigarette smoke. One night, he experiences a severe asthma attack that he cannot control with his aerosolized epinephrine spray. Ahmad is taken to the emergency department of the local hospital. He describes the sensation of a large man sitting on his chest while he is trying to breathe through a narrow straw. He has an incessant cough with thick, clear sputum. His chest examination is notable for bilateral expiratory wheezes and a prolonged expiratory phase. Laboratory tests show that his total white blood cell count is normal (8200 cells/μL), but there is an excess of eosinophils (9%).

The emergency medicine physician gives Ahmad albuterol, a bronchodilator, administered as a nebulized aerosol.

Ahmad's wheezing improves, although he also experiences tremulousness and a rapid pounding of his heart. The physician then administers an intravenous infusion of hydrocortisone, a glucocorticoid, to treat Ahmad's airway inflammation. Every 2 hours, Ahmad receives additional albuterol treatments by nebulizer.

QUESTIONS

1. What factors may have predisposed Ahmad to develop asthma?

   A. Ahmad is allergic to cats.

   B. Ahmad has a genetic atopic predisposition to asthma.

   C. Ahmad has a high concentration of T_H2 lymphocytes.

   D. Ahmad has a high concentration of eosinophils.

   E. Ahmad lives in a very cold environment.

2. Ahmad used an inhaled medication containing epinephrine to control his asthma symptoms. However, he had trouble concentrating after using this medication because it made him feel "nervous." When he used albuterol, he did not experience these symptoms. What is the explanation for this difference in adverse effects?

   A. Epinephrine is a stronger agent than albuterol.

   B. Epinephrine has an agonist effect on the β-adrenergic receptors in the central nervous system.

   C. Epinephrine is a nonselective adrenergic agonist.

   D. Albuterol has selective agonist action at the $β_1$-adrenergic receptor.

   E. Albuterol is metabolized and cleared more rapidly than epinephrine.

By the end of the night, Ahmad feels he can breathe comfortably again. On discharge from the emergency department, his mother is given a prescription for an inhaled steroid medication, fluticasone. Ahmad is instructed to use the fluticasone

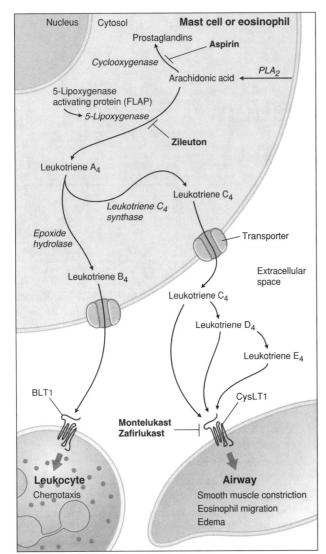

Figure 46-1. The Leukotriene Pathway in Asthma. Leukotrienes are some of the most potent bronchoconstrictors known and are important mediators of inflammation in the airway. Drugs that inhibit leukotriene production or receptor binding have a role in asthma therapy. Leukotrienes are formed when arachidonic acid is released from the inner leaflet of the plasma membrane by the action of phospholipase A_2 (PLA$_2$), and converted to leukotriene A_4 by the action of 5-lipoxygenase upon activation of the latter enzyme by 5-lipoxygenase activating protein (FLAP). Leukotriene A_4 is converted to leukotriene C_4 by the action of leukotriene C_4 synthase, and leukotriene C_4 is transported out of the cell. Leukotriene C_4 is converted to leukotriene D_4 and then to leukotriene E_4; all three of these cysteinyl leukotrienes binds to CysLT1 receptors expressed on airway smooth muscle cells, leading to bronchoconstriction and airway edema. Leukotriene A_4 is converted to leukotriene B_4 by epoxide hydrolase in mast cells and eosinophils. Leukotriene B_4 is transported out of the cell and binds to BLT1 receptors expressed on leukocytes, leading to leukocyte chemotaxis and recruitment. The leukotriene pathway can be inhibited by the 5-lipoxygenase inhibitor zileuton or by the CysLT1 receptor antagonists montelukast and zafirlukast. Adapted with permission from Drazen JM. Treatment of asthma with drugs modifying the leukotriene pathway. N Engl J Med 1999;340:197–206, Figure 1.

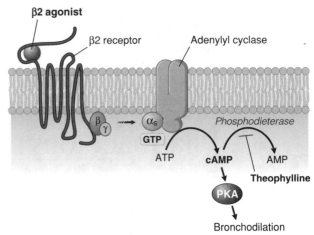

Figure 46-2. Mechanism of the β₂ Agonists and Theophylline. In airway smooth muscle cells, the activation of protein kinase A (PKA) by cyclic adenosine monophosphate (cAMP) leads to phosphorylation of a number of intracellular proteins and thus to smooth muscle relaxation and bronchodilation. Any therapy that increases the level of intracellular cAMP can be expected to lead to bronchodilation. In practice, this can be accomplished either by increasing the production of cAMP or by inhibiting the breakdown of cAMP. cAMP production is stimulated by β₂-agonist mediated activation of β₂-adrenergic receptors, which are G protein–coupled receptors. cAMP breakdown is inhibited by theophylline-mediated inhibition of phosphodiesterase. ATP = adenosine triphosphate; GTP = guanosine triphosphate.

sone inhaler twice daily, as well as an albuterol inhaler to replace his epinephrine spray. With his new medications, Ahmad has fewer attacks of asthma, but he continues to awaken several nights a week with asthmatic symptoms. He uses his albuterol inhaler several times every day to relieve his cough and wheezing. He finds that the steroid spray irritates his throat, and he is not as faithful in its use as he knows he should be.

3. Corticosteroids are a mainstay of preventive treatment for patients with asthma. Which of the following statements regarding the actions of corticosteroids is correct?
   A. Corticosteroids are administered in higher doses via inhalation because systemic absorption is negligible.
   B. Corticosteroids induce the production of inducible nitric oxide synthase, causing bronchial smooth muscle relaxation.
   C. Most inhaled corticosteroids bypass first-pass metabolism in the liver and can therefore cause systemic effects.
   D. Corticosteroids upregulate the transcription of antiinflammatory genes.
   E. Systemic corticosteroids can contribute to the development of osteoarthritis.

4. Ahmad found that the fluticasone spray caused local throat irritation and limited his compliance with this medication. What could Ahmad do to prevent this undesirable effect?

A. Spit it out.
B. Gargle with the spray solution.
C. Spray it into a paper bag and inhale deeply for several minutes.
D. Use a spacer to catch large spray droplets.
E. Take the medication with food.

At a check-up later in the year, Ahmad's new doctor recommends that he stop taking the theophylline tablets and instead prescribes a combination inhaler containing fluticasone and salmeterol, a long-acting bronchodilator. He also advises Ahmad to use albuterol when needed. With this new regimen, Ahmad finally feels that he is in control of his asthma, and he is able to play soccer and do better in school.

5. Ahmad was treated with oral theophylline. What is the mechanism of action of theophylline in the treatment of asthma, and how does this relate to its potential adverse effects?
A. Theophylline is a nonselective β-adrenergic agonist that can cause tachydysrhythmias and hypotension.
B. Theophylline is a nonselective adrenergic agonist that can cause hypertension and seizures.
C. Theophylline is an adenosine receptor antagonist that can cause diaphragmatic irritation and urticaria.
D. Theophylline is a phosphodiesterase inhibitor that can cause hepatic enzyme toxicity.
E. Theophylline is a phosphodiesterase inhibitor that can cause dysrhythmias, nausea, and vomiting.

6. Why are most asthma medications given by the pulmonary route rather than as pills?
A. Inhalation of the drug delivers it directly to the bronchioles and limits systemic adverse effects.
B. Asthma medications are not stable in the acidic environment of the stomach when administered in pill form.
C. In combination asthma therapy, the large number of pills to be taken to control symptoms would limit patient compliance.
D. Inhalation of the drug is technically easier than swallowing pills.
E. Oral administration of asthma medications prevents a sudden increase in the plasma concentration of the drug, and resultant toxicity.

7. Compared with corticosteroids, why do cromolyns and leukotriene inhibitors have a limited effect on overall lung function and symptom control in asthma?
A. Cromolyns only work for exercise-induced asthma.
B. Inhibition of leukotriene synthesis and action can trigger an immune response.
C. The inhibition of single pathways underlying the pathophysiologic process of asthma does not have a significant effect on the clinical disease.
D. Corticosteroids are more potent agents than cromolyns or leukotriene inhibitors.
E. Asthma cannot be controlled by cell-based inhibitors.

47

Integrative Inflammation Pharmacology: Gout

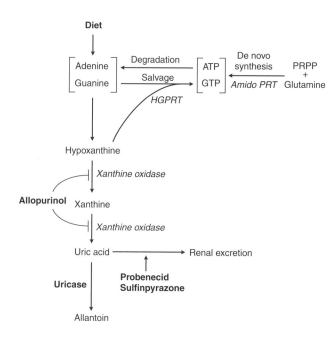

Figure 47-1. **Purine Metabolism.** Purines (adenine and guanine) can be formed via de novo synthesis or dietary salvaging. The de novo pathway utilizes the amino acid glutamine and phosphoribosyl pyrophosphate (PRPP) in a reaction catalyzed by amidophosphoribosyltransferase (amidoPRT). The salvage pathway converts dietary guanine or adenine to nucleotides. Hypoxanthine-guanine phosphoribosyltransferase (HGPRT) phosphorylates and ribosylates dietary adenine and guanine, creating the purine nucleotides used for DNA and RNA synthesis. Degradation converts all purines to xanthine and ultimately uric acid, which is excreted by the kidneys or gastrointestinal tract (not shown). Pharmacologic interventions that reduce plasma urate consist of reducing urate synthesis (allopurinol and its metabolite oxypurinol), increasing urate excretion (probenecid and sulfinpyrazone), or converting urate to the more soluble allantoin (uricase).

| TABLE 47-1 | Natural History of Gout |

Stage	Features	Pharmacologic Intervention
1 Asymptomatic hyperuricemia*	Plasma urate > 6.0 mg/dL in women; > 7.0 mg/dL in men	None
2 Acute gout	Acute arthritis Typically first metatarsophalangeal joint Excruciating pain	NSAIDs Colchicine Glucocorticoids
3 Intercritical phase	Asymptomatic hyperuricemia 10% may never have another acute attack	None
4 Chronic gout	Hyperuricemia Development of tophi Recurrent attacks of acute gout	Allopurinol Probenecid Sulfinpyrazone

*Note that the degree of hyperuricemia correlates with the likelihood of developing gout, but it is possible to develop gout without hyperuricemia. No pharmacologic intervention is indicated for asymptomatic hyperuricemia, but the cause should be investigated.
  NSAID-nonsteroidal antiinflammatory drug.

OBJECTIVES

■ Understand how disruption of normal purine metabolism causes gout.

■ Understand the pharmacology, uses, and adverse effects of agents used in the treatment of acute gout.

■ Understand the pharmacology, uses, and adverse effects of agents used in the management of chronic hyperuricemia and gout.

 CASE: PART 1

One morning, Mr. J., a 52-year-old man, awakens with excruciating pain in his great toe. Even the weight of the bedsheet is enough to make him want to scream; he is unable to put on a sock or shoe. Worried that something terrible has occurred, Mr. J. rushes to his doctor. Based on the history and physical findings, the physician diagnoses an acute attack of gout. The physician prescribes ibuprofen, which relieves the pain after 2 days.

QUESTIONS

1. Acute gouty arthritis occurs as a result of the inflammatory response to uric acid crystal deposition in the synovial fluid and tissues. Why was ibuprofen effective for Mr. J.'s acute attack of pain?

   A. Ibuprofen prevented cyclooxygenase-1 (COX-1)–mediated crystal deposition within the joints.

   B. Ibuprofen prevented COX-2 production of prostaglandins, which are associated with the inflammatory response to intraarticular crystals.

   C. Ibuprofen enhanced thromboxane-related crystal dissolution.

   D. Ibuprofen enhanced renal secretion of uric acid.

   E. Ibuprofen prevented COX-2 production of leukotrienes, which are associated with periarticular muscle contraction and spasm.

Mr. J. is well until 5 years later, when the symptoms recur and he treats himself with ibuprofen, successfully. Subsequently, he learns to anticipate the attacks, which slowly increase in frequency, until they occur once weekly. He uses ibuprofen at the first hint of pain. The morning after one of his attacks begins, Mr. J. goes to his doctor because the pain is not relieved with ibuprofen.

Focused examination reveals a swollen, red, and warm left knee, right midfoot, and right first metatarsophalangeal joint. There are 0.5-cm mobile nodules near the olecranon bilaterally and another at the inferior pole of the right patella. The rest of the exam is unremarkable. The physician aspirates Mr. J.'s left knee, revealing a cloudy yellow fluid that,

on microscopic examination, contains numerous leukocytes. Abundant needle-shaped microscopic crystals are also seen, some of them intracellular. An x-ray of the left knee is normal except for the presence of an effusion; a radiograph of the right foot shows an erosion of the distal first metatarsal.

2. Which of the following statements regarding uric acid deposition is correct?

   A. Uric acid crystals precipitate in joints when the plasma concentration of urate is greater than 7.0 mg/dL (in men).

   B. Uric acid crystals deposited in the renal tubules create tophi.

   C. Uric acid crystals deposit in the synovial tissues of joints, which are chronically under mechanical stress.

   D. Uric acid crystals deposit in the synovial tissues of joints, which are more peripherally located.

   E. Uric acid crystals deposit along the endothelial cell wall of peripheral vessels when the serum pH is acidic.

Mr. J. is treated with colchicine for 3 days and naproxen for 2 days. His condition improves rapidly.

3. How does colchicine reduce the inflammatory response during an acute attack of gout?

   A. Colchicine binds to tubulin and prevents the normal function of neutrophils and macrophages.

   B. Colchicine binds to COX-2 and inhibits its function within the periarticular space.

   C. Colchicine creates viscous mucus around uric acid crystals, limiting their local activation of complement.

   D. Colchicine binds to tubulin in gastrointestinal cells and inhibits their absorption of dietary urate.

   E. Colchicine binds to tubulin in the proximal renal tubule and prevents reabsorption of urate.

4. Which of the following is an adverse effect of colchicine use?

   A. seizures

   B. hypersensitivity reactions

   C. high urinary urate concentrations

   D. vomiting

   E. diarrhea

Three weeks later, Mr. J. returns to his physician while feeling well. He is given a prescription for allopurinol to take on a long term basis and one for colchicine to take during the first few months of allopurinol therapy.

5. Why did Mr. J. take colchicine during the first few months of treatment with allopurinol?

A. Coadministration of colchicine reduces the chance of precipitating acute gout.

B. Coadministration of colchicine enhances the renal secretion of urate.

C. Coadministration of colchicine activates allopurinol to oxypurinol.

D. Coadministration of colchicine inhibits xanthine oxidase.

E. Coadministration of colchicine reduces the deposition of urate in the renal tubules.

■ CASE: PART 2

One year later, Mr. J. is feeling so much better that he discontinues his use of allopurinol. He goes on vacation, where he enjoys meals of liver with anchovies and beer. One evening, he experiences a sudden onset of severe left flank pain, which feels like a stabbing in his side. The pain is associated with nausea and sweats. He visits the local clinic, where he is asked to give a urine sample. Much to his surprise and fright, he sees red blood in his urine. The clinic nurse establishes an intravenous line and administers intravenous fluids as well as intravenous ketorolac (a substituted phenylacetic acid nonsteroidal antiinflammatory drug) for pain, and prochlorperazine (a phenothiazine dopamine D2 antagonist) for nausea. Mr. J. feels improved after several hours of therapy and is counseled regarding his diet and told to restart his allopurinol.

QUESTIONS

1. Allopurinol is prescribed for the management of chronic gout. It decreases the concentration of urate in the blood. Which of the following mechanisms of action is responsible for the effect of allopurinol?

A. Allopurinol is an analogue of 5-phosphoribosyl-1-pyrophosphate (PRPP), allowing it to act as an inhibitor of de novo purine synthesis and decreasing purine metabolism to urate.

B. Allopurinol is an analogue of xanthine that prevents the normal function of oxypurinol in metabolizing urate.

C. Allopurinol is an analogue of xanthine that prevents the normal metabolism of xanthine to urate.

D. Allopurinol is an analogue of guanine that limits the breakdown of endogenous purines to urate.

E. Allopurinol is an analogue of xanthine oxidase that prevents its de novo synthesis of urate.

2. What is the likely cause of Mr. J.'s sudden severe flank pain?

A. tophaceous gouty deposits in the paraspinal muscles

B. uric acid stones obstructing the left ureter

C. chronically elevated urate precipitating acute renal failure

D. hypoxanthine and xanthine crystal deposition in the left kidney

E. uricase destruction of the left renal papillae

3. What is the rationale for the addition of probenecid in the pharmacologic management of chronic gout?

A. Probenecid inhibits the proximal renal tubule anion exchanger and decreases urate reabsorption in the proximal tubule.

B. Probenecid inhibits the proximal renal tubule H^+/K^+ ATPase pump and promotes active secretion of urate in the proximal tubule.

C. Probenecid inhibits prostaglandin-associated glomerular filtration of urate.

D. Probenecid reverses the normal action of the Na^+/H^+ ATPase pump in the proximal renal tubule, causing alkaline urine and enhanced urate excretion.

E. Probenecid "freezes" the enzymatic activity of xanthine oxidase in the proximal renal tubule and prevents formation of urate in the urine.

4. The formation of uric acid renal calculi is one potential adverse effect of uricosuric drugs. Another adverse effect of these agents is:

A. Sulfinpyrazone causes renal insufficiency.

B. Probenecid enhances renal elimination of penicillins.

C. Losartan causes renal hypertension.

D. Probenecid limits the renal elimination of penicillins.

E. Sulfinpyrazone causes accumulation of azathioprine.

5. In addition to liver, anchovies, and beer, which of the following are purine-rich foods?

A. tofu

B. dried beans

C. dark berries

D. whole grain breads

E. bananas

ANSWERS TO SECTION VI

CHAPTER 40 ANSWERS

CASE 1

1. **The answer is A.** The vascular reaction to tissue damage is one of the first events in the inflammatory response. Histamine is a vasoactive amine that is released in response to tissue damage. **Histamine mediates arterial and postcapillary venule dilation**, venous constriction, and **endothelial cell contraction**. This promotes blood flow to the area of damage, and increased capillary permeability allows inflammatory cells to migrate into the interstitium. The resulting exudate causes swelling and edema. Complement is activated by antigen–antibody interaction, interactions with foreign surfaces or complex carbohydrates, to trigger further inflammatory responses, including opsonization, chemotaxis, and formation of the membrane attack complex. Activated endothelial cells express intercellular adhesion molecules that promote adherence of leukocytes along the vascular endothelium. Antigen-presenting cells process and present antigenic fragments of foreign material to T cells.

2. **The answer is E.** Ibuprofen reduces the production of **prostaglandins** from arachidonic acid. Many of the products of the arachidonic acid pathway are proinflammatory. Interleukin-1 (IL-1) and tumor necrosis factor-α (TNF-α) are cytokines secreted by hematopoietic cells, which regulate leukocyte activity. C3b is a cleavage product of the complement cascade and an opsonin. Granzymes and perforins are cytotoxic proteins used by T cells to lyse infected cells. ICAMs are intercellular adhesion molecules expressed by activated endothelial cells, in order to promote leukocyte adhesion.

3. **The answer is C.** IL-1 and TNF-α are **interleukin** cytokines, which are two of the mediators responsible for the rise in Mark's temperature and fever. The membrane attack complex is a complex of proteins, a product of the complement cascade that forms large pores in the outer membrane of gram-negative bacteria, leading to cell lysis. Chemokines are cytokines that promote immune cell chemotaxis to areas of inflammation.

4. **The answer is C. Prevention of interleukin production would contribute to a lack of fever.** Inhibition of eicosanoid production would decrease several aspects of inflammation, including vasodilation, platelet activation, and fever, but not opsonization. Antihistamines reduce vasodilation and edema but do not affect leukocyte adhesion to endothelial cells. Inhibition of the complement cascade would have a general antiinflammatory effect, including a reduction in the production of opsonins, chemotaxis, and formation of the membrane attack complex. Nitric oxide is produced by endothelial cells. The major histocompatibility complex is a group of transmembrane proteins that bind and display protein fragments. They promote specificity of reaction to foreign antigens by the adaptive immune system.

5. **The answer is B. Innate immunity** is the initial stereotyped response to a foreign stimulus. This response includes the cells that secrete cytotoxic proteins, phagocytose bacteria, and amplify the inflammatory response by secreting cytokines. Adaptive immunity consists of specific responses intended to neutralize a particular foreign stimulus by activated cytotoxic T cells and antibody formation. Tolerance is a process by which immune cells mature in such a way that they do not recognize or attack native proteins. Anergy is the process by which immune cells lose reactivity and do not respond to antigenic stimuli.

CASE 2

1. **The answer is B. Mast cells** are tissue-resident granulocytes that contain histamine. Both mast cells and basophils bind IgE antibody and display IgE on their cell surface. If an exogenous antigen (such as urushiol) binds and crosslinks IgE, histamine is released. Cytotoxic and helper T cells are involved in the adaptive immune response to foreign antigens.

2. **The answer is D. Adaptive immunity** is characterized by an antigen-specific reaction to a foreign substance. In the case of poison ivy, an initial exposure to the urushiol antigen could cause a local contact dermatitis, but IgE antibodies are also formed in response to the presence of the antigen. On reexposure to urushiol

resins, the crosslinking of pre-formed IgE initiates the allergic response. In contrast, innate immunity is characterized by a stereotyped nonspecific response to a foreign antigen. Costimulation refers to the two-step process through which an immune response is triggered. Tolerance is the process through which developing immune cells mature in such a way that they do not recognize native proteins as foreign. Complement activation is one of the first innate mechanisms activated in response to a foreign antigen or tissue injury, and it amplifies the inflammatory response.

3. **The answer is A.** Corticosteroids exert multiple inhibitory effects on the inflammatory and immune responses, including limitation of cytokine release and **decreased leukocyte chemotaxis**, as well as decreased prostaglandin synthesis.

4. **The answer is E. Humoral immunity refers to the secretion of specific antibodies by differentiated B cells**, an important component of the adaptive immune response. (Cellular immunity refers to the actions of activated T cells as components of adaptive immunity.) Recruitment of basophils, phagocytosis of bacterial proteins, and presentation of bacterial protein fragments are all actions that occur as part of the initial, innate immune response to a foreign antigen. Angiogenesis, tissue repair, and scar formation are components of the resolution of the inflammatory response, mediated by the release of growth factors and cytokines.

5. **The answer is C.** Clinical signs of the inflammatory response include **pain** (dolor), redness (rubor), heat (calor), swelling (tumor), and loss of function (function laesa).

CHAPTER 41 ANSWERS

CASE 1

1. **The answer is B. Ibuprofen inhibits the action of COX and the production of prostaglandins.** Arachidonic acid, the precursor to the eicosanoid pathway, is released from cell membranes by the action of phospholipase A_2. Arachidonic acid is acted on by several enzymes that generate tissue-specific eicosanoids. The COX enzymes (particularly COX-2) convert arachidonic acid to prostaglandins, which can promote the inflammatory response. The LOX enzymes convert arachidonic acid to leukotrienes and lipoxins.

2. **The answer is D. Local COX-1 inhibition prevents the cytoprotective effect of prostaglandins on the gastric lining.** COX-1 is constitutively expressed in many tissues, where its production of prostaglandins is necessary for the maintenance of normal tissue function. In addition to NSAID-induced gastropathy, chronic use of NSAIDs can adversely affect renal blood flow and

cause renal ischemia, papillary necrosis, interstitial nephritis, and renal failure. Leukotrienes are products of the LOX enzyme pathway.

3. **The answer is A. TNF-α is a cytokine that enhances prostaglandin production and up-regulates COX-2 activity.** Both TNF-α and IL-1 are proinflammatory cytokines that promote and amplify the production of cellular and soluble mediators of inflammatory conditions. TNF-α inhibitors prevent further bone destruction and limit the symptoms of pain and joint swelling associated with rheumatoid arthritis. Isoprostanes are nonenzymatic products of arachidonic acid metabolism. They are potent vasoconstrictors that are associated with conditions of oxidative stress, including ischemic syndromes and atherosclerosis. Lipoxins are products of the LOX pathway. They modulate the inflammatory effects of leukotrienes and may be important in the resolution of inflammatory conditions.

4. **The answer is C.** The beneficial antiinflammatory effect of glucocorticoids is due to the production of **lipocortins and annexin derived peptides**. Lipocortins reduce prostaglandins in tissues by producing a local increase in annexins and annexin peptides that in turn act on specific lipoxin A4 receptors, which regulate phospholipase A_2 activity and limit the release of arachidonic acid, the precursor to the prostaglandin pathway. In addition, glucocorticoids also induce the formation of annexins (lipocortin and macrocortin), which block the proinflammatory response of leukocytes and promote the antiinflammatory activity of lipoxins. Finally, glucocorticoids repress COX-2 gene and enzyme expression. Isoprostanes are nonenzymatic vasoconstrictor products of arachidonic acid metabolism with no known role in inflammation. Infliximab is a TNF-α inhibitor.

5. **The answer is C. Aspirin is an irreversible COX inhibitor.** It nonselectively acetylates the active site of both COX-1 and COX-2, destroying the enzymes' cyclooxygenase activity. (This is in contrast to the other NSAIDs, which block the channel in COX where arachidonic acid would bind.) Aspirin-acetylated COX-2 remains enzymatically active and produces 15R-HETE from arachidonic acid, the precursor to the 15-epi-lipoxins, which are local-acting anti-inflammatory mediators. Salicylate similarly prevents the production of prostaglandins, thromboxanes, and prostacyclin. Reye's syndrome is a condition characterized by hepatic encephalopathy and liver steatosis, occurring in children with febrile illness treated with aspirin.

CASE 2

1. **The answer is E. COX-1 is constitutively expressed in many tissues, while COX-2 expression is induced under conditions of tissue injury or damage.** COX-1 has a primary role in protective and maintenance tissue functions. COX-2 is induced within hours of tissue injury in response to cytokine production and inflammatory conditions.

2. **The answer is B. COX-2 inhibitors prevent endothelial production of PGI$_2$ but do not prevent platelet production of TXA$_2$.** PGI$_2$ is a vasodilator and platelet inhibitor normally produced by endothelial cells. TXA$_2$ is a platelet-derived vasoconstrictor that promotes platelet aggregation and adhesion. The relative imbalance of these two mediators may be associated with the development of thrombotic events and atherosclerotic cardiovascular disease. Because platelets express primarily COX-1, the selective COX-2 inhibitors do not have the antiplatelet effect of the traditional NSAIDs. The specific COX-2 inhibition of normally protective, vasodilating endothelial cell products may disturb the local balance between PGI$_2$ and TXA$_2$, and promote local thrombosis and atherosclerotic disease. TXB$_2$ is an inactive metabolite nonenzymatically derived from TXA$_2$.

3. **The answer is A. Leukotriene-induced bronchoconstriction and mucus production** are inhibited by leukotriene antagonists such as montelukast and zafirlukast. Zileuton is an iron chelator that prevents the use of nonheme iron by 5-LOX, subsequently preventing the production of leukotrienes. It is also effective in promoting bronchodilation but has low bioavailability and liver toxicity, and is not widely used.

4. **The answer is D.** Chronic NSAID use may lead to the **inhibition of COX-2 derived eicosanoids, which may stimulate cell growth transcription factors**. Some human gastrointestinal tumors have been shown to express COX-2 (but not COX-1). It is hypothesized that COX-2–derived eicosanoids may bind to transcription factors that are involved in cell growth and differentiation, and provide excessive growth stimuli.

5. **The answer is D.** Acetaminophen overdose can cause **hepatic toxicity.** Acetaminophen is hepatically metabolized by conjugation. Its reactive intermediate is conjugated to glutathione, and when glutathione stores are depleted, this intermediate binds to hepatocytes, causing cell injury and destruction.

CHAPTER 42 ANSWERS

CASE 1

1. **The answer is A. Ellen is previously sensitized to environmental allergens.** Her prior exposure to allergens prompted the production of specific IgE antibodies. On reexposure every spring, these allergens cross-link IgE/Fc receptor complexes on sensitized mast cells. Mast cell degranulation releases histamine, which binds to its H1 receptors along the nasal epithelium. The resulting edema and inflammatory cascade cause nasal congestion, itching, sneezing, running nose, and tearing.

2. **The answer is B. Diphenhydramine shifts the H1 receptor to the inactivated state.** H1 antihistamines are inverse agonists of the H1 receptor. They bind to the inactive conformation of the receptor and shift the equilibrium toward the inactivated state, and reduce the effects of histamine. In contrast, histamine acts as an agonist for the active conformation of the H1 receptor.

3. **The answer is D. Diphenhydramine antagonizes the effect of histamine in the CNS.** Histamine may be important in the maintenance of wakefulness. As a first-generation H1 antihistamine, diphenhydramine is highly lipophilic and crosses the blood–brain barrier and antagonizes this normal effect of histamine in the CNS. The result is drowsiness, a common adverse effect of the first-generation H1-antihistamines.

4. **The answer is C. Loratadine is ionized at physiologic pH and does not cross the blood–brain barrier.** Other second-generation H1 antihistamines similarly are unable to penetrate the CNS. Because of their ionization, they have poor lipophilicity and do not cross the blood–brain barrier to interact with CNS H1 receptors. In addition, they have high protein binding and are not free to diffuse into the CNS.

5. **The answer is D. Altered drug metabolism** can result from cimetidine's inhibition of the P450 enzyme system. Drug–drug interactions with concomitantly administered drugs can lead to reduced drug metabolism, potentially toxic serum drug concentrations, and clinical toxicity. Sedation and dry mouth are potential adverse effects of the first-generation H1 antihistamines. Prolonged QT interval and ventricular dysrhythmias were associated with the second-generation H1 antihistamines, terfenadine and astemizole.

CASE 2

1. **The answer is A. Anaphylaxis is the systemic release of histamine by mast cell degranulation.** When an allergen is distributed systemically in a previously sensitized individual, it can stimulate mast cell and basophil release of histamine systemically. The life-threatening result is local and systemic vasodilation, with airway edema and shock and severe bronchoconstriction.

2. **The answer is C. Ingested penicillin tablets** are the likely cause of this patient's anaphylaxis, given his history of penicillin allergy and rapid onset of symptoms after ingesting unknown white tablets. The β-lactams, particularly penicillin, are the most common drug class associated with hypersensitivity reactions and anaphylaxis. The overall incidence of hypersensitivity is estimated to be approximately 5%, and 1% of penicillin hypersensitivity reactions are anaphylactic in nature.

3. **The answer is D. H1 antihistamines will reduce the histamine-induced vasodilation, edema, and bronchospasm** associated with the patient's anaphylactic symptoms.

4. **The answer is D. Inhaled β_2-receptor agonists will promote bronchial smooth muscle relaxation** and reduce bronchospasm and resistance to airflow. Although they are delivered directly to pulmonary β-receptors, they may have some crossreactivity at cardiac β_1-receptors, contributing to tachycardia. However, this secondary effect would be insufficient to improve this patient's hemodynamic status.

5. **The answer is C. Intravenous epinephrine** is the treatment for life-threatening anaphylaxis. As a nonselective adrenergic agonist, epinephrine reduces bronchospasm through its β_2-receptor agonist effect and improves blood pressure through its peripheral α_1-receptor agonist effect. Intravenous corticosteroids inhibit the transcription of genes for proinflammatory mediators. However, corticosteroid therapy does not produce a significant clinical response until about 6 hours after administration. Oral antihistamines would not be absorbed well in this setting of probable gastrointestinal edema and would not emergently treat anaphylaxis. Oral cromolyn is a prophylactic treatment for asthma that stabilizes mast cells and prevents their degranulation. Cromolyn has no role in the treatment of anaphylaxis. The treatment of anaphylaxis consists of removal of the offending antigen, emergent treatment for the anaphylactic reaction, airway management, and supportive care.

CHAPTER 43 ANSWERS

CASE 1

1. **The answer is B. G-CSF is a glycoprotein that stimulates the production of neutrophils** within the bone marrow. It is released by monocytes, macrophages, epithelial cells, and fibroblasts in the presence of infection. Locally, it stimulates neutrophil-mediated phagocytosis. GM-CSF has a broader effect than G-CSF and stimulates the differentiation of myeloid stem cells into eosinophils, monocytes or macrophages, and neutrophils. It also enhances the activity of mature leukocytes and promotes the differentiation of macrophages into Langerhans cells. Megakaryocytes form platelets under the promotion of thrombopoietin.

2. **The answer is C. Erythropoietin stimulates the differentiation of reticulocytes to erythrocytes.** Under conditions of hypoxia, hypoxia-inducible factor 1 alpha promotes the transcription of genes for erythropoietin in the kidney. Erythropoietin, a glycosylated protein, binds to its receptors in the bone marrow and promotes the differentiation of precursor cells in the erythroid lineage, specifically the differentiation of reticulocytes to erythrocytes. Myeloid cells are precursors of granulocytes, monocytes, and macrophages.

3. **The answer is D. Recombinant hematopoietic growth factors may have modified molecular structures that enhance their potency.** For example, the sialic acid groups attached to recombinant erythropoietin and darbepoietin enhance their potency and prolong their half-lives. Similarly, a G-CSF analogue has been conjugated to polyethylene glycol, which slows its metabolism, allowing for a more prolonged duration of action and less frequent administration. All recombinant hematopoietic growth factors are proteins, similar to their endogenous counterparts, and they must be administered parenterally.

4. **The answer is C. Recombinant human G-CSF can cause bone pain** that resolves with the discontinuation of the drug. GM-CSF is associated with fever, arthralgias, edema, and pleural and pericardial effusions. Recombinant erythropoietin has been associated with polycythemia and blood hyperviscosity when used by nonanemic patients. Erythropoietin and darbepoietin may induce hypertension. Autoantibodies against erythropoietin, and subsequent red cell aplasia, were reported in patients who received a particular formulation of recombinant erythropoietin between 1998 and 2003. Erythropoietin has been associated with a neuronal protective effect following periods of ischemia.

5. **The answer is D. Pancytopenia,** in which all hematopoietic cells lines are diminished, might be an indication for the administration of a general growth factor, such as stem cell factor.

CASE 2

1. **The answer is E. Hydroxyurea stimulates the expression of HbF-containing erythrocytes.** Hydroxyurea blocks cell division by inhibiting ribonucleotide reductase. Its efficacy in the treatment of patients with sickle cell disease may be related to its blocking the division of HbS-expressing erythroid precursors, and triggering a compensatory increase in HbF expression in order to maintain erythropoiesis. Sickle cell patients with increased HbF concentrations have less frequent painful crises and less severe anemia. Fetal hemoglobin consists of two alpha and two gamma chains. Adult erythrocytes contain HbA, which is comprised of two alpha and two beta globin chains.

2. **The answer is A. Hydroxyurea is associated with myelosuppression** and a potential increased risk of infection. Hydroxyurea also suppresses platelet production. Hydroxyurea has been used to treat patients with chronic myelogenous leukemia and polycythemia vera.

3. **The answer is D. Erythropoietin stimulates erythropoiesis of HbS-containing erythrocytes**, as well as that of HbF-containing cells. Its percentage increase in the concentration of HbF is therefore not as significant as that induced by hydroxyurea.

4. **The answer is D.** In Mr. O.'s case, measurements would show **erythropoietin elevated and reticulocyte count elevated**. In the setting of anemia and reduced oxygen-carrying capacity, erythropoietin will be elevated assuming the kidneys are functional. Erythropoietin stimulates precursor cells in the erythroid lineage, including reticulocytes to mature into erythrocytes.

5. **The answer is A. Interleukins control and stimulate white blood cell differentiation.** This family of regulatory proteins can acts as nonselective general growth factors. Some act specifically to enhance lymphocyte development and activation. Others stimulate the CFU-Mix cells, which subsequently become erythrocytes and megakaryocytes. Interferons are also regulatory proteins that modulate lymphocyte growth and activity. They also have antiviral actions and are used in the treatment of patients with hepatitis B and C.

CHAPTER 44 ANSWERS

CASE 1

1. **The answer is D. Cyclosporine prevents IL-2–mediated activation and proliferation of T cells.** It inhibits IL-2 production by activated T cells and the subsequent signaling of other lymphocytes. Anti-thymocyte globulin (ATG) is a preparation of rabbit-derived polyclonal antibodies directed against human T cells. Methotrexate is a folate analogue. Glucocorticoids downregulate the production of inflammatory cytokines. Eculizumab is an antibody against C5.

2. **The answer is E. Azathioprine's effects lack specificity, causing adverse effects.** Its actions affect all rapidly dividing cells, contributing to gastrointestinal and hematopoietic toxicity. However, it was the first immunosuppressant drug used after transplantation and is frequently a first-line agent. Azathioprine is a prodrug of 6-mercaptopurine, a purine analogue that is released when azathioprine reacts with sulfhydryl compounds. Azathioprine is less specific than the newer antimetabolites, mycophenolate mofetil and leflunomide. Leflunomide inhibits pyrimidine synthesis. Methotrexate is a folate analogue.

3. **The answer is C.** Symptoms of fever, myalgias, nausea, diarrhea, and drowsiness can occur after administration of OKT3. The symptoms are caused by OKT3 activation of T cells, resulting in the **cytokine release syndrome**. OKT3 is a mouse monoclonal antibody against human CD3, a membrane-signaling molecule on T cells. It depletes T cells via antibody-mediated activation of complement, and clearance of immune complexes. Because OKT3 is a mouse antihuman antibody, it can induce the formation of anti-OKT3 antibodies that reduce the drug's subsequent efficacy. Hyperacute transplant rejection occurs almost immediately after reperfusion of a transplanted organ because of the presence of preformed recipient antibodies, usually to blood type antigens of donor organs, or to cross-species transplanted tissue. Graft-versus-host disease is an alloimmune reaction that occurs when transplanted immune cells attack recipient cells. Induction therapy refers the administration of daclizumab in the weeks immediately after transplantation. Central tolerance is the process by which T and B cells mature in the thymus and bone marrow such that mature cells will not recognize self as foreign, and any autoreactive T- and B-cell clones are deleted.

4. **The answer is B.** The likely cause of Mrs. W.'s renal disease is **cyclosporine nephrotoxicity**. Cyclosporine is a specific inhibitor of T cells in that it inhibits interleukin-2 production, and its subsequent signaling of T cells. Its use is limited by severe adverse effects, including nephrotoxicity. This occurs because of cyclosporine promotion of interstitial fibrosis. Cyclosporine is also associated with the development of hypertension, hyperlipidemia, neurotoxicity, and hepatotoxicity. Alloimmunity occurs when immune cells recognize different major histocompatibility complex class I molecules on a tissue as foreign, and mount an immune response against that tissue. Inhibition of costimulation occurs then the second of two signals needed to activate immune cells is blocked, as by abatacept or belatacept.

5. **The answer is B.** Sirolimus (rapamycin) is isolated from the fungus *Streptomyces hygroscopicus*. It **inhibits protein synthesis and T-cell division** in the G1 phase. Its adverse effects include hyperlipidemia, leukopenia, and thrombocytopenia, but not nephrotoxicity. Sirolimus-eluting stents have been approved for the treatment of coronary artery disease. They are designed to prevent local coronary artery smooth muscle cell proliferation and in-stent restenosis after coronary stent placement.

CASE 2

1. **The answer is A. Budesonide will downregulate the expression of inflammatory cytokines and suppress prostaglandin production.** Glucocorticoids produce these broad antiinflammatory effects through their interaction with glucocorticoid response elements, which regulate gene expression. They are nonspecific immunosuppressant agents.

2. **The answer is D.** Because of azathioprine's powerful inhibition of normal immune cell function, an adverse effect of this therapy is increased **susceptibility to infection**. Patients should be alert to the development of infectious or constitutional symptoms, including fever, myalgias, generalized malaise, and nausea.

3. **The answer is C. Infliximab will undermine normal inflammatory responses to any infectious agents.** It is a partially humanized mouse antibody to human TNF-α, and it prevents the normal function of this cytokine, including the activation of T-helper cells,

elaboration of acute phase proteins, fever, and local containment of any inflammatory response. Patients being treated with infliximab are at risk for the development of serious infections that can progress to sepsis. Reactivation of latent tuberculosis has been reported in patients being treated with this agent.

4. **The answer is C. Cyclophosphamide, a DNA alkylating agent, is associated with the development of cardiotoxicity and bladder cancer** (as a result of its production of acrolein). Other adverse effects of cyclophosphamide include leukopenia and alopecia. Cyclophosphamide suppresses B-cell antibody production and has been used in the treatment of patients with systemic lupus erythematosus. Long-term use of glucocorticoids can cause weight gain, hypertension, osteoporosis, and diabetes, as well as suppress normal adrenal function. Cyclosporine can cause interstitial fibrosis and renal insufficiency. OKT3 can activate T cells and cause the cytokine release syndrome, characterized by fever, diarrhea, nausea, and drowsiness. Abatacept prevents costimulation and promotes anergy and apoptosis of T cells. Its major adverse effects include exacerbations of bronchitis in patients with chronic obstructive pulmonary disease, as well as increased susceptibility to infection.

5. **The answer is C. Methotrexate** is a folate analogue antimetabolite, which widely alters normal cell functions. It is both cytotoxic and antiinflammatory. Mycophenolate mofetil is a newer antimetabolite with specific action against lymphocytes. Tacrolimus specifically inhibits cell-mediated immunity through its inhibits of cytokine production. Infliximab is a specific antibody directed against TNF-α. OKT3 is a monoclonal antibody against human CD3 and promotes the specific depletion of T cells.

CHAPTER 45 ANSWERS

CASE 1

1. **The answer is C. Cigarette use impairs mucosal blood flow and limits bicarbonate production** by the pancreas. Impaired mucosal blood flow impairs the removal of acid, which has diffused across damaged mucus layers. NSAID use inhibits COX-1–mediated mucosal prostaglandin synthesis. (Prostaglandins are cytoprotective because they inhibit gastric acid secretion and enhance bicarbonate secretion, mucus production, cell turnover, and local mucosal blood flow.) NSAIDs may also potentiate pepsinogen secretion. This effect on pepsinogen by NSAIDs is independent of endogenous prostaglandin inhibition. Finally, NSAIDs also enter gastric epithelial cells, where they are trapped and cause local cell damage. *H. pylori* is a Gram-negative bacterium that is associated with non-NSAID–induced peptic ulcer disease. This bacteria attaches to the surface of gastric epithelial cells and elaborates virulence factors, which cause local cellular damage and promote an inappro-

priate inflammatory response. Increased gastrin secretion and decreased somatostatin and bicarbonate secretion are also associated with *H. pylori* infection. All of these factors promote local cellular damage and inhibit normal physiologic protective mechanisms. Caffeine ingestion is associated with increased gastric acid secretion. Other factors associated with the development of peptic ulcer disease include alcoholic cirrhosis, corticosteroid use, genetic predisposition, and psychological stress. Antacids do not promote gastrin cell proliferation; rather, they neutralize gastric acid.

2. **The answer is A. *H. pylori* produces and secretes damaging urease, lipase, and proteases.** The Gram-negative bacterium attaches to the surface of gastric epithelial cells, where it is able to survive by creating an alkaline buffer with ammonium hydroxide. It elaborates damaging virulence factors and elicits a T_H1 immune response, which promotes cytokine production and enhanced inflammation and epithelial cell damage. The number of antral somatostatin-secreting D cells is reduced in the setting of *H. pylori* infection, resulting in increased gastrin release. Cushing's ulcers are a result of gastric hyperacidity, caused by heightened vagal tone in patients with severe head injuries.

3. **The answer is B. *H. pylori* resistance to metronidazole has been reported in the United States** and is more common than clarithromycin resistance. Resistance is believed to be caused by three point mutations in *H. pylori*, and is of growing concern. The therapeutic regimen for *H. pylori* infection usually involves triple or quadruple therapy with a combination of antibiotics, a PPI, and bismuth (a protective coating agent that combines with mucus glycoproteins to form a barrier to protect cells from acid damage). Adverse effects of *H. pylori* therapy include hypersensitivity reactions to penicillins, nausea, headaches and superinfection with *Clostridium difficile*.

4. **The answer is E. PPIs irreversibly suppress acid secretion for 18 hours.** Their primary mechanism of action is through irreversible inhibition of the H^+/K^+ ATPase proton pump. They are indicated in the treatment of *H. pylori*–associated ulcers because they contribute to eradication of the infection by inhibiting the growth of the bacterium. This is why omeprazole was continued in addition to the rest of Tom's therapy for *H. pylori*-associated ulcer disease. PPIs are also used in the treatment of hemorrhagic ulcers because they support platelet aggregation and maintain clot integrity.

5. **The answer is E. Calcium carbonate binds gastric acid, forming calcium chloride and gas**, specifically carbon dioxide. All antacids neutralize gastric hydrochloric acid by binding to gastric acid and forming a salt and water. Aluminum-containing antacids can bind phosphate, causing hypophosphatemia. Magnesium-containing antacids can cause hypermagnesemia in patients with renal failure. Sodium bicarbonate can contribute to sodium retention. Calcium carbonate acts as an antacid as well as a calcium supplement, but may be constipating.

CASE 2

1. **The answer is A. H2 antagonists inhibit histamine binding to parietal cells and subsequent extrusion of hydrogen ions into the gastric lumen.** Histamine is one of three neurohormonal secretagogues (including gastrin and acetylcholine). Histamine binds to the H2 receptor on the basolateral membrane of parietal cells and through a cAMP-dependent process causes the H^+/K^+ ATPase pump to extrude H^+ into the gastric lumen. H2 antagonists reversibly and competitively block histamine binding to the H2 receptor. H2 antagonists also decrease gastrin- and acetylcholine-induced gastric acid secretion, indicating the importance of histamine in increasing or modulating the effects of cholinergic and gastrin-mediated acid secretion.

2. **The answer is D. Concurrent use of cimetidine and theophylline can cause tachyarrhythmias.** Cimetidine, the first H2 antagonist developed, has several drug–drug interactions. It inhibits the activity of hepatic P450 enzymes and the metabolism of several drugs, including theophylline, quinidine, phenytoin, and warfarin. Inhibition of these drugs' metabolism can lead to clinically significantly toxicity (tachyarrhythmias in the case of theophylline toxicity). Cimetidine is also an antagonist at the androgen receptor and can cause antiandrogenic adverse effects, including gynecomastia in men and galactorrhea in women. It is contraindicated for pregnant and nursing women because it crosses the placenta and is secreted into breast milk. Elimination of H2 antagonists is through both hepatic and renal mechanisms. Therefore, dosages of H2 antagonists should be decreased in the setting of liver failure or renal insufficiency. H2 antagonists compete for renal tubular secretion and can increase the concentrations of similarly eliminated drugs, such as procainamide. Ketoconazole uptake is reduced when it is administered with H2 antagonists because it requires an acidic gastric environment for absorption. PPIs are activated in the acid milieu of the stomach to their active form, a sulfenamide.

3. **The answer is E. PPIs are superior for healing NSAID-induced ulcers** and are indicated in patients who continue to use NSAIDs. PPIs are used to treat *H. pylori*–associated ulcers because they contribute to eradication of the infection. They are indicated for the treatment of hemorrhagic ulcers because they help maintain clot integrity.

4. **The answer is C. Both PPIs and H2 antagonists can be administered intravenously** to treat patients who are unable to take oral formulations. Both agents are hepatically metabolized and renally excreted. PPIs are contraindicated in pregnancy, while H2 antagonists (except cimetidine) are approved for use in pregnancy. Cimetidine can cause galactorrhea. Long-term PPI use is associated with enterochromaffin-like (ECL) and parietal cell hyperplasia in rats. Rats treated with PPIs for long durations have developed gastric carcinoid tumors. This has not been observed in humans.

5. **The answer is C. Sucralfate forms a viscous gel that coats and protects gastric epithelial cells.** It requires the acidic environment of the stomach to exert this protective effect. Colloidal bismuth is another coating agent often administered as part of a multidrug regimen for the treatment of *H. pylori*–associated peptic ulcers. Bismuth may also stimulate bicarbonate secretion and enhance mucosal prostaglandin secretion.

CHAPTER 46 ANSWERS

CASE 1

1. **The answer is B. Ahmad has a genetic atopic predisposition to asthma.** In such patients, an allergen, such as cat dander, can trigger an exaggerated response from T_H2 lymphocytes, and a cellular and humoral inflammatory response that includes the pulmonary infiltration by cells such as eosinophils. In these patients, environmental irritants, exercise, cold air, or infections can all trigger a hypersensitive bronchoconstrictive and hyperreactive inflammatory response.

2. **The answer is C. Epinephrine is a nonselective adrenergic agonist** that acts at both β- and α-adrenergic receptors. Its action at cardiac β_1-receptors causes tachycardia and palpitations, and its effects at peripheral α_1-receptors cause vasoconstriction and elevated blood pressure. These effects could cause Ahmad's feelings of "nervousness" after using an epinephrine-containing inhaler. In contrast, albuterol has a primarily selective agonist action at the β_2-adrenergic receptor, relieving bronchoconstriction. Overreliance on nonprescription epinephrine-containing inhalers for undiagnosed asthma has been associated with death.

3. **The answer is D. Corticosteroids upregulate the transcription of antiinflammatory genes** such as for the cytokines interleukin-10, -12, and -1 receptor antagonist. They also inhibit the transcription of proinflammatory genes. The resulting effect of their action includes a reduction in the number of inflammatory cells and damage to the airway epithelium, as well as a reduction in airway edema. When administered via inhalation, corticosteroids can be administered in smaller doses directly into the pulmonary bronchioles. This increases the amount of drug available at the target tissue and decreases systemic absorption. Newer inhaled corticosteroid preparations also undergo first-pass metabolism in the liver, further limiting systemic exposure to any drug that might be inadvertently swallowed during inhalation administration. Osteoporosis is one potential adverse effect of chronic systemic corticosteroid use.

4. **The answer is D.** Ahmad could relieve some of the oral discomfort and irritation he experiences with inhaled fluticasone by **using a spacer to catch large spray droplets**. Inhaled steroids can also cause oropharyngeal candidiasis from local deposition, and hoarseness secondary to deposition in the larynx. The use of a

spacer, or simply rinsing the mouth after administration, can minimize these symptoms.

5. **The answer is E. Theophylline is a phosphodiesterase inhibitor that can cause dysrhythmias, nausea, and vomiting.** Therapeutically, theophylline exerts a bronchodilating effect by preventing the breakdown of cAMP, resulting in bronchial smooth muscle relaxation. Inhibition of the phosphodiesterase isoenzyme IV in T lymphocytes can also contribute to immunomodulatory and antiinflammatory effects. Unfortunately, the nonspecific actions of theophylline on phosphodiesterase enzymes also contribute to its adverse effects of cardiac dysrhythmias, nausea, and vomiting. Theophylline is also an adenosine receptor antagonist. This antagonist effect can contribute to tachycardia, psychomotor agitation, gastric acid secretion, and diuresis. Because of its many nonspecific actions and narrow therapeutic index, theophylline is rarely used in the treatment of asthma.

6. **The answer is A. Inhalation of the drug delivers it directly to the bronchioles and limits systemic adverse effects.**

7. **The answer is C. The inhibition of single pathways underlying the pathophysiologic process of asthma does not have a significant effect on the clinical disease.** This is because the pathophysiology of asthma involves multiple inflammatory pathways. Therefore, inhaled corticosteroids remain a mainstay of therapy because of their overall antiinflammatory effects. Cromolyns are a prophylactic therapy in patients with allergic asthma associated with specific triggers, such as exercise.

CHAPTER 47 ANSWERS

CASE 1

1. **The answer is B. Ibuprofen prevented COX-2 production of prostaglandins, which is associated with the inflammatory response to intraarticular crystals.** Ibuprofen is a nonselective NSAID that inhibits the activity of both COX-1 and COX-2. Its effects at COX-2 prevent the formation of prostaglandins and thromboxanes, associated with the inflammatory response. Leukotrienes are products of the LOX enzyme metabolism of arachidonic acid. Uric acid crystal deposition in the first metatarsophalangeal joint (podagra) is a common first manifestation of gout (Stage 2 gout). The inflammatory reaction to crystal deposition consists of complement activation, release of chemotactic factors, and phagocyte and neutrophil recruitment and activation.

2. **The answer is D. Uric acid crystals deposit in the synovial tissues of joints that are more peripherally located.** Any variable that decreases the solubility

of urate (which is marginally soluble) can result in uric acid crystal deposition. Urate is less soluble at lower temperatures and in acidic environments. Crystal deposition tends to occur in cooler peripheral joints. Joint synovial fluid is more acidic than blood, favoring intraarticular crystal formation. Asymptomatic hyperuricemia (Stages 1 and 3 gout) can be present without the development of clinical gout. Conversely, it is possible to develop gout in the absence of hyperuricemia (defined as a plasma urate concentration greater than 7.0 mg/dL in men and greater than 6.0 mg/dL in women). Urate is secreted by the kidney and eliminated by the gastrointestinal tract. Deposition of uric acid crystals in periarticular tissues can create tophi, which also promote an inflammatory response and destruction of the synovial lining and cartilage.

3. **The answer is A. Colchicine binds to tubulin and prevents the normal function of neutrophils and macrophages.** Colchicine prevents tubulin polymerization and microtubule formation. Normal microtubule formation is necessary for chemotaxis and adhesion of neutrophils, phagocytosis of particles, trafficking of phagocytosed particles to lysosomes, and release of chemotactic factors. Because its mechanism of action also inhibits cell division, colchicine causes several adverse effects. Nonsteroidal antiinflammatory drugs inhibit COX.

4. **The answer is E. Diarrhea** is a common adverse effect of colchicine use. Because colchicine affects cell division, rapidly replicating cells such as the epithelial cells of the gastrointestinal tract are prevented from undergoing normal turnover. Diarrhea is a result. Other tissues that can be similarly affected include those of the hematopoietic and renal systems. Colchicine can also cause a peripheral neuropathy because of its inhibition of microtubule-dependent movement of nutrients along peripheral nerves.

5. **The answer is A. Coadministration of colchicine reduces the chance of precipitating acute gout** during the initiation of allopurinol therapy. Because allopurinol alters purine metabolism by inhibiting purine degradation, it can disrupt urate homeostasis and worsen or precipitate acute gouty arthritis. Therefore, allopurinol is coadministered with an NSAID or colchicine during the first several months of allopurinol therapy.

CASE 2

1. **The answer is C. Allopurinol is an analogue of xanthine that prevents the normal metabolism of xanthine to urate.** Gout is the result of an imbalance in the production and metabolism of purines (guanine and adenine). Metabolism of purines to hypoxanthine, xanthine, and urate is mediated by xanthine oxidase. This enzyme activity is inhibited by allopurinol, which is oxidized to oxypurinol, which subsequently "freezes" the normal activity of the enzyme's active site. PRPP is a ribose sugar that is the determinant of de novo purine synthesis.

2. **The answer is B.** Mr. J.'s sudden severe left flank pain (and gross hematuria) is caused by **uric acid stones obstructing the left ureter**. Uric acid is filtered and reabsorbed in the kidney, accounting for 65% of its elimination. High urinary urate concentrations, acidic urine, and dehydration can predispose individuals to the formation of urate stones in the kidney and ureter. Hypoxanthine and xanthine are moderately more soluble than urate and can be filtered in the kidney without forming stones. Uricase is an enzyme that oxidizes uric acid to allantoin, a compound easily excreted by the kidney. Humans do not produce endogenous uricase. It is available in the European Union as a protein purified from the fungus *Aspergillus flavus*. Rasburicase is available in the United States.

3. **The answer is A. Probenecid inhibits the proximal renal tubule anion exchanger and decreases urate reabsorption in the proximal tubule.** Probenecid is a uricosuric agent used in the treatment of chronic hyperuricemia in patients with gout. By enhancing the renal elimination of urate, probenecid shifts the balance between renal excretion and endogenous formation of urate, and lowers plasma urate concentrations.

4. **The answer is D. Probenecid limits the renal elimination of penicillins** and other organic anions. Therefore, although probenecid lowers plasma urate concentrations, it can cause an increase in the concentration of some drugs, necessitating an adjustment in drug dosage. Sulfinpyrazone has antiplatelet effects and can cause hematologic toxicity. Losartan is an angiotensin II receptor antagonist that also has uricosuric properties. Allopurinol inhibits the normal metabolism of purine analogues, such as azathioprine and mercaptopurine, both of which are also metabolized by xanthine oxidase.

5. **The answer is B.** Purine-rich foods include **dried beans**, sardines in oil, herring, organ meats, peas, spinach, asparagus, cauliflower, and mushrooms. Alcoholic beverages are also rich in purine.

VII

Fundamentals of Drug Development and Regulation

48

Drug Discovery and Preclinical Development

	Drug discovery		**Drug development**			
Phase	Target based Compound based	Lead optimization	Preclinical development	Phase I	Phase II	Phase III
Chemistry discovery						
Biology discovery	Target identification	Assay development and screening	Animal models of disease			
ADME	In vitro metabolism	Pharmacokinetics (animal)		(human)	Metabolism ⟶ Drug–drug interactions ⟶	
Toxicology	Screening	Preclinical	GLP toxicology ⟶		Development and reproduction	Carcinogenesis ⟶
Development chemistry						
Medical				Safety / Exposure	Efficacy / Dose selection	Registration trials

↑ IND   ↑ NDA

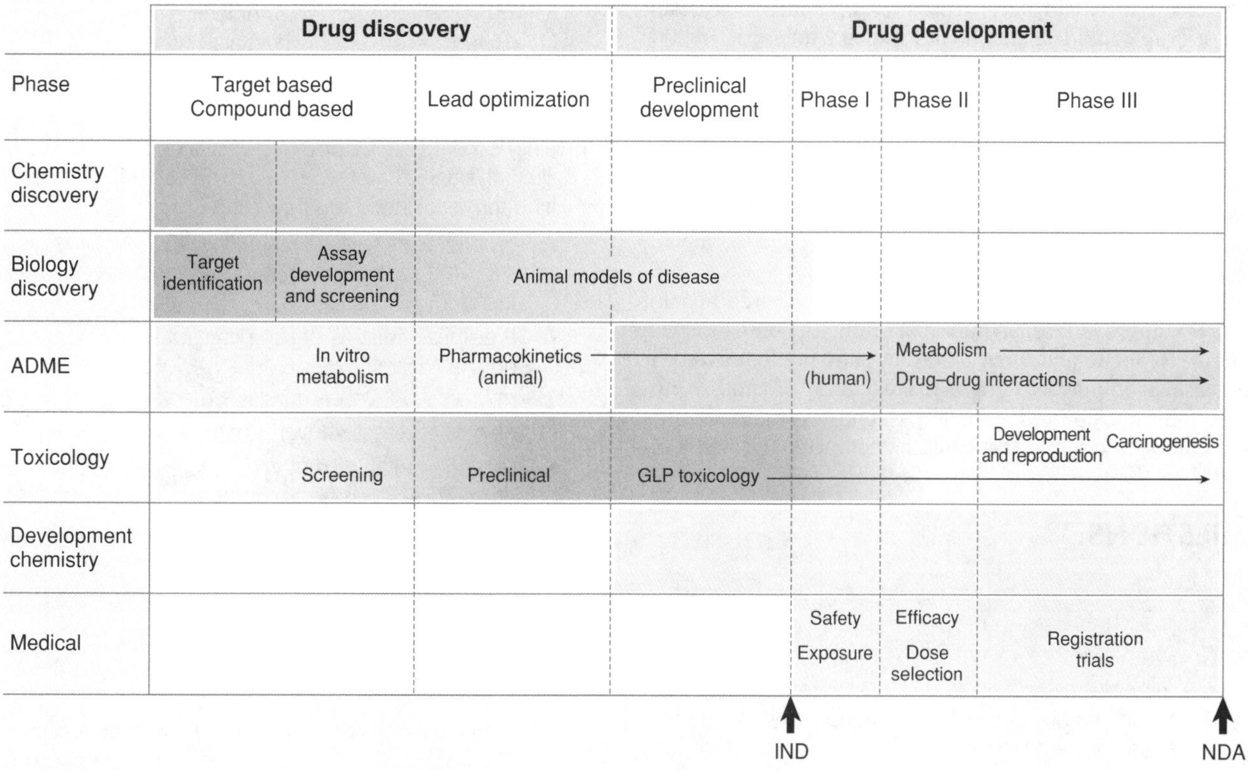

Figure 48-1. Sequence of Phases of Drug Discovery and Development. The important points to note are the general sequence of activities and the considerable overlap of functions with time. The process is highly interactive among several disciplines in an attempt to obtain the molecule with the greatest efficacy, fewest adverse effects, and greatest safety. The entire process from hit to drug approval can take 8 to 12 years and cost more than $1 billion. ADME = absorption, distribution, metabolism, and excretion; GLP = good laboratory practices; IND = investigational new drug application; NDA = new drug application.

OBJECTIVES

■ Understand the drug discovery process and phases of drug development.

 CASE 1

In 1987, researchers at Abbott Laboratories decided to target human immunodeficiency virus (HIV) protease in their search for a novel antiviral therapeutic. Abbott chose the protease because it is essential to HIV's replication and because it has an unusual substrate specificity (see Chapter

36, Pharmacology of Viral Infections). Because the natural substrate for the enzyme contains a phenylalanine–proline bond, a rare cleavage site for mammalian proteases, researchers reasoned that a drug that inhibits HIV protease would have relatively few adverse effects.

In 1989, crystallographers at Merck announced that they had elucidated the crystal structure of HIV protease. Based on the newly solved structure, researchers now knew that the viral protease was a symmetric dimer of two identical subunits. Using a molecular model, researchers at Abbott designed an analogue of the enzyme's natural substrate by replacing the proline in the natural sequence with a phenylalanine; this analogue was a symmetric molecule containing identical amino acids on each end of the structure. They also replaced the peptide bond in the center of the molecule with a functional group that mimicked the transition state of the enzymatic reaction, but was resistant to cleavage by the protease. Although this first molecule was a weak inhibitor of viral protease, the researchers used knowledge about the enzyme's structure to add additional functional groups to the molecule that would likely increase its potency. The result was a drug candidate that bound the enzyme with 10,000-fold higher affinity than the first structure; however, this candidate displayed poor pharmacokinetics.

Chemists continued to alter functional groups on the candidate drug until ritonavir, a highly potent molecule with acceptable pharmacokinetic properties, was created. Incidentally, studies of ritonavir in tissue culture showed that it inhibited a cytochrome P450 enzyme involved in the metabolism of other candidate protease inhibitors.

In 1996 (about 9 years after the initial research began), the FDA approved ritonavir for marketing. In 2000, based on pharmacokinetic and clinical studies showing that ritonavir increases the bioavailability (see Chapter 3) of another protease inhibitor, lopinavir, the FDA approved the marketing of a combination drug that contains both ritonavir and lopinavir.

QUESTIONS

1. What methods can researchers use to "discover" new drugs such as ritonavir?
   A. Synthesize natural products to make them biologically active.
   B. Modify natural products to enhance their affinity for a targeted receptor.
   C. Identify receptor targets and destroy them.
   D. Alter the molecular structure of biologic targets to fit current compounds.
   E. Test current libraries of compounds on diseased animals to find a "hit."

2. How can structural information about a molecular target help in the drug discovery process?
   A. Understanding the three-dimensional structure of an active site facilitates a "shotgun" approach to molecular screening of potential molecules.
   B. Identifying the three-dimensional structure of an active site negates the need for animal testing of potential molecules as future drugs.

   C. Identifying the three-dimensional structure of an active site allows for the design of a molecule to fit specifically into the site.
   D. Understanding the three-dimensional structure of an active site allows for its modification to fit known natural compounds.
   E. Crystallizing an active site along with its substrate can cure disease.

3. How do researchers evaluate drug candidates?
   A. They test potential molecules in diseased persons.
   B. They study potential genotoxicity in human fetuses.
   C. They test various formulations of the molecule to ensure that it can always be administered orally.
   D. They examine the metabolism of the molecule to predict potential drug–drug interactions and toxic metabolites.
   E. They compare potential molecules with natural compounds to ensure biologic activity.

4. How do drug development investigations help elucidate likely therapeutic features of a drug candidate, such as its pharmacokinetics and toxicities?
   A. Preclinical analysis of potential drugs ensures that a sufficient quantity of high-quality drug can be manufactured.
   B. Preclinical analysis of drug efficacy is conducted only on the most ill patients.
   C. Clinical studies of potential drugs must be conducted and tested over a minimum of 5 years.
   D. Clinical studies of drug toxicity are conducted after drug efficacy can be assured.
   E. Preclinical phase II trials are conducted to determine pharmacokinetics and toxicity in animal subjects.

5. The story of the development of ritonavir illustrates the process of:
   A. a compound-centered approach to drug design
   B. a natural analogue approach to drug design
   C. target-centered approach to drug design
   D. a phase III trial of drug design
   E. a "shotgun" approach to drug design

■ CASE 2

In the 1990s, cell adhesion molecules, which facilitate the adherence of circulating cells to endothelial cells, were identified. One of these molecules, the α4β1 integrin, was demonstrated on the surface of immune cells. α4β1 interacts with the vascular cell-adhesion molecule 1 (VCAM1) on the surface of endothelial cells. The binding of these molecules allows the adhesion of immune cells to the endothelium, and their subsequent penetration of the blood–brain barrier and entry into the central nervous system (CNS).

Researchers hypothesized that if the adhesion molecule, $\alpha4\beta1$, could be targeted, the entry of immune cells into the CNS could be prevented. This effect would have significant therapeutic possibilities in the treatment of autoimmune-associated diseases of the nervous system.

A monoclonal antibody to $\alpha4\beta1$ was developed and tested in rats. It was found to prevent the entry of autoimmune cells into the CNS, and to prevent the development of experimental autoimmune encephalitis, an animal model of multiple sclerosis. These encouraging results were the basis for the development of natalizumab, a humanized monoclonal antibody against the $\alpha4$ subunit of the $\alpha4\beta1$ integrin on immune cells.

QUESTIONS

1. The story of the development of natalizumab illustrates the process of:
   A. a compound-centered approach to drug discovery
   B. a combinatorial chemistry approach to drug discovery
   C. a target-centered approach to drug discovery
   D. a natural ligand approach to drug discovery
   E. a biological pathway approach to drug discovery

In clinical trials, natalizumab reduced the rates of disability in patients with multiple sclerosis and reduced the rate of relapse by 66%. Natalizumab was approved by the FDA in November 2004 for the treatment of patients with multiple sclerosis.

2. How did discovery chemistry and discovery biology interact in the production of natalizumab?
   A. A biological process was elucidated, for which chemical molecules were designed for biochemical testing of activity.
   B. Medicinal chemists prepared antibodies that were tested on multiple biological markers.
   C. Medicinal chemists determined the pK_A at which biological antibodies could function.
   D. Biologists measured the enzyme activity of the designated antibodies.
   E. A biological process was elucidated, and chemically altered to cure disease.

Three months after the introduction of natalizumab, it was linked to two cases of fatal progressive multifocal leukoencephalopathy (PML) in patients with multiple sclerosis. (PML is a rare, usually fatal viral infection of the CNS, caused by reactivation of the JC virus, an ubiquitous human polyomavirus, to which the majority of adults in Europe and the United States have antibodies.) Natalizumab was withdrawn, and all clinical trials were placed on hold as of February 2005 while the prior trial results were reviewed. On review, two cases of fatal PML occurred out of 1869 patients with multiple sclerosis treated with natalizumab for a median of 120 weeks. One additional case of PML was found of 1043 patients with Crohn's disease, after the patient received eight doses of the drug. Clinical trials were resumed in February 2006, and natalizumab was again approved in June 2006 by the FDA under a supplemental biologics license application. Natalizumab was reintroduced as monotherapy for relapsing forms of multiple sclerosis under a special, monitored drug registration and administration program, the TOUCH™ distribution program.

3. What is the relationship between preclinical animal and clinical human trials of new drugs?
   A. Animal studies cannot predict human adverse effects.
   B. Animal studies should be performed in models that mirror aspects of the targeted human disease.
   C. Animal studies should be performed for at least 120 weeks of drug therapy before human trials are initiated.
   D. Animal toxicity studies are regulated to prevent any deaths in subsequent human trials.
   E. Animal repeat-dose toxicity studies provide little data on the long-term effects of drugs in humans.

4. The physical and chemical characteristics of a drug are critical for knowing how best it can be administered, and how it should be stored. Which of the following statements regarding the chemical characterization of a drug is true?
   A. Mass spectrometry provides information on the three-dimensional structure of a drug.
   B. Nuclear magnetic resonance provides information on the molecular weight of a drug.
   C. The partition coefficient of a drug describes how well it distributes between an aqueous solvent and a hydrophobic solvent.
   D. A drug's solubility in oil solvents correlates with its enhanced bioavailability.
   E. X-ray crystallography characterizes the atomic composition of a drug.

5. Which of the following characteristics of a drug often require that it be administered parenterally, rather than enterally?
   A. The drug has no first-pass metabolism.
   B. The drug is acid insensitive.
   C. The drug is intended to act topically.
   D. The drug is water soluble.
   E. The drug is not water soluble.

49

Clinical Drug Evaluation and Regulatory Approval

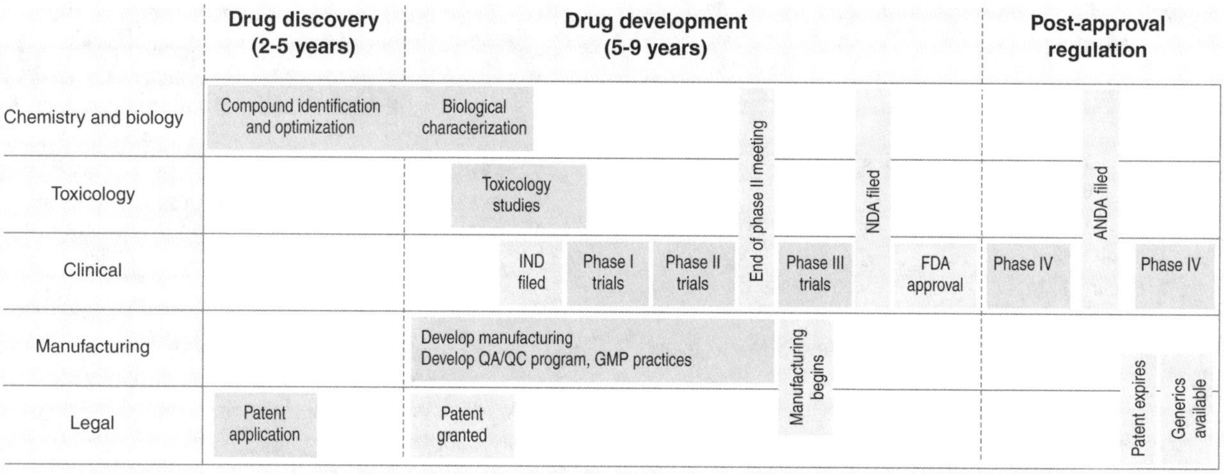

	Drug discovery (2-5 years)		Drug development (5-9 years)						Post-approval regulation	
Chemistry and biology	Compound identification and optimization	Biological characterization								
Toxicology		Toxicology studies				End of phase II meeting	NDA filed		ANDA filed	
Clinical			IND filed	Phase I trials	Phase II trials		Phase III trials	FDA approval	Phase IV	Phase IV
Manufacturing		Develop manufacturing Develop QA/QC program, GMP practices					Manufacturing begins		Patent expires	Generics available
Legal	Patent application	Patent granted								

Figure 49-2. Life Cycle of Drug Approval. The life cycle of approval for a new drug is complex, requiring an average of 11 years for completion. Drug discovery, discussed in Chapter 48, produces a new drug molecule. The first patents are usually filed at this stage and are granted several years later. The drug development process requires that biological characterization and toxicology studies in animals are conducted before an Investigational New Drug (IND) Application can be filed. In turn, an IND is required for the start of clinical trials. At the conclusion of successful clinical trials, a drug company files a New Drug Application (NDA), which is reviewed by the FDA. Once a drug is approved, it must be monitored for safety for the remainder of its lifespan (so-called phase IV). The first of the drug's patents expire 20 years after its application. Abbreviated New Drug Applications (ANDAs) can be filed before the original patent expires. Once a patent expires, generic versions of that drug can become available.

OBJECTIVES

■ Understand the process of drug evaluation and clinical drug development as it pertains to the drug approval process.

 ## CASE 1

Throughout the 1980s, Pfizer invested in research and development of a drug intended for the treatment of hypertension and angina. During clinical trials, the hoped-for efficacy was minimal; however, investigators (and subjects) observed that impotent men receiving the treatment were able to achieve erections. Pfizer subsequently patented this molecule for the treatment of erectile dysfunction (ED) and proceeded with its development. Between July 1993 and January 1997, 21 studies involving 3000 subjects ages 19 to 87 years were undertaken. In March 1998, Pfizer received approval from the Food and Drug Administration (FDA) to market sildenafil citrate as an oral therapy for ED. The drug was approved under the trade name Viagra®.

Sildenafil proved to be successful in treating ED. In addition, the drug offered patients greater convenience over existing treatments, which included an alprostadil pellet inserted into the urethra, an alprostadil injection administered directly into the base of the penis, and a constriction loop designed to slow venous outflow from the penis. Despite its widespread adoption, however, sildenafil was linked to a small number of deaths. In the 6 months following approval, a period during which more than six million prescriptions were dispensed, the FDA received reports of 130 deaths. Of these deaths, 77 were the result of cardiovascular events such as myocardial infarction, cardiac arrest, and coronary artery disease. Subsequent testing revealed conditions, situations, or drug interactions (e.g., concomitant use of nitrates) that represent contraindications to the use of sildenafil. As a result, the FDA ordered Pfizer to amend its label to include expanded warnings of potential cardiovascular adverse effects and drug interactions. In July 2005, the FDA reported in an alert that a small number of men lost eyesight in one eye sometime after taking sildenafil. This type of vision loss is called nonarteritic anterior ischemic optic neuropathy (NAION). The alert was followed by an additional update of the label and the labels of other drugs of the same class, vardenafil and tadalafil; the new labels gave a narrower description of the type of patients for whom sildenafil and other type V phosphodiesterase inhibitors are believed to be safe and appropriate.

QUESTIONS

1. What ethical standards govern the relationship between physicians and patients in clinical research?
   A. The clinical trial represents the best interests of the participant.
   B. The clinical trial must minimize the risks for the participants.
   C. The clinical trial must not continue if adverse events occur.
   D. The investigator must inform all participants when an adverse event occurs.
   E. The participant is not allowed to terminate their participation in a trial after they have assumed the risks and benefits of participating.

2. What is the purpose of informed consent in clinical trials?
   A. Informed consent assures that the investigator will not allow an adverse event to occur to a participant.
   B. Informed consent explains the benefits of the study to the participant.
   C. Informed consent explains the regulations regarding trial participation.
   D. Informed consent is a process in which participants are made aware of potential risks and benefits of a trial.
   E. Informed consent is not required for dying patients to participate in a study.

3. What testing must a drug undergo in order to gain approval for marketing?
   A. The drug must be tested for patient perceptions of palatability.
   B. The drug must be tested in all age groups and in gravid women to ensure safety.

C. The drug must be tested in three phases to ensure that all participants are blinded to the perceived effect of the drug.
D. The drug must be tested in three phases to rule out any placebo effect.
E. The drug must be tested in three phases with progressively increasing numbers of participants, and outcome measures.

4. Clinical studies proceed in three phases. Which of the following statements regarding Phase I, II, and III clinical trials of a drug candidate is correct?
   A. Phase I studies ascertain the pharmacokinetics of the drug in a small number of ill patients.
   B. Phase II studies ascertain the safety of a drug in ever-increasing dosages in several hundred healthy participants.
   C. Phase II studies are often nonblinded so that subjects can report any adverse effects quickly.
   D. Phase III studies ascertain specific clinical endpoints in several thousand patients with the disease of interest.
   E. Despite the progressive use of three phases of drug evaluation, the effects of the drug in the general population cannot be determined until the drug is approved for marketing.

5. A drug's approval depends on demonstrating that it is effective in improving primary clinical endpoints in Phase III studies. Which of the following is an example of a primary endpoint?
   A. total body tumor burden is decreased
   B. appetite improves
   C. serum glucose is lowered
   D. blood pressure is lowered
   E. mortality is decreased

■ CASE 2

Cyclooxygenase (COX) is an enzyme that plays an important role in the initiation of the prostaglandin synthesis cascade, and subsequently, inflammatory conditions. In the early 1990s, the cyclooxygenase-2 (COX-2) gene was discovered. It was found that COX-2 is an inducible enzyme and a mediator of the inflammatory response. This is in contrast to COX-1, which is constitutively expressed and responsible for many protective functions, particularly the maintenance of the gastrointestinal mucosal lining. Researchers hypothesized that a drug that selectively inhibits COX-2 while sparing COX-1 should be an effective antiinflammatory agent that does not have the potential adverse gastrointestinal side effects associated with COX-1 inhibition.

When the molecular structures of COX-1 and COX-2 were elucidated, substrates with specific antagonist activity at COX-2 were developed. Celecoxib and rofecoxib, the first specific COX-2 inhibitors, were developed and tested in animal models. They were found to decrease the inflammatory response in experimental animals without adversely affecting their gastrointestinal mucosa.

QUESTIONS

1. The trials of COX-2 inhibitors in animals are examples of:
   A. Preclinical animal studies of efficacy and toxicity
   B. Phase I trials of safety
   C. Phase II trials of efficacy
   D. Phase II trials of long-term primary endpoints
   E. Crossover placebo-controlled trials

On the basis of large-scale clinical trials, in May 1999, Merck received approval from the FDA to market rofecoxib as Vioxx® for the treatment of rheumatoid arthritis pain and inflammation. It was advertised as an antiinflammatory without gastrointestinal adverse effects. The drug quickly became very popular.

In November, 2000, the results of the VIGOR (Vioxx Gastrointestinal Outcomes Research) study were published, suggesting an association between the incidence of cardiovascular events and rofecoxib use. The VIGOR Study was a prospective, randomized, double-blind trial conducted in 8076 patients with rheumatoid arthritis. The study was designed to compare the incidence of serious gastrointestinal events associated with rofecoxib versus naproxen. The dose of rofecoxib studied was 50 mg/day, twice the FDA-approved dosage for long-term use. Patients at high risk for cerebrovascular and cardiovascular disease were excluded. The investigators noted a higher incidence of myocardial infarction (0.4% vs. 0.1%) in the rofecoxib group, and attributed this to a protective effect of naproxen as an antiplatelet nonselective nonsteroidal antiinflammatory drug (NSAID) and the lack of aspirin prophylaxis in a significant percentage of study participants.

2. The VIGOR study of rofecoxib and naproxen did not have a placebo arm. What is the utility of a placebo "control" in a study?
   A. A placebo control contributes to subject bias.
   B. A placebo control contributes to observer bias.
   C. A placebo control facilitates the interpretation of results as being attributable to drug effect, or to natural variations in disease.
   D. A placebo control facilitates the pharmacokinetic analysis of the study drug.
   E. A placebo control facilitates the interpretation of the "blinded" arm of the study.

The results of the APPROVe (Adenomatous Polyp Prevention on Vioxx) Trial were subsequently published in 2005. This was a prospective, randomized, double-blind, controlled trial conducted on 2586 patients with a history of colonic adenoma. The study was designed to determine the effect of 3 years of treatment with rofecoxib (25 mg/day) on the risk of recurrent neoplastic polyps of the large bowel. The incidence of thrombotic events (cerebrovascular, cardiovascular) was reported. The study was concluded early because of the incidence of adverse events in the rofecoxib group (hypertension, peripheral edema). Patients taking rofecoxib had a higher incidence and risk of serious thrombotic events, including acute stroke and myocardial infarction. The increased relative risk (1.92) of severe thrombotic events was apparent at 18 months of therapy.

3. When is an investigator required to terminate a clinical study before all clinical endpoints and outcomes have been measured?
   A. An investigator must terminate a study when a participant dies.
   B. An investigator must terminate a study when the risk of adverse effects on participants is perceived to be unacceptable.
   C. An investigator must terminate a study when the FDA considers it "not approved."
   D. An investigator must terminate a study when a participant complains to the FDA.
   E. An investigator must terminate a study when outcome measures of primary clinical endpoints show no drug effect.

The APC (Adenoma Prevention with Celecoxib) Study was also published in 2005. It was a prospective, randomized, double-blind study of 2035 patients with a history of colorectal neoplasia enrolled in a trial of low-dose (200 mg twice daily) versus high-dose (400 mg twice daily) celecoxib versus placebo for the prevention of colorectal adenomas. Celecoxib use was associated with a dose-related increase in the risk of myocardial infarction, sudden cardiac death, stroke, and heart failure: 3.4% high dose versus 2.3% low dose versus 1% placebo.

Given the results of these studies, in February 2001, the FDA Arthritis Advisory Committee met to discuss the association between rofecoxib and adverse cardiovascular events. The committee suggested a ''mandatory trial to assess cardiovascular risks or benefits of coxibs.'' In April 2002, the FDA instructed Merck to include a cardiovascular risk warning on the package insert for Vioxx®.

4. What is the purpose of the "black box" warning?
   A. The "black box" warning lists key safety information for drugs with certain safety risks.
   B. The "black box" warning summarizes all of the adverse events that have occurred in clinical trials of the drug.
   C. The "black box" warning contains toxicity information in the event of drug overdose.
   D. The "black box" warning lists safer, alternative drugs for use by patients who are at high risk of adverse effects.
   E. The "black box" warning provides readily understandable safety information translated into several languages.

In September 2004, rofecoxib was withdrawn from the market. More than 80 million patients are estimated to have taken the drug, accounting for drug sales profits of more than $250 billion annually. Since its withdrawal, a follow-up to the APPROVe Trial has been conducted to determine the incidence of adverse cardiovascular events in those patients who had participated in the original trial.

5. What was the purpose of the 1938 Food, Drug, and Cosmetic Act?

A. This act offers financial incentives to drug manufacturers that will develop orphan drugs.

B. This act mandates that dying patients must be included in compassionate use protocols.

C. This act supports the "off-label" use of drugs that are administered to dying patients.

D. This act provided for the creation of the FDA.

E. This act mandates that all drug manufacturers must obtain premarket approval from the FDA, contingent on the demonstrated safety of a new drug.

50

Systematic Detection of Adverse Events in Marketed Drugs

OBJECTIVES

■ Understand the rationale for postmarketing surveillance for adverse drug events.

■ Understand how pharmacoepidemiologic data are collected and analyzed to ascertain the relative risk or odds ratio of adverse events in marketed drugs.

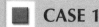

CASE 1

Edna C. is a 42-year-old woman with severe Type II diabetes. She has had difficulty complying with her insulin regimen, and on recent office visits, her hemoglobin A1c levels have been unacceptably high. Her physician has heard about an advance in the management of diabetes, a novel class of medications known as thiazolidinediones (TZDs). These drugs do not influence insulin secretion but instead enhance its action at target tissues. Eager to try and manage Ms. C.'s condition with this approach, her doctor prescribes the first drug in this class to be approved for clinical use, troglitazone (Rezulin®). Soon Ms. C.'s blood sugars and hemoglobin A1c levels decrease to near normal values and she experiences less polyuria and fatigue.

Three months after beginning troglitazone, Ms. C. complains of flu-like symptoms, nausea, and loss of appetite. Shortly thereafter, her husband notes that her complexion has become "sallow." Five days later, she is lethargic, and her skin is frankly jaundiced. Her total bilirubin level is 10.7 mg/dL (normal, 0.0–1.0 mg/dL), and her serum transaminase levels are 30 times the upper limit of normal. Within 1 week, she is comatose, and a diagnosis is made of fulminant acute hepatic necrosis, probably caused by troglitazone. An acceptable donor match is found, and Ms. C. undergoes a successful liver transplant.

Within weeks, similar case reports cause the manufacturer and regulatory authorities in most nations to suspend the use of troglitazone. It remains available in the U.S. market, where proponents argue that the public health benefits of potentially better diabetes control outweigh the relatively rare cases of hepatotoxicity that the new medication may cause. During this time, dozens of additional cases of troglitazone-induced liver failure are reported; 2 years later, it is withdrawn from the U.S. market.

Newer agents in the same class (pioglitazone, rosiglitazone) were introduced into practice after the withdrawal of troglitazone. Although similar to the older drug in their mechanism of action, they do not appear to present the same risk of liver damage, and they continue in widespread use. Ms. C. is doing well with her transplanted liver but requires chronic use of immunosuppressive drugs. Her diabetes is in excellent control on insulin and metformin.

QUESTIONS

1. How are drug risks ascertained before Food and Drug Administration (FDA) approval?
   A. Adverse effects in populations outside the United States are measured before FDA approval is given for a new drug.
   B. Large populations of clinical study volunteers are monitored for adverse effects for a minimum of 5 years.
   C. The incidence of adverse drug effects is noted in clinical trials and extrapolated to the general population.
   D. Toxicologic testing of drugs in animal models disqualifies all drugs with potential adverse effects from the approval process.
   E. Drugs that demonstrate efficacy compared with placebo are considered to be "low risk" in causing potential adverse effects.

275

2. What are the strengths and weaknesses of the pre-approval drug safety process?
   A. Strength: Clinical trial subjects accurately reflect the population of intended drug users.
   B. Strength: The mandated use of placebo-controlled clinical trials ensures future drug safety and efficacy.
   C. Strength: The duration of clinical trials is sufficient to measure beneficial "surrogate outcomes" of drug effect.
   D. Weakness: The incidence of a rare adverse drug effect is very difficult to measure in clinical trials.
   E. Weakness: Adequate clinical trials are difficult to perform because healthy volunteers are unwilling to be studied.

3. How do physicians and patients learn about the frequency and severity of adverse drug effects after approval?
   A. Physicians must enroll their patients in Phase IV studies of potential long-term adverse drug effects.
   B. Physicians must await the results of Phase IV studies of new drugs.
   C. Physicians access information from spontaneous reports to the FDA of adverse drug effects.
   D. Drug manufacturers require all patients to enroll in automated databases, which are periodically reviewed for adverse effects associated with new drugs.
   E. HMOs monitor adverse drug effects and cancel prescriptions when these effects occur.

4. How is the risk–benefit profile of a drug monitored after it is in widespread clinical use?
   A. Individual patients report any adverse effects to their primary care physicians.
   B. Individual patients report beneficial effects of drugs to the FDA.
   C. Cohorts of patients are followed to ascertain the benefits of a new drug.
   D. Case-control studies prospectively follow populations and quantify the hospitalizations in each group.
   E. Cohorts of patients are followed to determine the relative risk of the occurrence of an adverse effect.

5. Given that all medications have some adverse effects, how safe is "safe enough" in relation to a drug's benefits?
   A. A higher rate of potentially adverse effects might be acceptable if the drug is extremely efficacious in its therapeutic benefits.
   B. A statistical analysis of drug effects that reveals the incidence of adverse effects to occur less than once per 10,000 patients is acceptable as "safe."
   C. A comparison of the drug that reveals its rate of adverse effects to be significantly less than a competi-

tor drug, with a p value of <.05, is evidence of "safe enough."
   D. The FDA determines drug safety, based on individual patient profiles of comorbidities and potential confounding drug interactions.
   E. The risks and benefits of drug use are not able to be determined.

■ CASE 2

It is 1993. Yusa G. is a 33-year-old woman with a history of obesity since she was a teenager. She has a body mass index of 31 (normal, 18.5–24.9), a measure of body fat based on height and weight. Her primary care physician has counseled her for several years that she needs to lose weight to reduce her future risk of diabetes, dyslipidemias, heart disease, and arthritis. Despite attempts at dieting, Ms. G. has not been successful in reducing her weight. She has no great interest in exercise because simply walking around the block makes her feel short of breath.

Ms. G. has heard of the miraculous effects of a new diet drug combination, Fen-Phen. This combination of fenfluramine and phentermine was reported in a 1992 study from the University of Rochester to be more effective than diet and exercise in reducing weight. Ms. G. has read a summary of the study: More than 100 chronically obese patients took the drug combination, and they lost about 30 pounds on average! These people had no major reported adverse effects. Ms. G. calls her doctor to request a prescription for Fen-Phen.

QUESTIONS

1. Phentermine was approved by the FDA in 1959 as an appetite suppressant for the short-term (several weeks) treatment of chronic obesity. Fenfluramine was similarly approved by the FDA in 1973. Both are phenylethanolamines (amphetamine-like agents). How does the approval of these individual drugs for short-term use relate to their use and reported effects in combination?
   A. FDA approval of individual drugs implies that they are safe when used with other drugs.
   B. FDA approval of two individual drugs with similar therapeutic effects indicates that their combined effect will be synergistic.
   C. FDA approval of individual drugs is necessary for them to be subsequently used in combination.
   D. FDA approval of two individual drugs is not an indication of their safety when used in combination.
   E. FDA approval of two individual drugs with similar therapeutic effects includes an evaluation of their risk-benefit profile.

Ms. G.'s primary doctor, Dr. Lewis, is uncomfortable prescribing this combination of medications. She explains that this is an ''off-label'' use of the drugs. Their safety in combination has not been studied. Ms. G. is disappointed but agrees to another trial of an intensive diet and exercise regimen.

It is 1996. Despite her best efforts, Ms. G. has lost only 10 pounds in the past 18 months. She is exhausted by the stress of being overweight, and not being able to lose significant weight. She reads in the news that more than 6.6 million prescriptions have been written for Fen-Phen in the United States. She considers this information to be proof that Fen-Phen is ''safe enough'' for her! She visits a local clinic and obtains a prescription for Fen-Phen.

2. How does the annual number of prescriptions for a new drug relate to its efficacy and long-term safety?
   A. The number of prescriptions written for a new drug is not related to its long-term safety.
   B. The number of prescriptions written for a new drug is an indication of its proven long-term efficacy.
   C. The number of prescriptions written for a new drug is limited by the FDA to researchers who will closely monitor patients for adverse effects.
   D. The number of prescriptions written for a new drug is dictated by the pharmaceutical manufacturer's limited distribution of the drug.
   E. The number of prescriptions written for a new drug is not associated with the initial promotional advertising for the drug.

It is now 1997. Ms. G. loves the effects of her Fen-Phen. She has lost 45 pounds in the past 12 months and has not been back to Dr. Lewis. However, she reads a brief article in the newspaper that the Mayo Clinic has published a report of 24 obese patients who developed valvular heart disease, some requiring valve replacement. These patients had been taking the Fen-Phen combination diet aid. Over the summer of 1997, the FDA continues to receive reports of patients using Fen-Phen and dexfenfluramine (another related appetite suppressant) for prolonged periods and subsequently developing aortic and mitral valve abnormalities and primary pulmonary hypertension. In July 1997, the FDA issues a Public Health Advisory informing the public of potential adverse effects associated with Fen-Phen and dexfenfluramine. Ms. G. continues to take her diet pills. She has felt fine for the past year. However, she plans to discontinue Fen-Phen when she feels she has reached her desired goal weight.

3. What is one possible reason that these adverse effects were not revealed in clinical trials of the drugs?
   A. The clinical trials were performed outside of the United States and were not subject to FDA oversight.
   B. The clinical trials could not reproduce this effect, which was previously detected in animal models.
   C. The clinical trials measured inappropriate surrogate outcomes.

   D. The clinical trials did not have the authority to publish the data on adverse cardiac effects.
   E. The clinical trials were not of sufficient duration to detect this rare adverse effect.

In September 1997, the FDA requests a voluntary withdrawal of fenfluramine and dexfenfluramine from the U.S. market. Patients are advised to discontinue the use of these drugs in conjunction with an evaluation by their physician. Ms. G. is relieved that she seems to have suffered no ill effects from Fen-Phen. However, in early 1998, she develops lower extremity edema in her feet and shortness of breath when she walks. Frightened, she calls Dr. Lewis for an appointment and an echocardiogram.

As of 2006, phentermine is still available in the United States. Online advertisements for appetite suppressants have still promoted phentermine in combination with the selective serotonin reuptake inhibitor (SSRI) fluoxetine (Prozac®) as Phen-Pro. This combination of drugs has not been approved by the FDA and is considered an ''off-label'' use of these medications.

4. As a result of a cohort study of a new drug, the relative risk of developing a particular adverse outcome is calculated to be 3. What does this mean?
   A. Patients using the new drug are able to take only one third of the directed dose before they develop an adverse outcome.
   B. Patients using the new drug are three times more likely to develop an adverse outcome.
   C. Patients using the new drug may take it up to three times daily before they develop an adverse outcome.
   D. Patients not using the new drug have three times the risk of developing an adverse outcome.
   E. Patients not using the new drug can take up to three times the recommended dose before they experience an adverse outcome.

5. How can biological advances specifically improve drug monitoring for safety?
   A. Biological advances allow for the evaluation of large numbers of patients.
   B. Biological advances further the development of drugs that have few adverse effects.
   C. Biological advances stimulate the development of nondrug therapies for chronic illness.
   D. Biological advances further the development of antidotes for drug toxicity.
   E. Biological advances allow for earlier and more accurate prediction of potential toxicities associated with new drugs.

ANSWERS TO SECTION VII

CHAPTER 48 ANSWERS

CASE 1

1. **The answer is B.** There are numerous methods by which researchers can identify and test potential new drugs. One is to **modify natural products to enhance their affinity for a targeted receptor.** Because many natural compounds are biologically active, modifying their structure or creating semisynthetic analogues can create more specific, active molecules. Identifying receptor targets and elucidating their molecular structure also allows researchers to develop specific molecules targeted to biologic receptor sites. Screening current libraries of compounds in assays based on the drug target can identify multiple potentially active compounds that can subsequently be tested more rigorously, and refined for specific activity at the targeted site.

2. **The answer is C. Identifying the three-dimensional structure of an active site allows for the design of a molecule to fit specifically into the site.** Nuclear magnetic resonance and x-ray crystallography can allow researchers to study the shape of the active site, and design and modify a small number of molecules to enhance their specific affinity for the site. In contrast, a "shotgun" approach to molecular screening of molecules might test many nonactive and less specific molecules, before identifying those with the greatest potential as future drugs.

3. **The answer is D.** Promising lead molecules are tested before choosing the most likely drug candidates for clinical development. Molecular testing may include an examination of **the metabolism of the molecule to predict potential drug–drug interactions and toxic metabolites.** Various formulations of the molecule are studied to ensure that it can be administered in a manner that achieves the greatest bioavailability. Genotoxicity is studied *in vitro*. Potential molecules are tested in animal models of human disease. This phase of potential drug evaluation does not involve human testing.

4. **The answer is A. Preclinical analysis of potential drugs ensures that a sufficient quantity of high quality drug can be manufactured.** The preclinical phase of drug development also includes animal toxicology and pharmacokinetic studies, and preparation of regulatory documents. Clinical development includes the preparation for drug studies conducted in various patient populations and disease states.

5. **The answer is C.** The development of ritonavir illustrates the process of a **target-centered approach to drug design**. Researchers at Abbott Laboratories targeted the HIV protease because it is essential to HIV replication and does not have a substrate analogue in mammals. After the crystal structure of the HIV protease had been elucidated, researchers could design an analogue of the enzyme's natural substrate that would act at the targeted site, while having few adverse effects in patients. In contrast, a compound-centered approach to drug design starts with the analysis of a specific compound, with intentions to refine it for potential drug use.

CASE 2

1. **The answer is C.** The development of natalizumab illustrates **a target-centered approach to drug discovery**. After the adhesion molecules, $\alpha4\beta1$ and VCAM1, were identified, researchers targeted $\alpha4\beta1$ for antibody development.

2. **The answer is A. A biological process was elucidated, for which chemical molecules were designed for biochemical testing of activity.** In other words, the molecular process of immune cell adhesion to endothelial cells was elucidated. Specific monoclonal antibodies to an adhesion molecule were designed and tested for activity against the adhesion molecule.

3. **The answer is B. Animal studies should be performed in models that mirror aspects of the targeted human disease** in order for the results to be predictive of drug effects in humans. Animal studies may need to be performed over a short or prolonged period of testing, depending on the time necessary to produce a measurable outcome of therapy. Animal

repeat-dose toxicity studies provide information on clinical, chemical, and histologic effects of various drug dosages on all organ systems. Animal toxicity studies are a critical component of assessing the potential risks to clinical trial subjects and are regulated by the Good Laboratory Practices. Animal studies can predict many, but not all, human adverse effects.

4. **The answer is C. The partition coefficient of a drug describes how well it distributes between an aqueous solvent and a hydrophobic solvent.** This information helps predict how well the molecule will cross biologic membranes. Mass spectrometry provides information on the drug's molecular weight. Nuclear magnetic resonance provides information on the types and patterns of chemical bonds in the drug. X-ray crystallography characterizes the three-dimensional structure of the molecule. A drug's solubility is measured in multiple solvents, especially water, to provide information on its bioavailability.

5. **The answer is E. The drug is not water soluble.** Although some hydrophobic drug molecules can be administered orally, in most cases, if a drug is poorly soluble in water, it will need to be administered parenterally. Other drug characteristics that favor parenteral administration include a high first-pass metabolism, instability in the gastrointestinal tract, and drugs that are macromolecules or proteins.

CHAPTER 49 ANSWERS

CASE 1

1. **The answer is B. The clinical trial must minimize the risks for the participants.** Provisions must be made for the overall care of the patient. The investigator must terminate the trial when the risks become incompatible with the goals of the trial. Adverse events must be reported to an ethics or safety committee. Investigators must ensure fair and equitable participant selection. These ethical principles, which were established by the International Conference on Harmonization and the Declaration of Helsinki, govern the ethical relationship between investigators and trial participants.

2. **The answer is D. Informed consent is a process in which participants are made aware of potential risks and benefits of a trial.** With this information, a participant can decide voluntarily whether or not to participate in a trial. Patient participants with a poor prognosis must also understand that the results of the research may not directly benefit them, but may benefit future patients.

3. **The answer is E. The drug must be tested in three phases with progressively increasing numbers of participants and outcome measures.**

4. **The answer is D. Phase III studies ascertain specific clinical endpoints in several thousand patients with the disease of interest.** They study drug safety, dosage, and effectiveness. Because the number of participants in Phase III studies is large, these study results can usually be extrapolated to the general population. Phase II studies involved several hundred patients with the disease of interest and assess drug safety over various dosage regimens, as well as preliminary effectiveness. Phase I studies evaluate drug safety and tolerability in a small number of healthy subjects. The results of each phase of drug testing critically inform the design of the subsequent clinical trials.

5. **The answer is E. Mortality is decreased.** This is a primary clinical endpoint. Primary clinical endpoints include such outcomes as survival, improvements in patient functioning, and improvements in patients' perception of their wellness. Surrogate or secondary endpoints include measurable markers such as decreased disease or tumor burden, reduction in plasma markers such as glucose or low-density lipoprotein cholesterol, and changes in cardiovascular measurements such as blood pressure or cardiac output.

CASE 2

1. **The answer is A.** The trials of COX-2 inhibitors in animals are examples of **preclinical animal studies of efficacy and toxicity.**

2. **The answer is C. A placebo control facilitates the interpretation of results as being attributable to drug effect or to natural variations in disease.** In the case of the VIGOR trial, the difference between rofecoxib and naproxen in their association with adverse cardiovascular events was attributed to a protective effect of naproxen. Without a control arm to the study, this finding could not be confirmed to be truly the result of a protective effect of naproxen, versus the baseline incidence of disease in this study population, versus an adverse effect of rofecoxib. The use of placebo helps to eliminate subject bias. Observer bias can be countered by blinding the study drug and placebo.

3. **The answer is B. An investigator must terminate a study when the risk of adverse effects on participants is perceived to be unacceptable.**

4. **The answer is A. The "black box" warning lists key safety information for drugs with certain safety risks.** The FDA may also require drug sponsors to create medication guides that are distributed to patients and communicate potential safety information in readily understandable language.

5. **The answer is E. This act mandates that all drug manufacturers must obtain premarket approval from the FDA, contingent on the demonstrated safety of a new drug.** This was in response to the poisoning and deaths of Americans in 1937 after they consumed an untested antibiotic product that contained diethylene glycol. The Orphan Drug Act of 1983 allows the FDA to offer financial incentives to drug manufacturers who will develop orphan drugs for rare diseases. Compassionate use protocols allow promising investigational therapies to be used on extremely sick patients who are not eligible to participate in an ongoing trial. The "off-label" use of a drug refers to its use for indications not approved by the FDA. The Pure Food and Drug Act of 1906 prompted the creation of the federal agency that eventually became the FDA.

CHAPTER 50 ANSWERS

CASE 1

1. **The answer is C. The incidence of adverse drug effects is noted in clinical trials and extrapolated to the general population.**

2. **The answer is D. Weakness: The incidence of a rare adverse drug effect is very difficult to measure in clinical trials.** Although the duration of clinical trials may be sufficient to measure beneficial "surrogate outcomes" of drug effect, these metrics may not reflect the intended clinical outcomes of new drugs or potential long-term adverse effects. Many clinical trials are performed with individuals, who may not accurately reflect the population of actual drug users. Placebo-controlled clinical trials of new drugs may not be feasible for ethical reasons.

3. **The answer is C. Physicians have access to information from spontaneous reports to the FDA of adverse drug effects.** Spontaneous reporting is one of the most heavily relied-upon sources of drug information. However, the majority of drug-associated adverse effects are never reported. Automated health care utilization databases provide information about large populations of patients, including their prescription use and their hospitalizations. Patient registries may keep track of well-defined populations of drug users and any drug-associated adverse effects they may experience, but they are not regularly mandated by the FDA. Phase IV postmarketing studies of new drugs are sometimes requested of drug manufacturers to address unanswered

questions pertaining to a new drug's effect or safety. However, the FDA cannot mandate that Phase IV studies be completed.

4. **The answer is E. Cohorts of patients are followed to determine the relative risk of the occurrence of an adverse effect.**

5. **The answer is A. A higher rate of potentially adverse effects might be acceptable if the drug is extremely efficacious in its therapeutic benefits.** Postmarketing studies of drug risks are not usually mandated in the United States. Head-to-head comparisons of drug benefits and potential adverse effects are rarely performed prospectively on large populations of drug users.

CASE 2

1. **The answer is D. FDA approval of two individual drugs is not an indication of their safety when used in combination.** Although both phentermine and fenfluramine had been approved by the FDA based on individual drug efficacy and safety studies, the combination had not been evaluated in clinical trials or submitted to the FDA for approval.

2. **The answer is A. The number of prescriptions written for a new drug is not related to its long-term safety.** In fact, initial sales of new drugs are heavily influenced by marketing campaigns directed toward physicians and consumers in order to maximize sales during the launch period of the new drug.

3. **The answer is E. The clinical trials were not of sufficient duration to detect this rare adverse effect.** The duration of many clinical trials is based on a demonstration of drug efficacy and does not necessarily predict potential adverse effects associated with long-term or chronic use of the drug. As a result, rare or uncommon adverse effects may not be detected during clinical trials.

4. **The answer is B. Patients using the new drug are three times more likely to develop an adverse outcome** as compared to patients not taking the drug.

5. **The answer is E. Biological advances will allow for earlier and more accurate prediction of potential toxicities associated with new drugs,** specifically related to pharmacogenomic differences in patient populations. Earlier prediction of potential adverse drug effects will facilitate the surveillance of potentially at-risk populations that use new drugs.

VIII

Poisoning by Drugs and Environmental Toxins

51

Poisoning by Drugs and Environmental Toxins

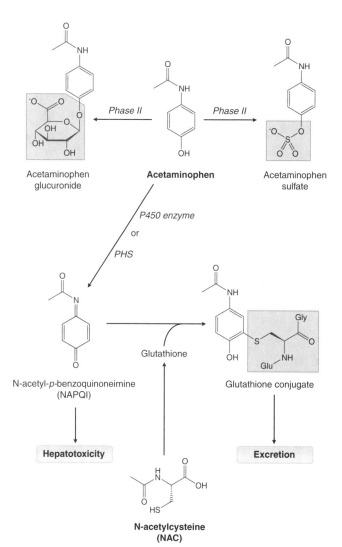

Acetaminophen
glucuronide

Phase II ← Acetaminophen → Phase II

Acetaminophen
sulfate

P450 enzyme
or
PHS

N-acetyl-*p*-benzoquinoneimine
(NAPQI)

Glutathione

Glutathione conjugate

Hepatotoxicity

Excretion

N-acetylcysteine
(NAC)

Figure 51-1. Mechanism of Acetaminophen Poisoning and Treatment. Acetaminophen is not toxic by itself but can be converted to toxic metabolites in the liver by the oxidative action of P450 enzyme or prostaglandin H synthase (PHS). Most acetaminophen is conjugated to sulfate or glucuronate via conjugation (phase II) reactions. However, a small amount is oxidized to N-acetyl-*p*-benzoquinoneimine (NAPQI), which can bind to hepatic proteins and cause

OBJECTIVES

■ Understand the mechanisms by which some xenobiotic agents can cause toxicity.

■ Understand how to reduce or reverse the toxicity associated with some xenobiotic agents.

CASE 1

The W. family is out of money. Times are difficult, with few opportunities in the sheet metal industry. After a few months of trying to make ends meet, Mr. W. decides to stop paying the electricity bill. Instead, he borrows a propane generator from a friend who works in the air conditioning business. Mr. and Mrs. W. and their teenage son set up the generator in the garage attached to the house, so no one will be able to see that they are using it as a source of electricity. That night, they gather together in the living room to watch television.

The next morning, a neighbor knocks on the front door, but there is no response. He looks in the living room window, and to his horror sees three people lying motionless on the couch. He calls the police, who break down the door and confirm that all the family members have died, including the two dogs and a cat.

centrolobular necrosis (hepatotoxicity). NAPQI can be conjugated to glutathione to form the nontoxic glutathione conjugate. In cases of acetaminophen overdose, glutathione is depleted, and NAPQI is free to cause hepatotoxicity. N-acetylcysteine (NAC) can be administered as an antidote. NAC, which is a metabolic precursor for glutathione, repletes hepatocellular glutathione levels and thereby prevents NAPQI-induced hepatotoxicity.

QUESTIONS

1. In this case, what was the likely cause of the deaths of the W. family members and their pets?
A. propane
B. carbon dioxide
C. hydrochloric acid
D. carbon monoxide
E. carbon tetroxide

2. Why were the family members not alarmed by any symptoms of the toxin?
A. The toxin is heavier than air.
B. The toxin is odorless and colorless.
C. The toxin cannot be detected by any household screening alarms.
D. The toxin causes muscle weakness and paralysis.
E. The toxin causes immediate disability and death.

3. Which routine laboratory test(s) could confirm the likely cause of death?
A. urinary carbon levels
B. oxyhemoglobin concentration
C. deoxyhemoglobin concentration
D. carboxyhemoglobin concentration
E. methemoglobin concentration

4. What was the likely source of the toxin in this case?
A. improperly operating propane generator
B. propane generator fueled with carbon monoxide
C. automobile exhaust in the garage
D. inadequate electricity generation for television function
E. "tight building" syndrome

5. Oxygen therapy is the antidote to the poisoning illustrated in this case. The use of oxygen to treat carboxyhemoglobin is an example of:
A. chelation
B. buffering
C. enzyme inhibition
D. restoration of an active site
E. adsorption of a toxin

 CASE 2

Your new neighbor's dilapidated garage sits on your property line. You suspect that the paint, which is flaking off its exterior walls, is lead based. Your neighbor tells you that he is going to strip and remove the paint because his wife is pregnant with their first child and he has heard that lead is bad for babies. He states he will rent a heat gun to do the job. "By the way," he says, "do you mind if I need to step in your vegetable garden to get at part of the garage wall?" You recall that the 3-year-old boy who previously lived in your neighbor's home was treated for lead poisoning. He used to play in a sandbox next to the garage.

QUESTIONS

1. What is the most important source of environmental lead today?
A. pewter drinking goblets
B. calcium supplements that contain lead-contaminated crushed bone
C. flaking lead paint
D. leaded gasoline exhaust
E. soft water

2. What are the possible effects of lead in exposed persons?
A. acute intermittent porphyria in teenagers who sniff leaded gasoline
B. painful peripheral neuropathy in smelter workers
C. encephalopathy in toddlers who eat paint chips
D. macrocytic anemia in pregnant women
E. hypotension in battery recycling workers

3. Why are infants and young children at greater risk for lead toxicity at lower blood levels than adults?
A. Infants have larger brains.
B. Toddlers have more hand-to-mouth activity.
C. Children absorb lead through the skin more efficiently.
D. Adults do not absorb lead through the gastrointestinal tract.
E. Adults store more lead in the soft tissues.

4. Which of the following laboratory measurements might suggest lead exposure?
A. amino acidemia
B. heme-positive stools
C. folate deficiency
D. decreased δ-ALA excretion in urine
E. increased erythrocyte protoporphyrin

5. Treatment for lead toxicity includes removal from the source of exposure, adequate nutrition and vitamin supplementation, and in some cases, chelation of lead. Which of the following is used to chelate lead?
A. deferoxamine
B. trientine
C. dimercaptosuccinic acid
D. lewisite
E. dithiocarb

ANSWERS TO SECTION VIII

CHAPTER 51 ANSWERS

CASE 1

1. **The answer is D. Carbon monoxide** poisoning was the likely cause of death in this case. Carbon monoxide is the leading cause of poisoning morbidity and mortality in the United States. It is a chemical asphyxiant that causes tissue hypoxia and ischemia through its pharmacologic effects on heme-containing molecules. Propane is an easily liquefied, simple, aliphatic hydrocarbon found in natural gas and petroleum. It is often used as a fuel. As a gas, it is a simple asphyxiant that displaces oxygen from the environment.

2. **The answer is B. The toxin is odorless and colorless,** and therefore it provides no warning signs to victims. It has a similar gas density to air and diffuses evenly in an enclosed environment, such as a garage or an attached house. Carbon monoxide can be detected by specific household alarms. Carbon monoxide causes nonspecific, vague symptoms referable to its deleterious effects on tissue oxygenation, especially of the brain and heart. Symptoms include headache, nausea, malaise, drowsiness, and reduced exercise capacity. At high concentrations of exposure, symptoms include loss of consciousness, seizures, myocardial ischemia, pulmonary edema, and ventricular dysrhythmias.

3. **The answer is D.** The diagnosis of carbon monoxide exposure can be made by the measurement by co-oximetry of an elevated **carboxyhemoglobin concentration** in heparinized blood samples. Pulse oximetry detects oxyhemoglobin and deoxyhemoglobin, but not carboxyhemoglobin.

4. **The answer is A. An improperly operating propane generator** was the source of carbon monoxide in this case. Carbon monoxide is a product of incomplete combustion of carbon-based fuels. Automobile exhaust also contains carbon monoxide and can contribute to poisoning when exhaust is not ventilated from an enclosed space, such as a garage.

5. **The answer is D.** The displacement of carbon monoxide from hemoglobin by oxygen is one example of **restoration of an active site**. Hyperbaric oxygen or 100% normobaric oxygen displace carbon monoxide from its binding site on hemoglobin and hasten the reactivation of oxygen-carrying hemoglobin. Oxygen administration may also limit the cascade of inflammatory damage caused by carbon monoxide in the brain.

CASE 2

1. **The answer is C.** The most important source of environmental lead today is **flaking lead paint** from homes built before the 1950s. Lead was added to paint to make its color brighter and to enhance its durability in bad weather conditions. Therefore, older homes, especially in New England, are still sources of lead because of flaking paint and contaminated soil and dust. Leaded gasoline was a major source of environmental lead from the 1920s through the 1970s, when tetraethyl lead additives were finally banned. By the 1970s, when lead poisoning cases peaked, 350,000 tons of tetraethyl lead had been produced worldwide. Tetraethyl lead use is responsible for 98% of environmental lead pollution. Lead was once used in the manufacture of pewter drinking goblets. Some calcium supplements that contain crushed bone may also contain lead if the source bone was contaminated with lead. Soft water enhances the dissolution of lead from older plumbing solder, contaminating household water. Other sources of lead that have caused toxicity include alternative medicines and folk remedies.

2. **The answer is C.** Lead toxicity can cause **encephalopathy in toddlers who eat paint chips.** Small children efficiently absorb lead from the gastrointestinal tract. One paint chip can contain up to 200 mg of lead, which is sufficient to cause a sudden increase in absorbed lead, which is transported in erythrocytes, distributed to soft tissues including the brain, where it can cause acute encephalopathy. Sniffing leaded gasoline can contribute to lead-induced peripheral neuropathy. Smelter workers and battery recyclers are occupationally exposed to lead and are at risk for peripheral motor neuropathy (classically, wrist drop), chronic renal disease, and hypertension. Mobilization and redistribution of lead from bone stores can occur during pregnancy, leading to potentially toxic blood levels. Normochromic or hypochromic anemia and constipation can occur at elevated lead levels. Lead exposure is associated with spontaneous abortion.

3. **The answer is B. Toddlers have more hand-to-mouth activity** and are more likely to ingest lead-contaminated dust and paint chips. In addition, infants and young children are at greater risk for lead toxicity than adults because they absorb lead from the gastrointestinal tract five to 10 times more efficiently than adults. For example, 30% to 50% of ingested lead is absorbed from the gastrointestinal tract in children compared with only 10% in adults. Nutritional deficiencies of iron, zinc, or calcium, high fat intake, inadequate caloric intake, and vitamin D all enhance lead absorption. As compared to adults, small children do not distribute as much lead to bone, where it can be stored for years in a relatively inert form (half-life of more than 20 years). Finally, infants and children younger than age 2 years have a less well-developed blood–brain barrier, which does not protect the brain from lead exposure.

4. **The answer is E. Increased erythrocyte protoporphyrin** can result from lead exposure. Lead inhibits heme synthesis at several steps. It inhibits the actions of δ-aminolevulinic acid dehydratase, leading to an accumulation of δ-aminolevulinic acid in blood and urine. Lead also inhibits ferrochelatase, preventing the incorporation of iron into protoporphyrin. Lead binds to mitochondria in glomeruli and in renal tubules and causes proximal tubular dysfunction. A Fanconi-like syndrome can occur, with glycosuria, aminoaciduria, and hyperphosphaturia. Persistent exposure can lead to irreversible interstitial fibrosis and renal failure.

5. **The answer is C. Dimercaptosuccinic acid** is a water-soluble derivative of dimercaprol that can be administered orally, and is much less toxic than other chelators. It mobilizes lead from soft tissue stores but does not allow redistribution into the brain during chelation therapy. In contrast, dimercaprol is administered parenterally in a peanut oil base. Indications for its administration include encephalopathy. Calcium disodium-EDTA (ethylenediaminetetraacetic acid) mobilizes lead from bone and the kidneys, but when used alone, it may allow the redistribution of lead into the central nervous system. It is also a nonspecific chelator of other metals, including zinc, copper, iron, cobalt, and manganese. It is administered intravenously and can potentially cause renal toxicity. Deferoxamine is used to chelate iron. Dithiocarb is used to chelate nickel. Treatment for lead exposure depends heavily on the remediation of environmental sources of lead, alteration of behaviors that enhance exposure, and chelation of body lead. Abatement of a lead-contaminated environment should only be performed by qualified persons.

IX

Frontiers in Pharmacology

52

Pharmacogenomics

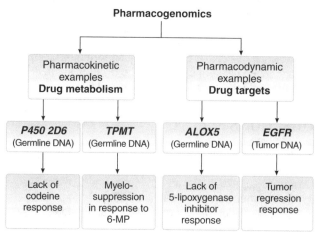

Figure 52-1. Pharmacokinetic and Pharmacodynamic Pharmacogenomics. The figure depicts the major pharmacokinetic (drug metabolism) and pharmacodynamic (drug target) examples described in this chapter. Shown are the affected gene *(in italics)*, whether germ-line or somatic (e.g., tumor) DNA is involved, and the clinical response observed in the presence of the variant allele(s). *P450 2D6*, cytochrome P450 2D6 gene; *TPMT*, thiopurine S-methyltransferase gene; *ALOX5*, 5-lipoxygenase gene; *EGFR*, epidermal growth factor receptor gene; 6-MP, 6-mercaptopurine.

OBJECTIVES

■ Understand principles of pharmacokinetic and pharmacodynamic variations in drug effects.

■ Understand how pharmacogenomics can affect the therapeutic and toxic effects of drugs and consequently influence the optimum choice of drug for individual patients.

 CASE 1

Robert H. is shoveling snow one wintry morning in Minnesota when he slips and falls on a patch of ice. He immediately feels pain in his left hip and is unable to stand. He is brought to the hospital, where x-rays reveal that he has fractured his hip. He undergoes surgery the next day and is discharged to a rehabilitation hospital 3 days later. After less than 24 hours at the rehabilitation hospital, Mr. H. develops the sudden onset of pleuritic chest pain. He is taken to the emergency department, where a CT scan with intravenous contrast reveals a pulmonary embolus. He is treated with heparin, and warfarin is started at a dose of 5 mg each day with a target international normalized ratio (INR) of 2.0-3. Mr. H. is discharged back to his rehabilitation hospital and referred to his local physician. When the initial INR is measured, it is 6.2, a value associated with an increased risk of hemorrhage. He was taking no other medication that might interfere with plasma levels of warfarin. The physician advises Mr. H. to stop taking warfarin for 2 days. After multiple attempts at adjusting his dose of warfarin, Mr. H. eventually reaches a stable INR of 2.5 taking 1 mg of warfarin each day.

QUESTIONS

1. What additional laboratory information could most assist in deciding how to anticoagulate Mr. H.?
   A. purity analysis of Mr. H.'s warfarin
   B. Mr. H.'s *CYP2C9* genotype
   C. Mr. H.'s *CYP2D6* genotype
   D. Mr. H.'s renal function
   E. Mr. H.'s hepatic concentration of vitamin K epoxide reductase complex

2. How would the above information have helped in the selection of Mr. H.'s initial warfarin dose?

- **A.** If Mr. H.'s warfarin were impure, a larger dose could be administered.
- **B.** If Mr. H. has the *CYP2C9*2* or *CYP2C9*3* genotype, a smaller dose could be administered.
- **C.** If Mr. H. has the *CYP2D6*1* genotype, a larger dose could be administered.
- **D.** If Mr. H. has diminished renal function, a smaller dose could be administered.
- **E.** If Mr. H. has a high concentration of vitamin K epoxide reductase complex I, a smaller dose could be administered.

3. What molecular mechanisms might be responsible for the apparent sensitivity of Mr. H. to warfarin?

- **A.** Mr. H. has the *CYP2C9*1* wild-type variant allele.
- **B.** Mr. H. has the *CYP2D6*1* variant allele.
- **C.** Mr. H. has an inactive haplotype of vitamin K epoxide reductase complex I.
- **D.** Mr. H. has excessive concentrations of vitamin K epoxide reductase complex I.
- **E.** Mr. H. has the *CYP2C9*3* variant allele.

4. The most common factor associated with pharmacogenetic variation in an individual's response to a medication is:

- **A.** genetic variation in target protein expression
- **B.** genetic variation in absorptive capacity for polar molecules
- **C.** genetic variation in catalytic enzyme synthesis
- **D.** genetic variation in thiopurine S-methyltransferase activity
- **E.** gender

5. Which of the following statements regarding genetic variation in *CYP2D6* is correct?

- **A.** Different ethnic groups have different frequencies of both the "poor metabolizer" and "ultra-rapid metabolizer" *CYP2D6* phenotypes.
- **B.** The *CYP2D6* enzyme is a member of the family of microsomal conjugating enzymes responsible for the phase II metabolism of drugs.
- **C.** The discovery of the *CYP2D6* polymorphism is a research breakthrough, but is not clinically relevant because most drugs are metabolized by conjugation.
- **D.** "Ultra-rapid metabolizers" have only one functioning copy of the *CYP2D6* gene.
- **E.** "Poor metabolizers" for *CYP2D6* are frequently overdosed on cough medication.

 CASE 2

You are working in a family practice clinic. You note that there is some variability in your patients' blood pressure response to the antihypertensive agent, clonidine. In fact, when you examine your patients' charts based on ethnicity, you note that African American patients seem to achieve somewhat better blood pressure control on clonidine as compared to Caucasians. You decide to research the literature to find information on the ethnic differences in drug efficacy and patient sensitivity.

You find the following information: Genetic polymorphisms can affect an individual's response to a drug. Recent investigation has revealed polymorphisms in human adrenoceptor genes, including the α_2-adrenoceptor, a G protein–coupled receptor that is expressed in the varicosities of sympathetic neurons innervating vascular smooth muscle. Activating the α_2-adrenoceptor stimulates a second messenger cascade system, which subsequently inhibits neuronal voltage-gated calcium channels. The result is autoreceptor-mediated inhibition of norepinephrine release.

QUESTIONS

1. A single nucleotide polymorphism (SNP) in the α_2-adrenoceptor (Asn251 to Lys251) is found with an allele frequency of 4% in African Americans and 0.4% in European Americans. How might such a polymorphism alter the potency or efficacy of clonidine, an α_2-adrenoceptor agonist used to treat hypertension?

- **A.** The SNP could be associated with an increased G protein–stimulated signaling for a given level of receptor binding by clonidine.
- **B.** The SNP could be associated with enhanced norepinephrine synthesis.
- **C.** The SNP could be associated with decreased α_2-adrenoceptor degradation by clonidine.
- **D.** The SNP could be associated with a decreased synthesis of α_2-adrenoceptor.
- **E.** The SNP could be associated with an increased synthesis of α_2-adrenoceptor.

2. Another polymorphism (Del301-303) has three glutamate residues deleted from the third intracellular loop of the α_2-adrenoceptor. This change results in complete loss of agonist-induced receptor desensitization. How might this polymorphism affect a patient's long-term response to clonidine?

- **A.** The dose of clonidine necessary to achieve blood pressure control would need to be reduced over time.
- **B.** The dose of clonidine necessary to achieve blood pressure control would need to be increased over time.
- **C.** The action of clonidine at the receptor would not be attenuated over time.

D. The action of clonidine at the receptor would be attenuated over time.

E. The patient would develop increased sensitivity to the effects of clonidine over time.

3. Mechanisms by which genetic variations can alter pharmacodynamics include which of the following?
   A. alterations in enzyme degradation
   B. alterations in DNA binding to enzymes
   C. alterations in DNA binding to target proteins
   D. alterations in receptor protein quantity
   E. alterations in gene modification in somatic cells

4. Genetic variations in enzyme activity can be associated with seemingly "idiosyncratic" reactions to some drugs. The genetic variation in the production of the enzyme, glucose 6-phosphate dehydrogenase, puts some ethnic groups at higher risk for which of the following drug-associated reactions?

A. anaphylaxis
B. red cell aplasia
C. Coombs-positive hemolytic anemia
D. oxidant-induced hemolytic anemia
E. hypoxia-induced erythrocyte sickling

5. Which of the following is one example of the application of pharmacogenomics in choosing certain drugs for specific patient populations based on genetic differences in the response to a drug?
   A. the use of sulfonamides in patients with glucose 6-phosphate dehydrogenase deficiency
   B. the use of a hydralazine combination antihypertensive in African Americans
   C. the use of isoniazid in patients with a slow-acetylator phenotype
   D. the use of acetaminophen in Caucasians
   E. the use of azathioprine in patients with inflammatory bowel disease

53

Protein-Based Therapies

▪ CASE 1

M.R. is a 55-year-old traveling salesman who presents to the emergency department of a small rural hospital with left chest pain and lightheadedness. The pain started suddenly 1 hour ago when he was carrying a large box. At first, M.R. felt as if he was going to pass out, but the pain and lightheadedness improved at rest and eventually resolved after 20 minutes. M.R. denies any other symptoms, and he has no history of medical problems. He takes no medications, he is not a smoker, and his father died unexpectedly in a car accident at age 53. On physical examination, M.R. is afebrile with a heart rate of 100 bpm, blood pressure of 150/90 mm Hg, and respiratory rate 16 breaths/min. His pulse-oximeter displays 96% on a nasal cannula with oxygen flowing at 2 L/min. He appears to be comfortable, and the remainder of his physical examination is notable only for an S4 heart sound. There is no evidence of fecal occult blood. His ECG demonstrates sinus tachycardia with no ST segment elevation. His chest x-ray is normal. His STAT chemistry panel shows normal sodium, potassium, chloride, bicarbonate, blood urea nitrogen, and creatinine levels. Cardiac biomarkers and coagulation studies are pending. M.R. is given aspirin, metoprolol, and sublingual nitroglycerin on his arrival in the emergency department.

On admission to the hospital, his troponin T returns at 1.34 ng/mL (normal 0–0.1 ng/mL), and he develops 2-mm ST-segment depression in leads V1–V3 when he has chest pain. At this time, he is also given heparin, abciximab, and clopidogrel, and his chest pain resolves. His clinical course is stable overnight.

The next day, however, M.R. develops crushing substernal chest pain and diaphoresis, and his ECG shows 4-mm ST-segment elevation in leads V2–V4. Because cardiac catheterization is not available at the regional cardiac center

for at least 4 hours, M.R. is given tenecteplase in the coronary care unit, and his aspirin, metoprolol, nitroglycerin, heparin, and clopidogrel are continued. He stabilizes on this regimen.

After an otherwise uneventful 5-day hospitalization, M.R. is transferred to the regional cardiac center for catheterization with a diagnosis of unstable angina that evolved into an ST elevation myocardial infarction. Outpatient plans include cardiac rehabilitation and treatment with aspirin, metoprolol, enalapril, spironolactone, and sublingual nitroglycerin as needed.

QUESTIONS

1. By what mechanism does abciximab act?
   A. Abciximab is a monoclonal antibody that reduces inflammatory responses associated with tumor necrosis factor α within coronary arteries.
   B. Abciximab is a monoclonal antibody that clumps and destroys aggregating platelets at the site of clot formation.
   C. Abciximab is a monoclonal antibody that prevents fibrinogen binding to platelets and platelet aggregation.
   D. Abciximab is a recombinant protein that prevents clot formation by inhibiting thrombin.
   E. Abciximab is a liposomal delivery system that delivers antibodies against fibrin to areas of developing clot.

2. How could abciximab augment the function of clopidogrel and aspirin in this case?
   A. Abciximab also prevents platelet aggregation through a third mechanism of action.
   B. Abciximab makes the antagonist effects of aspirin on cyclooxygenase more potent.
   C. Abciximab prevents the metabolism of clopidogrel.
   D. Abciximab makes platelets more sensitive to the effects of aspirin and clopidogrel.
   E. Abciximab destroys platelets so there is a reduced requirement for aspirin and clopidogrel.

TABLE 53-1   A Functional Classification of Protein-Based Therapies

Group I: Protein Therapeutics with Enzymatic or Regulatory Activity

Ia: Replacing a protein that is deficient or abnormal

Factor VIII	Beta-glucocerebrosidase	Pancreatic enzymes (lipase, amylase, protease)
Factor IX	Laronidase	Lactase
Insulin	Agalsidase beta	Adenosine deaminase
Insulin analogues (lispro, aspart, glargine)	Alpha-1-proteinase inhibitor	Pooled immunoglobulins
Growth hormone (GH)		

Ib: Augmenting an existing pathway

Erythropoietin	Type I alpha-interferon	Tissue plasminogen activator (tPA), alteplase
Darbepoetin alfa	Interferon alpha-2a (IFNα-2a)	Reteplase (deletion mutein of plasminogen activator (rPA)
Granulocyte colony stimulating factor (G-CSF)	Peginterferon alfa-2a	Tenecteplase
Granulocyte-macrophage colony stimulating factor (GM-CSF)	Interferon alfa-2b (IFNα-2b)	Factor VIIa
Interleukin-11 (IL-11)	Peginterferon alfa-2b	Drotrecogin alfa (activated protein C)
Human follicle stimulating hormone (FSH)	Interferon beta-1a (rIFN-β)	Teriparatide (human parathyroid hormone 1-34)
Human chorionic gonadotropin (HCG)	Interferon beta-1b (rIFN-β)	Exenatide
	IFN-gamma	Platelet-derived growth factor (PDGF)
	Interleukin-2 (IL-2), epidermal thymocyte activating factor (ETAF), aldesleukin	Trypsin
		Nesiritide

Ic: Providing a novel function or activity

Papain	L-asparaginase	Lepirudin
Collagenase	PEG-asparaginase	Streptokinase
Dornase alfa, human deoxyribonuclease I		Etanercept

Group II: Protein Therapeutics with Special Targeting Activity

IIa: Interfering with a molecule or organism by binding to it and thereby blocking its function or targeting it for degradation

Rituximab	Alefacept	Omalizumab
Alemtuzumab	Efalizumab	Palivizumab
Cetuximab	Infliximab	Enfuvirtide
Bevacizumab	Anakinra	Abciximab
	Muromonab-CD3	Ovine digoxin immune serum, Fab fragment
	Daclizumab	Pegvisomant
	Basiliximab	

IIb: Stimulating a signaling pathway

Trastuzumab	Tositumomab

IIc: Delivering other compounds or proteins

Gemtuzumab ozogamicin	I-131 tositumomab

Group III: Protein Vaccines

IIIa: Protecting against a deleterious foreign agent

HBsAg	OspA

IIIb: Treating an autoimmune disease

Glatiramer acetate (formerly copolymer-1)
Anti-Rh IgG

IIIc: Treating cancer

Currently in clinical trials

Group IV: Protein Diagnostics

DPPD	Growth hormone releasing hormone (GHRH)	Thyroid stimulating hormone (TSH)
HIV antigens	Secretin	Glucagon
Hepatitis C antigens		

3. By what mechanism does tenecteplase act?

  A. Tenecteplase is a recombinant variant of growth factor that enhances the production of plasmin.

  B. Tenecteplase is a monoclonal antibody that targets fibrinogen and prevents the formation of fibrin in clots.

  C. Tenecteplase is a monoclonal antibody that coats platelets and causes lysis of clots.

  D. Tenecteplase is a genetically engineered derivative of tPA that binds to plasminogen and causes lysis of fibrin in clots.

  E. Tenecteplase is a genetically engineered derivative of streptokinase that inactivates thrombin.

4. Which of the comparative statements about tenecteplase and heparin is correct?

  A. Tenecteplase, but not heparin, can cause life-threatening hemorrhage.

  B. Neither tenecteplase nor heparin is related to an endogenous molecule.

  C. Tenecteplase, but not heparin, is indicated in acute myocardial infarction.

  D. Tenecteplase activates an enzyme; heparin is an enzyme.

  E. Tenecteplase promotes the dissolution of clot; heparin prevents clot propagation.

5. Which of the following statements regarding protein-based therapy is correct?

  A. Protein-based therapy is not as specific as small-molecule drug therapy.

  B. Protein-based therapy commonly elicits an immune response.

  C. Protein-based therapies are considered experimental by the Food and Drug Administration.

  D. Protein-based therapies can be used to treat genetically determined diseases.

  E. Protein-based therapies require the production of molecules in animal and bacterial species.

■ CASE 2

You are working in the emergency department when a 32-year-old woman, Kathleen O., is brought by ambulance after a motor vehicle crash. Mrs. O. was a restrained driver who was struck on the driver's side by another vehicle. Her car skidded and rolled over once down a shallow embankment. She had no loss of consciousness and was easily extricated from the damaged vehicle by paramedics. She arrives on a backboard in spinal immobilization to protect her cervical spine. She is crying and very upset. She tells you that she is 10 weeks' pregnant and wants to know if there may have been some injury to the baby. A trauma evaluation is performed, including routine laboratory testing and imaging.

Mrs. O. reports that she feels a small amount of spotting on her underwear, and a pelvic examination does reveal a small amount of pink discharge coming from the closed uterine os. A pelvic ultrasound demonstrates an intact uterus with a normal appearing intrauterine pregnancy and normal fetal heart activity. The remainder of Mrs. O.'s trauma evaluation reveals no other injury. Her laboratory evaluation is also reassuring. However, you find that her blood type, sent with the routine trauma labs, is type A, Rh(D) antigen negative. You confirm with her that this is her first pregnancy.

Based on Mrs. O.'s presentation, you cannot exclude the possibility of a small degree of fetomaternal hemorrhage as a result of this trauma.

QUESTIONS

1. If Mrs. O. is Rh(D) antigen negative and her fetus is Rh(D) antigen positive and there has been some mixing of fetal and maternal blood as a result of this trauma, what could be the result in Mrs. O.?

  A. Mrs. O. could develop antibodies to her own erythrocytes.

  B. Mrs. O. could develop antibodies to her fetus' erythrocytes.

  C. Mrs. O. could suffer an anaphylactic reaction.

  D. Mrs. O. could suffer a transfusion reaction to Rh(D) negative erythrocytes in the future.

  E. Mrs. O. could develop an autoimmune disease.

2. If Mrs. O. is Rh(D) antigen negative and her fetus is Rh(D) antigen positive and there has been some mixing of fetal and maternal blood as a result of this trauma, what could be the result in the fetus?

  A. The fetus could develop antibodies to the Rh(D) antigen.

  B. The fetus could develop antibodies to maternal proteins and be unable to nurse after birth.

  C. The fetus could suffer hemolysis as a result of maternal anti-Rh antibodies.

  D. The fetus could suffer bone marrow aplasia as a result of maternal anti-Rh antibodies.

  E. The fetus could suffer a transfusion reaction to Rh(D) erythrocytes in the future.

3. You explain to Mrs. O. that, based on her Rh typing, she should have therapy to prevent future harm to the fetus. This therapy and its intended effect are:

  A. exchange transfusion to exchange any Rh(D) positive blood for Rh(D) negative blood

  B. transfusion with Rh(D) positive blood to induce desensitization to foreign Rh antigens

  C. hepatitis D vaccine to prevent sensitization to all D antigens

  D. anti-Rh(D) immunoglobulin to prevent sensitization to Rh(D) antigens

  E. vitamin D to prevent the formation of antibodies against all D antigens

4. Administration of the above therapy is a form of:
   A. protein replacement therapy
   B. vaccination
   C. enzyme inhibition
   D. immunoadhesion
   E. antigenic neutralization

5. Which of the following is a protein-derived vaccine?
   A. purified protein derivative (PPD)
   B. etanercept
   C. OspA
   D. secretin
   E. L-asparaginase

54

Drug Delivery Modalities

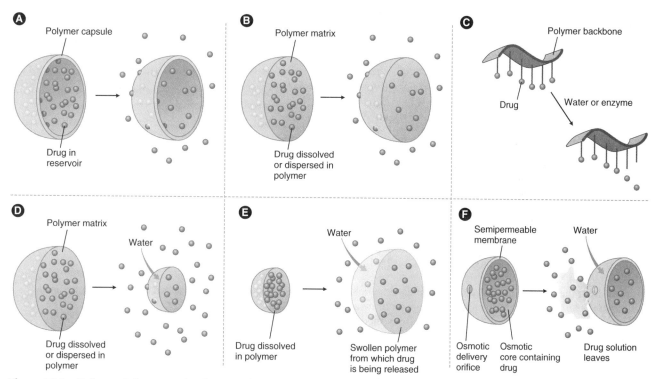

Figure 54-1. Polymer Release Mechanisms. In all panels except **C**, the simplified diagrams represent polymeric systems in cross-section. The most common release mechanism is diffusion, whereby the drug migrates from its initial location in the polymer system to the polymer's outer surface and then to the body. Diffusion can occur from a reservoir (**A**), in which a drug core is surrounded by a polymer film, or from a matrix (**B**), where the drug is uniformly distributed through the polymeric system. Drugs can also be released by chemical mechanisms such as cleavage of the drug from a polymer backbone (**C**) or hydrolytic degradation of the polymer (**D**). Exposure to a solvent can also activate drug release. For example, the drug can be retained in place by polymer chains; upon exposure to environmental fluid, the outer polymer regions begin to swell, allowing the drug to diffuse outward (**E**). An osmotic system in the form of a tablet with a laser-drilled hole in the polymer surface (**F**) can provide constant drug release rates. Water diffuses through the semipermeable membrane into the tablet along its osmotic gradient, swelling the osmotic core inside the tablet and forcing drug solution out through the hole. Combinations of the above approaches are possible. Release rates can be controlled by the nature of the polymeric material and the design of the system.

OBJECTIVE

■ Understand the therapeutic advantages and limitations of novel drug delivery systems.

 CASE 1

March 1988: M.F. is 13 years old. His parents begin to notice that he is tired much of the time, despite getting plenty of sleep. He can no longer participate on his school's track team because he becomes exhausted in the middle of races, the same races he had often won less than 1 year earlier. Also, M.F. complains of being thirsty constantly and, as a result, consumes large quantities of water. M.F. goes to his family physician, who measures his blood glucose level at 650 mg/dL (approximately six times the normal level) and makes an initial diagnosis of Type I diabetes mellitus. The diagnosis is confirmed in the hospital, where M.F.'s physicians stabilize his blood glucose and develop an insulin therapy regimen. He is taught how to draw a drop of blood from his fingertip to measure his blood glucose and how to give himself subcutaneous injections of insulin. Each day, M.F. injects recombinant human insulin before breakfast and before dinner.

January 1997: Throughout high school and most of college, M.F. rarely monitors his glucose levels and purposely keeps them higher than recommended. He wants to be as ''normal'' as possible, which for him means never allowing his glucose level to fall so low as to require food in the middle of a class or at other unusual times. As M.F. becomes older, he begins to appreciate that avoiding the long-term consequences of poorly controlled diabetes—atherosclerosis, retinopathy, nephropathy, and peripheral neuropathy, among others—is worth the inconvenience of better control. He switches to a four injection per day regimen and begins checking his blood glucose four to five times every day. Eventually, he switches from multiple subcutaneous injections (MSI) to continuous subcutaneous insulin infusion (CSII) with an insulin pump. The pump delivers a constant basal level of insulin that can be supplemented with bolus injections before meals, thereby more closely approximating the body's normal control of blood glucose levels.

September 2014: Back in 1997, M.F. used his insulin pump for only about 3 months, deciding that the small machine he needed to keep constantly attached to his body was not compatible with his active lifestyle or self-image. He resumed MSI therapy for several more years, until he began participating in human trials for a new, implantable insulin delivery system. Now a 2-year supply of insulin is incorporated into a polymer matrix that can be implanted in the subcutaneous fat of the abdomen. A device in M.F.'s wristwatch constantly measures his glucose levels transdermally and transmits instructions to a magnetic oscillator implanted near the polymer delivery system. The dosing advantages of the insulin pump are thus achieved without M.F.'s feeling limited or tied to a machine in any way. He simply has the polymer system replaced every 2 years and makes minor daily adjustments to the programmed delivery parameters in his wristwatch device. M.F. is looking forward to receiving a transplant of pancreatic beta cells developed from his own stem cells that will cure his diabetes.

QUESTIONS

1. Why is oral administration of insulin not practical?
   A. Insulin is too large a molecule to be absorbed across the gastrointestinal mucosa.
   B. Insulin is an acidic molecule that becomes ionized in the small intestine and unable to be absorbed.
   C. Insulin is extensively metabolized by the liver on first pass through the portal circulation.
   D. Insulin does not have membrane transporters to fa-

cilitate its absorption across the gastrointestinal mucosa.
   E. Insulin is a peptide drug that is degraded in the intestinal tract.

2. By what other routes can insulin be administered?
   A. transdermal
   B. rectal suppository
   C. subcutaneous injection
   D. sublingual dissolution
   E. intrathecal

3. A dry powder aerosol inhaler has been approved for the pulmonary delivery of insulin. What is one advantage of delivering drug molecules, such as insulin, via the lungs?
   A. The lungs do not have an acidic environment.
   B. The lungs have a large number of proteolytic enzymes, which activate prodrugs.
   C. The lungs absorb drugs locally and limit their systemic distribution.
   D. The lungs have large absorptive surface areas.
   E. The lungs have minimal numbers of inflammatory cells to phagocytose drug molecules.

4. How can polymers be used to optimize and simplify the administration of some drugs?
   A. Gradual diffusion of drugs from polymer reservoirs provides for a controlled release of drug into the body.
   B. Polymer reservoir systems can facilitate diffusion of large and small drug molecules.
   C. Polymer systems never degrade and can be reused indefinitely.
   D. Polymer matrices can accommodate a large volume of drug.
   E. Polymer matrices are composed of lipid bilayer membranes that are not recognized as foreign antigens and do not elicit an immune response.

5. How do polymer chain reservoir delivery systems differ from liposome-based delivery systems?
   A. Polymer–drug complexes can target drug delivery to specific tissues.
   B. Polymer-based drug delivery systems cannot accommodate large volumes of drug.
   C. Polymer–drug complexes can circulate intravenously.
   D. Polymer-based systems are taken up by the reticuloendothelial system.
   E. Polymer–chain reservoirs contain lipids.

CASE 2

Megan D. is a 41-year-old woman with end-stage metastatic cervical cancer and chronic abdominal pain. She is taking oxycodone (a synthetic opioid) 10 mg orally every 4 to 6 hours and a fentanyl transdermal patch dose of 600 μg/hour to control her pain. (Fentanyl is also a synthetic opioid analgesic with a high potency [about 80–100 times morphine] that was first introduced in the United States in 1968.)

QUESTIONS

1. What is the most important benefit of transdermal fentanyl compared with oral oxycodone for pain control?
   A. Transdermal fentanyl causes more rapid peak drug levels and rapid analgesia.
   B. Oral oxycodone is difficult to swallow in pill form.
   C. Oral oxycodone is hepatically metabolized to toxic metabolites.
   D. Transdermal fentanyl allows for slow, sustained drug delivery.
   E. Transdermal fentanyl is metabolized more slowly than oral oxycodone.

2. What is the major barrier to the absorption of transdermal fentanyl?
   A. stratum basale
   B. stratum lucidum
   C. stratum corneum
   D. stratum spinosum
   E. dermis

Ms. D.'s mother cares for her at home. She washes her daily and changes her fentanyl patches every 2 days using the following method: She removes the patches without touching the center of the adhesive surface, washes her daughter's skin with soap and water, removes any residual adhesive with her fingernails, sprays the skin site with fluticasone propionate, a corticosteroid, to decrease skin irritation, applies a new patch, and holds her hand over it for 20 seconds to promote good adherence. She rinses her hands with warm water using no soap.

One month after Ms. D.'s mother begins changing the fentanyl patches, her mother has redness and a burning irritation of her hands. Ms. D.'s mother becomes very somnolent in the afternoons and has depressive symptoms, no energy, lack of appetite, and gradual weight loss. Five months later, she begins using gloves while changing her daughter's fentanyl patches, and she subsequently develops the following symptoms: irritability, jitteriness, abdominal cramping, and some loose stools. These symptoms last for about 4 to 6 weeks, until she returns to her baseline health.

3. What is the most likely explanation for Ms. D.'s mother's symptoms?
   A. Fentanyl-induced contact dermatitis and systemic iontophoresis.
   B. Transdermal absorption of residual fentanyl, opioid effects, and withdrawal.
   C. Anaphylactoid reaction to transdermally absorbed fentanyl.
   D. Fentanyl-induced cavitation of the lipid bilayers of the skin on her hands.
   E. Transdermal absorption of residual fentanyl, resulting in hepatic toxicity.

Ms. D.'s brother, Morris D., is a 44-year-old construction worker with a work-related back injury and chronic back pain. His pain is controlled with a transdermal fentanyl patch dose 75 μg/hour. He is working as a counselor at a basketball summer camp. After several days of outdoor activities in high heat, he is noted by his boss to become lethargic and difficult to arouse after a nap. An ambulance is urgently called, and Mr. D. is resuscitated with intravenous naloxone, an opioid antagonist. He develops symptoms of opioid withdrawal. In the hospital, Mr. D.'s fentanyl patch is removed, and his withdrawal symptoms are treated. He returns to his baseline mental status within 48 hours.

4. What conditions affect the absorption of transdermally delivered drugs?
   A. Hot, moist conditions increase drug absorption.
   B. Ultrasound damage to skin tissue decreases drug absorption.
   C. Electrical stimulation of skin tissue decreases drug absorption.
   D. Exercise decreases drug absorption.
   E. Hyperhidrosis decreases drug absorption.

5. Several months later, Ms. D., whose pain has progressed, is found dead with three 600-μg/hour fentanyl patches on her chest. How might the simultaneous use of multiple transdermal patches cause toxicity?
   A. Multiple patches enhance analgesia and do not cause toxicity.
   B. Multiple patches can cause life-threatening skin necrosis.
   C. Multiple patches can disrupt the renal elimination of active drug metabolites.
   D. Multiple patches can inhibit the hepatic metabolism of the drug.
   E. Multiple patches can cause an excessive accumulation of the drug.

ANSWERS TO SECTION IX

CHAPTER 52 ANSWERS

CASE 1

1. **The answer is B.** Knowledge of **Mr. H.'s *CYP2C9* genotype** could assist in planning his anticoagulation. Warfarin is metabolized predominantly by *CYP2C9*. The gene for *CYP2C9* is highly polymorphic, such that the variant alleles are associated with different levels of enzyme activity and, therefore, different rates of drug metabolism. Patients who carry an allele associated with reduced enzyme activity are at risk for supratherapeutic warfarin levels, overanticoagulation, and hemorrhage. CYP2D6 is not responsible for warfarin metabolism. Warfarin acts at the vitamin K epoxide reductase complex I. It is not eliminated by the kidney.

2. **The answer is B. If Mr. H. has the *CYP2C9*2* or *CYP2C9*3* genotype, a smaller dose could be administered.** These alleles are associated with decreased enzyme activity, compared to the wild-type *CYP2C9*1* allele and, therefore, a reduced rate of warfarin metabolism.

3. **The answer is E. Mr. H. has the *CYP2C9*3* variant allele.** This allele is associated with approximately 5% of wild-type enzyme activity. Patients with reduced metabolizing capacity may have an increased sensitivity to warfarin. In addition, patients with the vitamin K epoxide reductase complex I haplotype associated with the *CYP2C9* genotype may also be at increased risk for hemorrhage.

4. **The answer is C. Genetic variation in catalytic enzyme expression** is the most common factor responsible for pharmacogenetic variations in an individual's response to medications. Thiopurine S-methyltransferase is one example of an important drug-metabolizing enzyme with genetic polymorphism.

5. **The answer is A. Different ethnic groups have different frequencies of both the "poor metabolizer" and "ultra-rapid metabolizer" *CYP2D6* phenotypes.** For example, 5% to 10% of Caucasians and 1% to 2% of East Asians are "poor metabolizers." In contrast, the "ultra-rapid metabolizer" phenotype occurs in 13% of the Ethiopian population. Knowledge of ethnic variations in pharmacogenetic parameters may allow for "tailored" drug therapy, improved efficacy, and reduction of the incidence of adverse effects in patient populations. The *CYP2D6* enzyme is a member of the family of microsomal oxidative enzymes responsible for the phase I metabolism of drugs. Many drugs are metabolized by *CYP2D6*, including some antidysrhythmics, neuroleptics, analgesics, and antidepressants. "Ultra-rapid metabolizers" may have up to 13 copies of the *CYP2D6* gene.

CASE 2

1. **The answer is A. The SNP could be associated with an increased G protein–stimulated signaling, for a given level of receptor binding by clonidine.** This SNP would increase the efficiency of coupling of the α_2-adrenoceptor to downstream effector molecules. This would result in an increase in the apparent potency of clonidine, suggesting that lower doses should be used in patients with this allele. Depending on the extent of receptor reserve, the SNP could also be associated with an increase in the efficacy of clonidine, again suggesting that lower doses should be used in patients with this allele.

2. **The answer is C. The action of clonidine at the receptor would not be attenuated over time.** The most common desensitization mechanism involves G protein receptor kinases (GRKs) such as βARK-1. This enzyme is activated by Gβγ, leading to phosphorylation of the third intracellular loop/C-terminal of the receptor; in turn, receptor phosphorylation recruits β-arrestin to the receptor. The arrestin–receptor complex interferes with G-protein activation and limits the signaling by receptor agonists (e.g., clonidine). Loss of this inactivation process would minimize steady-state inactivation of the α_2-adrenoceptor in response to clonidine treatment.

3. **The answer is D. Alterations in receptor protein quantity** are one way that genetic variations may im-

pact an individual's response to drugs. For example, persons who have multiple repeats in the variant allele for *ALOX5* show a greater response to the asthma medication, zileuton. The amount of receptor protein synthesized may be dictated by genetic differences in the promoter regions and in the actual transcription of the gene.

4. **The answer is D. Oxidant-induced hemolytic anemia** can occur in patients who have deficient levels or inactive forms of the enzyme, glucose 6-phosphate dehydrogenase. There is genetic variation in the production of the enzyme, such that 10% to 20% of African Americans have reduced enzyme activity.

5. **The answer is B. The use of a hydralazine combination antihypertensive in African Americans** is one example of the application of pharmacogenomics in "tailoring" certain drugs to specific patient populations, based on genetic differences in the response to a drug. In contrast, sulfonamides can cause erythrocyte oxidant stress and hemolysis in patients with glucose 6-phosphate dehydrogenase deficiency, and should be avoided in patients with this enzyme deficiency. Azathioprine is used therapeutically in patients with inflammatory bowel diseases but can place slow acetylators at increased risk for drug toxicity because of a reduced capacity to metabolize the drug. Similarly, slow acetylators are at increased risk for isoniazid-associated hepatic toxicity.

CHAPTER 53 ANSWERS

CASE 1

1. **The answer is C. Abciximab is a monoclonal antibody that prevents fibrinogen binding to platelets and platelet aggregation.** Infliximab is a monoclonal antibody against TNF-α that is used in inflammatory conditions such as rheumatoid arthritis. Lepirudin is a recombinant protein based on the natural protein, hirudin, that inhibits thrombin.

2. **The answer is A. Abciximab also prevents platelet aggregation through a third mechanism of action.** Aspirin irreversibly inhibits platelet COX-1 and thereby prevents the formation of platelet-derived thromboxane, a vasoconstrictor and activator of platelets. Clopidogrel inactivates the platelet adenosine diphosphate receptor and inhibits adenylyl cyclase production of cyclic adenosine monophosphate (cAMP), preventing platelet aggregation. Clopidogrel is used in combination with aspirin to inhibit platelet activation. The addition of abciximab to this regimen further reduces platelet aggregation.

3. **The answer is D. Tenecteplase is a genetically engineered derivative of tPA that binds to plasminogen and causes lysis of fibrin in clots.** Tenecteplase has a greater specificity than endogenous tPA for binding to plasminogen, and therefore causes more efficient fibrinolysis. Alteplase is a recombinant form of tissue plasminogen activator. Reteplase is a genetically modified form of recombinant tPA. Streptokinase is a tissue plasminogen activating protein produced by group C β-hemolytic streptococci.

4. **The answer is E. Tenecteplase promotes the dissolution of clot; heparin prevents clot propagation.** Tenecteplase is a recombinant derivative of tPA that activates plasminogen to plasmin in order to lyse clots. Heparin is related to an endogenous glycosaminoglycan that enhances the activity of antithrombin III and prevents clot formation and clot extension. Both agents may be indicated in acute myocardial infarction, and both agents can cause life-threatening hemorrhage.

5. **The answer is D. Protein-based therapies can be used to treat genetically determined diseases.** Protein-based therapy is typically much more specific then small-molecule drug therapy. Because the body produces many proteins that are used as therapies, protein-based therapies do not commonly elicit an immune response.

CASE 2

1. **The answer is B. Mrs. O. could develop antibodies to her fetus' erythrocytes,** specifically to the Rh(D) antigens on the surface of the fetal cells. The "Rh" stands for rhesus, the monkeys in which the antigens were first discovered. Approximately 15% of the U.S. population does not have the Rh antigen on their erythrocytes. There is some ethnic variability in the incidence of Rh-negative status: 15% to 20% of Caucasians, 5% to 10% of African Americans, and fewer than 5% of persons of Chinese or American Indian descent are Rh negative. There are several different Rh antigens. In persons who have Rh-positive erythrocytes, the Rh antigen is designated "D." If a Rh-negative mother with a Rh-positive fetus has mixing of fetal erythrocytes with her blood, she may become sensitized to the Rh antigen, which is seen as foreign, and develop antibodies against the fetus' erythrocytes. Maternal Rh sensitization can occur as a result of fetomaternal hemorrhage in the setting of spontaneous miscarriage, induced abortion, trauma, or during delivery. Rh-negative women can also develop antibodies to the Rh antigen as a result of transfusion of Rh-positive blood.

2. **The answer is C. The fetus could suffer hemolysis as a result of maternal anti-Rh antibodies.** Maternal IgG antibodies to the Rh antigen can cross the placenta, coat fetal erythrocytes, and induce their destruction. The result in the fetus or newborn can be hemolytic anemia (erythroblastosis fetalis), elevated bilirubin level, and jaundice. Severe Rh incompatibility can lead to kernicterus as a result of bilirubin deposition in the brain, and to hydrops fetalis (a life-threatening form of severe anemia, fetal heart failure, edema, and respiratory distress and circulatory collapse in the newborn). As little as 1 ml of fetal blood entering the maternal circulation has been reported to be sufficient to induce maternal antibodies. However, some Rh-negative mothers do not develop Rh antibodies.

3. **The answer is D.** This therapy is **anti-Rh(D) immunoglobulin**, and its intended effect is **to prevent sensitization to Rh(D) antigens.** This immune globulin was approved in the late 1960s. Its use has reduced the risk of maternal-fetal Rh incompatibility from 10% to 20%, to less than 1% in the United States. Anti-Rh(D) immunoglobulin is generally administered to Rh-negative mothers between 28 and 32 weeks of gestation and again within 72 hours of delivery. It is also administered under conditions in which fetomaternal hemorrhage may have occurred. This therapy prevents maternal sensitization to the ongoing pregnancy, and to future pregnancies with Rh-positive fetuses. Exchange transfusion has been used to treat newborns with severe Rh incompatibility-induced hemolytic anemia. Transfusion with Rh(D) positive blood can sensitize Rh-negative persons and induce the formation of anti-Rh antibodies.

4. **The answer is E.** Administration of the above therapy (anti-Rh(D)-immunoglobulin) is a form of **antigenic neutralization.**

5. **The answer is C. OspA** is a protein-derived vaccine for Lyme disease. Purified protein derivative (PPD) is a noninfectious protein component of *Mycobacterium tuberculosis* that is used to determine whether an immunocompetent person has had previous infection with *M. tuberculosis*. Etanercept is a fusion of two human proteins that is used to neutralize the inflammatory effects of TNF in inflammatory diseases. Secretin is a recombinant protein that stimulates pancreatic secretions and gastrin release. It is used to diagnose pancreatic exocrine dysfunction or gastrinoma. L-asparaginase is purified from *Escherichia coli* and is used to lower the serum concentration of asparagine in patients with acute lymphoblastic leukemia, the cells of which require exogenous asparagine to survive.

CHAPTER 54 ANSWERS

CASE 1

1. **The answer is E. Insulin is a peptide drug that is degraded in the intestinal tract.** Intact peptide and protein drugs are poorly absorbed because of proteolysis in the gastrointestinal tract. Currently, they must be administered parenterally.

2. **The answer is C. Subcutaneous injection** and intravenous infusion are both parenteral methods of insulin administration. Research has also focused on intranasal insulin spray and pulmonary delivery of insulin.

3. **The answer is D. The lung has a large absorptive surface area**, the alveoli. The tissue lining of the alveoli is very thin, facilitating diffusion of molecules. A limited number of proteolytic enzymes are present in lung tissue to degrade drugs before their absorption. Depending on the particle size, aerosolized drug particles may escape clearance by alveolar macrophages. Finally, aerosolized drugs can act locally on pulmonary tissue and can be absorbed systemically in a noninvasive manner.

4. **The answer is A. Gradual diffusion of drugs from polymer reservoirs provides for a controlled release of drug into the body.** However, polymer reservoirs can only facilitate the diffusion of a small volume of drug. Polymer chains can accommodate only small amounts of drug.

5. **The answer is B. Polymer-based drug delivery systems cannot accommodate large volumes of drug**, therefore limiting the dose per unit volume administered. In contrast, liposomes have a high drug-carrying capacity. Both drug delivery systems can be used in active targeting of specific tissues for drug delivery: the polymer-drug conjugate can be linked to tissue-specific antibodies; the liposome-based delivery systems can also deliver antibodies to specific tissues. Liposomes can be protected from the immune system by attaching moieties such as polyethylene glycol, which increase their hydrophilicity.

CASE 2

1. **The answer is D. Transdermal fentanyl allows for slow, sustained drug delivery.** The transdermal fentanyl delivery system was approved by the Food and Drug Administration (FDA) in 1990 and is designed to deliver a controlled release of drug in order to maintain a constant therapeutic concentration. It avoids the peaks and troughs of drug concentrations associated with periodic oral administration of short-acting drugs, such as oxycodone. It is used to treat patients with chronic, stable pain. The patch consists of four layers: a polyester film backing; the gel drug reservoir (fentanyl, hydroxyethylcellulose and 0.1 mL of alcohol/$10cm^2$ to enhance the rate of drug flow and increase the permeability of the skin); a membrane that controls the rate of fentanyl delivery; and a silicone adhesive, which also contains fentanyl. A depot of drug concentrates in the outer layers of the skin, from which it is slowly absorbed into the systemic circulation. The amount of fentanyl released per hour is proportional to the surface area of the patch. The serum concentration of drug slowly increases and

reaches a plateau 12 to 24 hours after the patch is applied to the skin.

2. **The answer is C. The stratum corneum**, the outermost layer of the epidermis, is the major barrier to transdermal drug absorption. The other layers of the epidermis, in order of superficial to deep, include the stratum lucidum, stratum granulosum, stratum spinosum, and stratum basale.

3. **The answer is B.** Ms. D.'s mother experienced **transdermal absorption of residual fentanyl, opioid effects, and withdrawal.** Some amount of fentanyl remains in used patches, ranging from 28% to 84% of the original concentration, which is sufficient to cause serious toxicity and death. Because some unpredictable amount of active drug remains in used patches, gloves should be worn when the patches are removed to prevent secondary opioid intoxication in caregivers. Discarded patches are a potential source of fentanyl for misuse and abuse, and should be disposed of under safe, secure conditions.

4. **The answer is A. Hot, moist conditions increase drug absorption.** Anything that can increase the passive diffusion of fentanyl across the epidermis could be expected to enhance drug absorption. Conditions such as excessive heat exposure (e.g., hot temperatures, exertion, hot tubs and saunas, fever) increase blood flow to the skin and subsequent drug delivery from the epidermal depot. Skin breakdown or irritation may also enhance the diffusion of drug from the patch through the skin. Sonophoresis is the use of ultrasound to enhance dermal drug absorption. Iontophoresis is the use of low-voltage electrical pulses applied locally to enhance dermal drug absorption.

5. **The answer is E. Multiple patches can cause an excessive accumulation of the drug**, toxic opioid concentrations, and subsequent respiratory depression and death. As the therapeutic use of the fentanyl patch has increased in the treatment of chronic pain, reports of abuse and subsequent toxicity have also increased. Fentanyl extracted from transdermal patches has been administered for abuse purposes via inhalation, oral ingestion and swallowing, oral transmucosal (licking or chewing), and intravenous injection. Because fentanyl is highly lipid soluble, the amount of drug inhaled and absorbed through the pulmonary vasculature after the use of "fentanyl smokes" is large and causes central nervous system toxicity within seconds. In 2005, the FDA issued an alert regarding serious adverse events related to narcotic overdose in patients using the fentanyl transdermal patch for pain control.